The Complete Guide to Psychiatric Drugs, Revised and Expanded Edition

Straight Talk for Best Results

Edward H. Drummond, M.D.

John Wiley & Sons, Inc.

BST

Published by John Wiley & Sons, Inc., Hoboken, New Jersey
Published simultaneously in Canada

Limit of Liability/Disclaimer of Warranty: The information contained in this book is not intended to serve as a replacement for professional medical advice. Any use of the information in this book is at the reader's discretion. The author and the publisher specifically disclaim any and all liability arising directly or indirectly from the use or application of any information contained in this book. A health care professional should be consulted regarding your specific situation.

For general information about our other products and services, please contact our Customer Care Department within the United States at (800) 762-2974, outside the United States at (317) 572-3993 or fax (317) 572-4002.

Wiley also publishes its books in a variety of electronic formats. Some content that appears in print may not be available in electronic books. For more information about Wiley products, visit our web site at www.wiley.com.

Library of Congress Cataloging-in-Publication Data:
Drummond, Edward H., date.
  The complete guide to psychiatric drugs : straight talk for best results / Edward Drummond.— Rev. and expanded ed.
      p. cm.
  Includes bibliographical references (p.   ) and index.
  ISBN-13 978-0-471-75062-8 (pbk.)   MAR '07
  ISBN-10 0-471-75062-X (pbk.)
    1. Psychotropic drugs—Handbooks, manuals, etc.   2. Psychopharmacology—Handbooks, manuals, etc.   I. Title.

RM315.D87 2006
615'.788—dc22   2006040951

10 9 8 7 6 5 4 3 2 1

To Amy, Rosa, and Mikey

CONTENTS

Acknowledgments

I again thank most of all my wife and two children for their love and support through the process of writing. I also want to express my appreciation to Jay Couture and Wassfy Hanna, M.D., who have supported me for many years at the clinic where I put what I say in this book into practice; Shannon Miser-Maven, my agent; and Tom Miller, my editor at John Wiley.

Who Should Read This Book?

This book is intended to help patients and their families use psychiatric medication knowledgeably, safely, and to best advantage. Psychotherapists and other health professionals who work with people with psychiatric problems will find a practical reference for all aspects of the use of psychiatric medication.

Part I describes what is known and unknown about psychiatric problems and medications. It will give you the information you need to distill the facts from the misconceptions popularized in the media. This will give you a solid foundation on which to base decisions you make about medication. Part II guides you through the process of determining whether or not you should try medication. Part III describes different psychiatric disorders and their treatment. The full range of treatments beneficial for each disorder is described, with the focus on how to get the most out of medications. Part IV describes how to best use medication if you decide it may help you. It then describes each medication in detail. Strategies for managing side effects are described.

This book is not a replacement for a physician. Never start or stop a drug without consulting your doctor.

PART I

The Myths about Medication

CHAPTER 1

Psychiatric Drugs—Poison or Panacea?

Unhappy all her life, a thirty-one-year-old woman has felt good, alive, *normal,* only in the last few months since she's been taking Prozac. A middle-aged man feels trapped in a cycle of anxiety and addiction to Xanax. The parents of a teenage boy with hallucinations think their son is calmer on clozapine, but he feels like a zombie. Teachers are thrilled with the effects of Ritalin on a fourth-grader, but his mother worries about how it affects his personality. The daughter of an elderly woman with Alzheimer's disease hopes Cognex will help her mother's failing memory but worries about the doctor's warning that it can cause liver problems.

One in four people in the United States will suffer from depression at some point in their lives, one in five from anxiety. Millions more experience debilitating symptoms from schizophrenia, bipolar disorder, attention deficit disorder, and other psychiatric problems. More than thirty million people in the United States consume billions of dollars worth of psychiatric medications such as Prozac, Ritalin, Xanax, clozapine, and lithium. However, most people suffering from psychiatric problems receive no treatment.[1]

There is a great deal of information about psychiatric problems and drugs in the media. Pharmaceutical companies have developed many new psychiatric drugs in the last decade, which they promote at public events and in popular magazines. Celebrities like Mike Wallace, Patty Duke, William Styron, and Lawton Chiles have gone public with their problems and their experiences with medication. Many people not in the public eye have told their stories on television, in print, and on radio talk shows. Television shows like *Frontline* and *Sixty Minutes* have focused on psychiatric problems such as attention deficit disorder, posttraumatic stress disorder, and the debate over the reality of sexual abuse.

Some media stories on television and in print have praised the use of medications. Many doctors have welcomed the drugs with open arms, ignored the problems with drug treatment, and dropped other effective forms of treatment. Third-party payers such as HMOs and managed-care organizations promote the use of drugs over other forms of treatment. Some people take medication in the hope that it will be a panacea that will solve every aspect of their distress.

Other people have heard things that make them worry that psychiatric medication could poison them. They recall the "mind-numbing" tranquilizers used in mental hospitals in the 1950s. They remember Miltown and Equanil, used to treat depression and anxiety in the 1950s and '60s, drugs that are now seen as having damaged the lives of people who used them. They don't want to get addicted to medication, as they may know has happened to millions of people who take benzodiazepines like Valium and Librium (and their newer cousins Klonopin, Xanax, and Ativan). They've heard the reports that Prozac might have made some people commit suicide. They've heard that too many children are prescribed Ritalin.

Does Prozac transform people and make them happy? Does it make some people commit suicide? Is Ritalin appropriate for people with attention deficit disorder or is it used by schools as a cheap way to contain rambunctious children? Are Klonopin and Xanax good treatment for people with panic disorder and anxiety, or are they addictive drugs that need to be avoided at all costs? Is Clozaril a "miracle" for schizophrenia or does it just turn a person into a compliant zombie? Are medications a poison we should avoid or a panacea that can cure every ill?

Much of the information presented in the media is one-sided, distorted, or outright wrong. The media need to sell stories and the truth gets lost in the rush to tell you something exciting, especially if the truth involves complex details. Most people are skeptical of what they hear or read, but have no place to turn for accurate information about psychiatric disorders and proper treatment. Although some people are knowledgeable about psychiatric problems and medications used in their treatment, many possess only fragmentary information that is often inaccurate. These people often receive poor care and continue to be quite distressed. Many patients in psychological pain turn to their family physician for help, unaware that the vast majority of physicians do not have the training, time, or inclination to perform a comprehensive psychiatric assessment and are woefully ignorant of the full range of treatments that can be used to help a person in distress.

If you are depressed, anxious, or having a psychological problem, you may be as perplexed about what to do as the people described above. You may wonder whether there is medication that will cure the problem or whether it will help at all. You may be concerned that medication will cause side effects or damage your body. You may be unsure whether it will be harmful in some way that you may not be able to notice right away. You may worry about getting addicted. You may wonder whether psychiatric medications will interact unfavorably with medications that you need for a medical problem. You may want to know whether there are treatments other than medications that might help you.

I have long been troubled by the difficulties people experience when they consider psychiatric medication. I know that most people aren't familiar with psychiatric problems and the medications used in their treatment. I also know that when people feel distressed enough to see a psychiatrist, their problems may impair their concentration and sap their willpower to do anything but get through the day. Trying to manage their distress, talk to a doctor they've never met before about intimate details of their lives, understand what the doctor is saying about their problems, learn about the different treatment options, and decide between different medicines that are completely unknown is extremely difficult! It is no wonder that many people say to the doctor, "I'll do whatever you say," and take whatever prescription is handed out.

This can be a big mistake. Although your doctor cares about you, you do yourself no favors to give up control of your treatment. Psychiatric problems are not like other medical problems such as a broken leg or pneumonia where the best treatment has been determined by scientific studies. There are too many subjective, personal aspects of our psychological makeup and problems to use such a cookbook approach. You can be helped, but not by haphazardly planned and poorly administered treatment.

It's important that you know that there really *are* good treatments if you have a psychiatric problem. Our understanding of psychiatric problems like depression, anxiety, schizophrenia, and bipolar disorder and the treatments that have been developed for them are vastly superior to what we had fifty, twenty, and even ten years ago. That is the good news, the good, important news that should give you hope.

But how do you make sense of the information that is out there? Are psychiatric diagnoses accurate or even useful? What is a "chemical imbalance"? Why are psychiatric drugs suddenly so popular? Are they safe? Your questions about psychiatric problems and the medications used to treat them are valid ones.

I am asked these questions every day by my patients. I've spent a great deal of time in my work with thousands of patients over the last fifteen years to give people accurate answers to these very sensible questions. I've learned that almost everyone wants to know their diagnosis and understand their problems. They want to know about medications and how to use them most sensibly. They don't want a lot of psychobabble—they want the facts in a clear, straightforward manner.

You *can* learn what you need to know about psychiatric problems and the medications used to treat them. You'll learn that medications are neither a poison nor a panacea, but a powerful tool that *may* help you. You will be rewarded many times over by knowledge that will help you make an informed judgment about treatment. Then you can be sure that the decision you make about medication will be the right one for you.

Since you won't know which is the right treatment or medication until an accurate diagnosis is made, our first step will be to understand those symptoms and make a diagnosis. And that runs us smack dab into the problem that everyone who considers psychiatric medication must face: how to make an accurate diagnosis.

CHAPTER 2

The Truth about the "Accurate Diagnosis"

Although we may all think that we know what a diagnosis is, the term is actually used in a variety of different ways. Sometimes a diagnostic term describes the main symptom in a word derived from Latin or Greek, such as asthma (Greek for "panting") or diabetes (Greek for "to go through," and applied to disorders of excessive urination). Sometimes it's a term that describes the part of the body that isn't working correctly, such as "heart failure" or "broken leg." Sometimes the term describes the cause of the illness, such as "the flu," referring to the influenza virus. No matter where it comes from, however, the purpose of a diagnosis is to communicate the essential aspect of whatever ails a person.

Is there a one- or two-word "diagnosis" for your problems, one that will communicate the essential aspect of what is troubling you? The medical and psychiatric professions promote the idea that an accurate diagnosis is possible. This is a myth! It is a dangerous myth that pigeonholes you and your difficulties into a one- or two-word label. It ignores the complexity of the causes of your distress and limits the understanding of what is happening to you and inside of you. Most important, the myth of the "accurate diagnosis" severely narrows treatment options for many psychiatric problems and has contributed to the excessive use of medication prevalent in our country today.

Let's confront this myth. Let's look at what a diagnosis really is, how it has been applied to psychiatric problems, and how little we actually know about most psychiatric disorders. This will help you to build a good foundation for understanding your psychiatric problems and what you should do about them.

The Three Components of a Diagnosis

The word *diagnosis* derives from the Greek language and means, literally, "to know through," or to know fully. Three aspects of an illness need to be understood before one can say that an illness is fully understood. The *etiology* is the cause of the illness. The *pathogenesis* is the process by which the etiology produces the symptoms of the illness. The *syndrome* is the set of symptoms that occur in the individual.

These three aspects are most easily seen in the understanding and description of a physical illness. For example, the etiology of the common cold is a rhinovirus.

The pathogenesis is a combination of the actions of the virus and the body's reaction to the virus. When a rhinovirus implants in the cell of a person's throat, it uses the cell's machinery to replicate itself. The cell begins to break down as its processes go awry under the onslaught. When it finally collapses, hundreds of rhinovirus copies are released that go on to infect other cells in the host and, sometimes, other people. As soon as the virus gets into the cells, however, the body begins to mobilize its defenses. It sends other cells through the blood to the area to try to kill the virus. These cells send out messages to tell the body to heat up so the invader can be more easily killed. Some specialized cells make chemicals that attach themselves to the virus and then pick up the virus that is attached to the chemical and kills it. The body sends extra fluids so the cells can clean up and restore the body's integrity more easily. As a result of the viral attack and the body's defense, a person experiences the syndrome that is familiar to all of us: fever, sore throat, and a runny nose.

The common cold is relatively well understood because our technology is good enough to identify the etiology (viruses can actually be seen under an electron microscope, and their chemical composition can be determined through genetic testing), people have studied and understood the process of infection and inflammation for many decades and understand a great deal of underlying biochemistry and physiology, and throats can be looked at over and over again to follow the whole process.

Most illnesses, however, are not as completely understood as a sore throat. There are some illnesses that have a clear etiology, but the pathogenesis remains a mystery. For example, excessive radiation can cause certain kinds of cancer, but we have no idea how this occurs. Sometimes we don't know the etiology, but we have a good understanding of the pathogenesis. We don't know the etiology of diabetes, but we know only too well the problems people have if their sugar is too high: excessive urination of sugar and other blood chemicals that, if unchecked, can result in coma and even death.

Sometimes we know part of the etiology and pathogenesis but do not have a complete picture. For example, we know that some of the reasons people have heart attacks include smoking, high blood pressure, obesity, high cholesterol, high-fat diet, and intense exertion. Physicians understand some cellular mechanisms of the pathogenesis, such as the tendency of the cells lining the walls to take cholesterol into themselves if there is a lot of cholesterol in the bloodstream. This causes the cell to swell so there is less room for blood to get through. If sudden exertion causes the heart to need more oxygen, not enough blood can get through the narrowed space. As the heart continues to beat quickly, the muscle cells cramp up and develop pain. If the lack of oxygen is prolonged and severe enough, the cells may even die (i.e., from a heart attack).

As much time, money, and effort as we spend on heart disease, however, there is still much that we don't know. How does smoking worsen the problem, and why doesn't everyone who smokes get a heart attack? Why do some people with high blood pressure never have heart attacks? Why do some people have heart attacks without much fat in their arteries? Why do some people have heart attacks but feel no pain? Even the diagnosis "heart attack" or, more specifically, a "myocardial infarction," has several different types, can be mild, moderate, or severe, and can have different consequences to an otherwise healthy forty-year-old or a seventy-year-old with diabetes, high blood pressure, and kidney problems. Our understanding of the etiology, pathogenesis, and even the syndrome of heart disease is incomplete.

Medical problems that occur in people are too complex to fully capture, "to know through," in one or two words. Let's not confuse what a diagnosis really should be—a full understanding of an illness—with a one- or two-word label that we use as a shorthand phrase to refer to the etiology, pathogenesis, and syndrome.

Diagnoses in Psychiatric Disorders

We usually have at least a partial explanation for a physical disorder because we know a lot about how the body works. There is a lot we don't know, but it is unusual for a person to experience physical symptoms that cannot be at least partially understood.

Psychiatric disorders are vastly different from physical disorders, however, because our understanding of how the normal brain works is incomplete. We know a fair amount about how the brain interacts with the rest of the body. We know a great deal about how the brain makes muscles move. We know much about the way the brain connects with the five senses of sight, hearing, feeling, taste, and smell. We know very little, however, about the neurological processes of learning, memory, thoughts, reasoning, and consciousness, and the production of emotions.

How much do we really know about psychiatric disorders? Can we accurately describe the syndromes? Do we know the etiology or pathogenesis for any psychiatric disorder? Can we make an "accurate diagnosis"? This is a crucial question to ask if you are going to make a sensible decision about medication, though it is one that many patients and health care providers avoid. Let's look at how much is known about several of the most common psychiatric disorders.

Panic Attacks   A panic attack, also called an anxiety attack, is a discrete period of intense subjective anxiety accompanied by physical symptoms such as palpitations, shortness of breath, sweating, tremor, nausea, and fears of dying, having a heart attack, or going crazy. Panic attacks often begin suddenly and may last from a few minutes to a few hours. Panic disorder (PD) is the diagnostic label generally applied to people with the syndrome of panic attacks.

Psychiatrists have been debating the etiology of PD throughout this century. The psychoanalytic viewpoint became popular with Freud's investigations and theories at the turn of the century. The analysts believed that panic attacks were a manifestation of unconscious conflicted feelings such as the drive for sex and the internal prohibitions against it. They believed that people with PD could be helped primarily through therapy aimed at uncovering unconscious feelings. Many people benefited from psychoanalysis. Many people disliked this form of treatment, however, because it required meeting with the analyst four or five times a week for many years.

In the last twenty years it has been demonstrated that PD is more frequent in people who have had stressful experiences. For example, people who have been the victims of sexual abuse have a higher rate of PD, as well as other forms of anxiety and depression. People who undergo life-threatening experiences as adults, such as extreme weather events, disasters, or combat in war also experience a higher rate of PD. Children whose parents die, divorce, or abuse alcohol have a higher rate of PD and anxiety as adults. Psychiatrists and therapists who focus on stressful life experiences often recommend psychotherapy in which the person tries to acknowledge and put into perspective the anxiety and other feelings that arise from these experiences. Different forms of psychotherapy have been helpful to many people with PD, although some people continue to suffer debilitating symptoms.

In an effort to find more effective treatments, some psychiatrists focused on biological investigations. These researchers discovered that PD appears to run in families. They observed temperamental differences among newborns and infants and found that a small minority showed moderate to marked shyness. They demonstrated that panic attacks could be induced by an injection of lactate, a chemical produced by the body during exercise, only in people with panic disorder. They found that medications such as Imipramine and Nardil ameliorated panic attacks. Finally, they demonstrated that benzodiazepines such as Valium and Xanax helped panic attacks, apparently by working on a unique receptor in the brain called the benzodiazepine receptor. The psychiatrists with a biological orientation proposed medications as the only needed treatment.

Among the psychiatrists proposing a biological etiology of panic attacks was David Sheehan, a Harvard psychiatrist and author of *The Anxiety Disease.* He stated that "the central problem here [anxiety] springs from some source inside the individual's body, rather than a response to a situation outside the person. . . . In this anxiety disease, as in all diseases, nature has malfunctioned in some way."[1] Unfortunately for the proponents of the biological model, however, the "malfunction" has yet to be determined, in spite of a great deal of work. No specific genetic defect or biological abnormality leading to panic disorder has been identified.

Because of our ignorance about the true etiology of panic disorder, these different groups continue to argue about what constitutes the best treatment and recommend different things to patients, some promoting drugs and others psychotherapy. The treatment you receive depends on the orientation of your psychiatrist, not on a solid foundation of knowledge about the etiology and pathogenesis of the disorder itself.

Attention Deficit/Hyperactivity Disorder   It has been known for many years that some children, primarily boys, have pronounced difficulties with inattentiveness, impulsivity, and hyperactivity. Many such children cause difficulty for their families and schools to the point that they are brought to their doctors to investigate whether something is wrong with them. These children have been categorized in the scientific literature as abnormal and given a diagnostic label, even though much of their behavior falls within the normal range. The first term applied was hyperkinetic behavior syndrome.[2] This label was replaced by hyperactivity, and then minimal brain disease. The current term for the syndrome is attention deficit/hyperactivity disorder (ADHD).

Parents and professionals disagree on whether the syndrome of ADHD even exists, and, in fact, there are no reliable diagnostic tests or procedures that definitively determine the presence or absence of ADHD. The label is generally applied when a child manifests inattentiveness, hyperactivity, and impulsivity at home or school and scores abnormally on behavior checklists filled out by parents, teachers, and health care providers. The scales rely on subjective interpretations of such behaviors as "often talks excessively," "has difficulty playing quietly," "has difficulty awaiting turns in games," "has difficulty remaining in seat when required to do so," "often doesn't listen," and "often interrupts or intrudes on others."[3]

There is no accepted agreement about the etiology or pathogenesis. One group sees the behavior as biologically based. This group points to genetic evidence that demonstrates that the diagnosis appears to run in families. They note that there is a higher incidence of ADHD in identical twins, who share the exact same genetic material, than in fraternal twins, who share only the same amount of genetic material as any two siblings. This group tends to see medication as the first line of treatment.

Skeptics of the diagnosis and illness model of ADHD point out, with some validity, that rating scales measuring behaviors such as those listed above show the value that the raters place on compliance, docility, and being "good," rather than the validity of these behaviors as diagnostic of any disorder. They believe that there is nothing particularly wrong with these children except a society that does not accept this kind of behavior. They believe that the diagnosis of ADHD "medicalizes" and "pathologizes" normal behavior, labeling the children as deficient or ill when there is no justification for it. This group of people generally works to change the environment in which these children find themselves to one where their natural strengths can flourish. They vigorously oppose medication.

A third group believes these children have real difficulties that set them apart from other children. Although this group concedes that some of these children are more energetic, they feel that stress in the child's life, such as parental conflict, death, illness, or substance abuse, substantially contributes to the troubling behaviors. These people feel that the best treatment involves therapy aimed at helping the child cope with the stress more effectively and teach them more appropriate ways of behaving; These people focus on elaborate behavior plans for the child and the adults around them and are generally opposed to medication.

Once again, different theories abound and lead to vastly different treatments. Should you move your child to a different school, start a behavior plan, or start Ritalin? You will get very different answers depending on whose opinion you seek.

Obsessive-Compulsive Disorder   The syndrome of obsessive-compulsive disorder (OCD) is characterized by time-consuming intrusive unwanted thoughts (obsessions) such as fears of contamination or a desire to have things in a certain order, and repetitive behaviors (compulsions) such as handwashing. It is extremely distressing and disabling to affected individuals, whose symptoms can develop in childhood or adulthood and wax and wane throughout the rest of their lives.

The etiology and pathogenesis are unknown. The early psychoanalysts focused on internal conflicts and recommended psychoanalysis. Behaviorally oriented psychologists believe that the thoughts and behaviors satisfy some psychological need of the person. They use behavior modification techniques to help the person develop other methods of gaining relief. Improvements in the symptoms from medicines like Prozac and Luvox have recently led to theories that stress a biological abnormality. Each of these theories appears to have some validity, and each treatment has helped some people. However, recent work suggests that the exacerbations of the symptoms of some children with OCD may be related to infection by the streptococcus bacteria.[4] These researchers suggest that people with OCD may benefit from prophylaxis with antibiotics.

So is psychoanalysis, behavior modification, Luvox, or an antibiotic the treatment of choice? You will receive very different treatment depending on whose office you walk into, primarily because we are unable to make an "accurate diagnosis."

Schizophrenia   Schizophrenia is a lifelong illness that usually begins in the teen years or the twenties. The syndrome consists primarily of psychotic thoughts such as delusions (false beliefs), hallucinations (false perceptions), and paranoia, although there are often disturbances in a person's emotions and behavior as well. The presence or absence of some of these symptoms in a person leads some observers to apply the label of schizophrenia and others to apply different ones. For example, some clinicians apply the term "delusional disorder" if the delusion could have some basis in reality, such as a belief that one is being poisoned or followed. Some people apply the term "schizoaffective disorder" if there are pronounced alterations in mood, such as depression. Depending on the diagnostic label applied, different treatments and medications are recommended.

There is no accepted etiology of schizophrenia although there have been many theories. For centuries people believed that people with schizophrenia were possessed by demons because of their bizarre thoughts and behavior. Infection with syphilis and masturbation were considered as late as the turn of the century. Theories ascribing schizophrenia to a genetic abnormality or stressful life experiences began to emerge around the turn of the century. In the 1950s, '60s, and '70s, many people believed that stress put on children by parents caused schizophrenia. Some believed that the "schizophrenogenic" mother was the source of the problem. Naturally the treatment was to help the child to separate from the family. Murray Bowen, an author and clinician working at this time, even put whole families into the hospital in order to facilitate such a separation. Some psychiatrists, notably Peter Breggin, author of *Toxic Psychiatry* and a long-term critic of the psychiatric profession, believe that schizophrenia is a "psychospiritual" crisis that calls for psychotherapy not medications.[5] As medications emerged that were more effective than therapy, and as abnormalities in the brains of people with schizophrenia were documented, the notion that schizophrenia was caused by stress and could be cured by psychotherapy lost favor.

There appears to be a genetic component because relatives of schizophrenia have a higher rate of schizophrenia themselves. Genes cannot be the whole story because of the differing rates of schizophrenia in identical (monozygotic) twins. While fraternal (dizygotic) twins share only the same number of genes as any two siblings, monozygotic twins have exactly the same genes. However, monozygotic twins have only a 50 percent concordance rate for schizophrenia; in other words, when one twin has schizophrenia, the other has only half a chance of having schizophrenia. This means people with the same genes do not necessarily get schizophrenia. There must, therefore, be some factor other than genes that contributes to the development of schizophrenia.

Some research suggests that a viral infection of the mother during the second trimester of pregnancy may cause schizophrenia. Higher rates of schizophrenia were found in offspring of mothers who were in their second trimester of pregnancy during the influenza epidemic in 1957 in Finland, but not during the epidemics of 1918 or 1957 in Scotland.[6]

The pathogenesis of schizophrenia is unclear as well. Although there are abnormalities in the size of different areas of the brain and the levels of some of the chemicals in brain cells of people with schizophrenia, it isn't known how these relate to the production of the syndrome. For almost a century the hallmark of people with schizophrenia was the deterioration of intellectual capacity and functioning throughout the course of their lives. It was believed that the illness itself caused progressive brain damage. This contributed to the hopelessness felt by patients, their families, and clinicians. This hopelessness led to extreme treatments such as insulin therapy, electroshock therapy, lobotomy, and long-term institutionalization of people with schizophrenia.

In fact, many people with schizophrenia, once stabilized on medication, can make a remarkable recovery and go on to establish intimate relationships, raise children, achieve steady employment, and find meaning and deep satisfaction in their lives. Since medications don't cure schizophrenia, many observers now believe that the illness of schizophrenia does *not* cause progressive brain damage, and that the deterioration seen previously was due more to the inadequate support and treatment people received for the illness. In other words, the theory of the deteriorating brain, believed to be the hallmark of the pathogenesis of schizophrenia, turns out not to be true. My own experience is that the vast majority of people with schizophrenia function with increasing success as their lives progress.

The unfortunate truth is that we don't know what causes schizophrenia or even what the illness is. Although many forms of treatment have proved beneficial, no treatment has a solid theoretical foundation.

Bipolar Disorder   The syndrome of bipolar disorder was first noticed in the 1800s. It was given the name manic-depressive illness because extended periods of depression, with its attendant lethargy, dysphoria, hopelessness, tearfulness, poor appetite, and suicidal thoughts, alternate with extended periods of manic symptoms of elation, grandiose thinking, rapid speech, accelerated thoughts, and hyperactivity. Sometimes manic thinking can include hallucinations and delusions. There are often extended periods of normal mood and good functioning.

In the middle of the twentieth century in the United States, psychiatrists believed anyone with psychotic symptoms had schizophrenia, even those with mood swings characteristic of bipolar disorder. As a result, the frequency of bipolar disorder appeared quite low. It became apparent in the 1960s and '70s, however, that the rate of diagnosis of bipolar disorder and schizophrenia in this country was much lower than in Europe. In the 1970s, it was found that people with bipolar disorder experienced a marked improvement on lithium while those with schizophrenia did not. Upon more rigorous diagnostic assessment, it was apparent that the American psychiatric practice of ascribing a diagnosis of schizophrenia to anyone with psychotic symptoms was simply not valid.

There is no psychological or laboratory test that reliably demonstrates the presence or absence of the syndrome of bipolar disorder. As a result, the threshold at which the diagnosis of bipolar disorder is applied to an individual is unclear. Some clinicians reserve it for people with severe mood swings that result in hospitalization. Some apply it to individuals who have any substantial variability in their moods, as is sometimes seen in people who have been sexually abused, or those who experience rapid mood shifts over the course of a day.

The etiology of bipolar disorder is unknown, although studies of families and twins strongly suggest a genetic component. Several researchers have made claims in recent years of specific genetic defects in people with bipolar disorder. These reports have not been confirmed by other investigators.

The pathogenesis of bipolar disorder is unclear. There is uncertainty about when bipolar disorder even begins. It was believed for many years that people first experienced symptoms of bipolar disorder in their twenties or early forties. It has become clear in recent years, however, that these time periods were picked primarily because that is when people were first hospitalized and diagnosed. Careful listening to adults with bipolar disorder revealed that many had mood swings as teenagers and even children. With the increasing availability of psychiatric treatment in recent years for children, more and more are seeking help for symptoms that suggest bipolar disorder. Although they don't have the euphoria that is characteristic of adults, they show marked irritability, impulsivity, and impaired judgment. Medications used in the treatment of bipolar disorder appear to help their distress. As a result, the diagnosis of bipolar disorder is now frequently given to children, something almost unheard of twenty years ago.

The confusing aspect about this is that many adolescents are irritable, aggressive, and impulsive because they are upset about their life circumstances. In recent years some of these teenagers have found their way into psychiatric hospitals, labeled with the diagnosis of bipolar disorder and placed on medications. Some psychiatric hospitals made a practice of admitting adolescents in distress, using the diagnosis of bipolar disorder inappropriately in order to increase their billing to insurance companies. This practice was so widespread that the federal government finally intervened, charging the hospitals with fraud and assessing fines of millions of dollars. Many of these children did not have bipolar disorder at all, but were acting inappropriately because of stresses in their families, with their friends, and at school. They needed therapy to help them deal with their lives.

So, who has bipolar disorder, and how can you be sure? There are enormous stakes involved both for patients who are prescribed medicines and providers whose financial well-being depends on the answers.

The "Chemical Imbalance" Theory

The current fad in making diagnoses is the "chemical imbalance" theory. The term "chemical imbalance" is drawn from the Biological Model of the mind, which proposes that psychiatric disorders are caused by abnormalities in the biological makeup of the brain.

Two trends contributed to the rise of the Biological Model and the "chemical imbalance" theory. First, starting in the 1950s, medications were developed that improved specific symptoms of many psychiatric illnesses. The first was Thorazine, which decreased the intensity of the hallucinations and delusions of people suffering from schizophrenia. Drug companies then developed and marketed medicines that treated other psychiatric problems. Benzodiazepines like Valium and Xanax decreased anxiety. Tofranil and Elavil, first marketed in the 1960s, and Prozac, Zoloft, and Paxil released in the 1980s helped millions of people with depression.

As technology improved, our understanding of how these medicines worked in the brain grew tremendously. New theories of psychiatric problems emerged based on how the medicines worked. For example, it appeared that the effect of Thorazine was due to its ability to block the effects of dopamine, a neurotransmitter important to brain function (see Appendix A). This gave rise to the theory that schizophrenia was caused by an excess of dopamine, commonly termed the *dopamine hypothesis*. Researchers proposed that depression was due to a deficit in norepinephrine, the *catecholamine hypothesis,* based on the knowledge that different antidepressants raised levels of norepinephrine in the brain. Lithium fixed the highs and lows of Bipolar Disorder, which perhaps was caused by a periodic excess or deficiency of a brain chemical. All the theories proposed an excess or a deficiency of a brain chemical, that is, a "chemical imbalance."

The development of new medicines was complemented by other research findings. These findings, and the way they dovetailed with the understanding of how drugs worked, strengthened belief in the "chemical imbalance" theory of the Biological Model.

For example, other findings supported the dopamine hypothesis of schizophrenia. Amphetamines produced an excess of dopamine and also led to psychotic symptoms. Dopa, a drug used in Parkinson's disease, is converted to dopamine in the body and can also produce hallucinations and delusions. Other drugs with widely different chemical structures that also blocked dopamine were as effective as chlorpromazine.

Other research appeared to confirm a biological etiology of depression. It was discovered that some people with depression have lower levels of the breakdown products of norepinephrine in the urine, implying that there is less in the brain. Depressed people with low levels of 5-hydroxyindoleacetic acid, the breakdown product of serotonin, were found to be at greater risk for suicide.[7]

As the evidence began to pile up, drugs became increasingly popular. Their popularity was not due solely to their effectiveness, however. Different groups advanced their own separate agendas, using the "chemical imbalance" theory as a protective umbrella, but contributing to the increased use of medication beyond what was justified by the evidence. Capitalizing on the market for psychiatric medications, the pharmaceutical industry promoted drugs far more aggressively than ever before to doctors and, recently, even to the public. Third party payers (TPPs) like insurance companies, health maintenance organizations, and managed care organizations offered drugs because they were the cheapest form of treatment. Some psychiatrists increasingly concentrated their practice on the prescription of medications to preserve their patient base and income, as TPPs have refused to pay for psychotherapy and hospitalization. Family practitioners, internists, and pediatricians increasingly prescribed psychiatric medications as well. Finally, many patients used drugs for relief rather than other forms of treatment that are more costly, take more time, and are more difficult than taking medication.

This rush to medication, however, overlooks the enormous holes in the "chemical imbalance" theory derived from the Biological Model. Research has documented the presence of biological abnormalities in many psychiatric disorders, but there is no specific evidence that any of these abnormalities is the *cause* of any disorder. It may appear that the gaps are about to be filled in. In fact, however, there are many lines of reasoning against a pure biological etiology of psychiatric disorders.

First, no biological etiology *has* been proven for any psychiatric disorder (except Alzheimer's disease, which has a genetic component) in spite of decades of research. Second, life experiences contribute to the development of some psychiatric disorders. For example, parental loss prior to the age of 18 leads to an increased risk of developing panic disorder and different phobias as adults.[8] Third, non-biological treatments effectively treat some psychiatric disorders. For example, a combination of practice with relaxation techniques, two to three months of cognitive-behavioral therapy, and attention to lifestyle changes can ameliorate panic attacks in many people. These facts, and others, strongly suggest that "abnormal biology" is not the sole cause of psychiatric disorders.

A more accurate model for the etiology of psychiatric disorders is the *Biopsychosocial* Model. This model proposes that three main areas of life interact to cause psychological problems: 1) Our *biology* through our genes, brain chemistry, medical conditions and drugs; 2) the unique constellation of feelings, desires, thoughts, and behaviors that makes up our own unique *psychology;* and 3) the events and people in our *social* experience that shape our life.

This model is more complex, obviously, which is one reason it is less popular. However, it offers far more to help you than the narrow view that only biology matters because it clarifies that many aspects of your life may be contributing to your distress. This gives you the opportunity to help your problems in *many* different ways, not just with medication. Diet, exercise, different forms of psychotherapy, constructive activities, and healthy relationships with others can be enormously helpful to you no matter what the problem.

So don't accept the myth that we can make an "accurate diagnosis." No one or two word label is the unquestionable "truth." Neither should you believe that your problems are due solely to a "chemical imbalance." No theory fully captures you, your life experience, or your problems. This doesn't mean that depression, hallucinations, and anxiety don't exist. But we need to recognize the difference between what we really know and what are merely hopeful theories, between the truth and what we merely think may be true.

Take the time to educate yourself about the symptoms you're experiencing, the different ways people have understood them in the past and currently, and the treatments that have been tried. Learn what is true and what is not true, what is known and what is merely guessed at. Only then can you make a sensible choice about medications and other treatments. In the next section, I'll describe what you need to consider to help you make that choice sensibly, knowledgeably, and correctly.

PART II

Is Medication for You?

CHAPTER 3

What to Discuss with Your Doctor *before* You Start Medication

It is important to consider many aspects of your life in order to arrive at an appropriate understanding of your problems, the context in which they are occurring, and what treatments would be best. Although it is reasonable to start with the idea of "I'm depressed and maybe Prozac would help me," that is merely a starting point. Many more issues need to be understood in order to know whether medication makes sense for you.

There are six domains you should discuss with your doctor in order to determine whether you should take medication. You need to weigh the information in each area in order to determine whether medication makes sense for you. There is no foolproof way to do this. The issues are not reducible to numbers that can be added, with medication prescribed if a certain score is reached. There is no single factor that overrides all the others. Carefully weigh *all* of the issues, and clarify in your mind which ones you will base your decision on.

Can Medication Help?

1. Know who you are

2. Establish the presence of a specific psychiatric syndrome

3. Assess the factors that shape psychiatric syndromes

4. Make a *complete* diagnosis

5. Know your treatment preferences

6. Create your treatment plan

---

1. Know Who You Are

In the assessment and treatment of any psychiatric problem a number of basic facts about yourself should be taken into consideration.

Age   Your age shapes the symptoms you are having, the way you may view them, and the treatment choice. Feelings of intense anxiety in a six-year-old starting school, a sixteen-year-old going on a first date, and a twenty-six-year-old going to the market have very different meanings and different consequences. The six-year-old needs encouragement and perhaps some visits to the school with friends before it starts. The sixteen-year-old needs some words of support and perhaps some advice about how to handle issues of money, sex, and curfew. The twenty-six-year-old may need an involved treatment program of psychotherapy, relaxation techniques, and medication.

Hallucinations in a teenager and an eighty-year-old mean different things as well. Although both need full psychiatric and medical evaluations, the teenager may need medication, help with friends and school, and psychotherapy, while the senior citizen may need only some supportive changes around the house.

Gender   Males and females do not experience psychiatric symptoms in the same way. For example, women are most troubled by the loss of an important relationship in their life through death, separation, or conflict, while men tend to feel most distressed when their ability to achieve and maintain satisfying employment is impaired. Treatment wishes can be quite different. For example, couples therapy may be enormously important to a woman whose main concern is a disruption in her relationship with her husband, while individual and group therapy may be more appropriate for a man who is having difficulty getting along with others and has lost a series of jobs.

Relationship Status   A person's marital status significantly influences the treatment choices for any psychiatric problem.

If your relationship with your partner is largely supportive, then it can be helpful for the partner to know what specific disorder you have and the treatments that will help you, how long they will go on, and how likely they are to be effective. Sometimes the partner can help to evaluate the effect of a particular treatment.

If there are problems in the relationship, and it appears that the relationship is the primary problem, then therapy directed at sorting out the source of the problem and resolving it satisfactorily is essential to a return to good health. If the psychiatric problem is primary, then it is essential to treat the problem as rapidly as possible and help the partner to understand that it may take some time for the symptoms to resolve before the relationship can improve.

Medications can have a variety of side effects that can alter your functioning in a number of ways. Many psychiatric medications can cause or exacerbate difficulties in your sexual relationship with your partner. It is important to explore treatment options that will minimize difficulties between you and your partner.

Employment   Psychiatric problems can both be caused by work and affect your work performance.

People who are anxious or depressed find it difficult to concentrate on their work and maintain a high level of performance. It's important to address your symptoms quickly in order to help you function well as soon as possible.

Are you so distressed that you are not able to work? It may be that medication and therapy are insufficient, and that you need vocational rehabilitation or other job support services to help you get back into the workforce.

Sometimes medications can cause side effects that impair a person's concentration, level of alertness, and coordination. I once worked with a man suffering from relatively severe anxiety who wanted to hold off on medication. He could not tolerate any loss of coordination, fatigue, nausea, or light-headedness because he worked in a construction job where any slight mistake would endanger both him and his coworkers. We agreed that psychotherapy was a more sensible treatment than medication.

Is work itself the source of your difficulties? Are you having difficulty because your work conditions are leading you to feel extremely stressed? Is the problem you, or are the requirements of the job unreasonable? Sometimes it makes more sense to change vocations than engage in psychiatric treatments when the main problem is actually the job itself.

Cultural Heritage   Almost all the cultures of the world are present in the United States to some degree. Many hold very different beliefs about health and illness, the theoretical basis for treatment, and the possible effectiveness of medications. Even the standard model of "objective, scientific" Western medicine has come under increasing question as alternative treatments appear to hold more promise than Western medicines in the treatment of some illnesses. For example, acupuncture has found increasing acceptance in the West to aid in the relief of pain, even though the theoretical foundation of acupuncture, that of an underlying energy circulating around the body that can be redirected by the insertion of pins, appears without validity to most Western scientists.

Depending on your own cultural heritage, you may experience a specific syndrome of psychological distress that is well known to you, but may be unknown to your doctor. Examples of such syndromes include such things as *ataque de nervios* among Latinos, *ghost sickness* among some Native American tribes, *koro* among Southeast Asians, and *zar* among North Africans. You may also hold beliefs that are directly contradictory to those of Western medicine and the possible benefits of psychiatric medication. It is important to communicate these beliefs to your doctor if you are in distress and are considering any form of psychiatric treatment.

However, you should also open your own mind to the possibility that there are effective treatments for your current difficulties that may work for you, even though they were pioneered through Western scientific thought and medical practices. I have seen people from China, Cambodia, East Africa, Puerto Rico, Argentina, and Native Americans benefit from medications, psychotherapy, and changes in diet, exercise, and lifestyle that were foreign to their own culture.

Religion   Religious beliefs affect how we see the difficulties we are experiencing and what we think will help us. For many of us, the behaviors and rituals encouraged by our faith help us to withstand the vicissitudes of life. These include celebrations of positive events such as births and weddings, as well as mourning rituals around death. Meditation by practitioners of Hinduism and Buddhism, the curing ceremonies of Native Americans, and prayer by Christians are long-standing practices that offer support when things appear most bleak.

There are times, however, when religious practices alone are not enough to alleviate distress. For example, most cultures these days recognize that a person suffering terrifying hallucinations and delusions is experiencing an illness, not a crisis in faith or a possession by the devil.

If you are experiencing psychiatric symptoms and are considering treatment that appears to be in conflict with your beliefs, you owe it to yourself to carefully consider both viewpoints. Most people find that they can remain faithful to their religious beliefs while still getting some practical help from physicians and caregivers in the form of treatment such as counseling and medication.

Personality   You have your own unique constellation of feelings, thoughts, and behaviors that make up your personality. These play a role in any psychiatric problem you experience. For example, if you are the kind of person who needs to be in control, it may be hard for you to experience symptoms of anxiety in which you feel as if your body is out of control. Your personality will also affect your choice of treatments. If you intensely dislike feeling out of control, you may want medication because you see it as the fastest way to get your unruly body to behave. On the other hand, you may not want to depend on an outside force that controls you.

There are so many different ways of understanding a person's personality that there is no easy way to sum yourself up. Decide for yourself what characteristics about your thoughts, feelings, and behaviors are most important to you, what effect they have on your psychiatric problem, and how they affect your treatment choice. Although your insight into yourself may not be perfect, don't be afraid to try to describe yourself psychologically. It is an essential part of understanding *you* and shouldn't be neglected in your assessment of the nature of your difficulties and the treatment you need.

2. Establish the Presence of a Specific Psychiatric Syndrome

The most important issue is to determine whether there is a psychiatric disorder present, and if so, which one. This is a complex issue, and it generates considerable disagreement. Some people believe any deviation from normal behavior is part of a psychiatric syndrome, while others believe that even the most extreme forms of thought and behavior are normal variations.

It is important to educate yourself about what disorder you may or may not have so that you can make the best use of treatment. Too many people are given a diagnosis based on one or two symptoms and are then given medication that may not even help. Don't let this happen to you. Learn about the psychiatric problem that you are having and the full range of treatments available.

There are three parts to any psychiatric syndrome: the main problem, its associated symptoms, and its effect on you and those around you.

Describe the Main Problem   Most people are able to describe their difficulties with words like "nerves," "depression," "mood swings," or "memory problems." Sometimes it's hard to boil down all the feelings, behaviors, and difficulties in your life into one or two words, especially if the problems are more related to your behavior than your feelings. Usually, however, there is one problem that is most troubling and that leads you to consider psychiatric treatment. Medical doctors call this the *chief complaint,* and organize their interview, physical exam, and laboratory tests around it. Common examples of chief complaints are things like chest pain, cough, or fever.

Psychiatric chief complaints are usually feelings, behaviors, or difficult life circumstances. Feelings such as anxiety, depression, or excessive anger are common. Behaviors like insomnia, forgetfulness, or alcohol abuse often lead people to come for help. The loss of a relationship or changes in health or work often lead people into treatment as well.

Describe the Associated Symptoms   The associated symptoms complete the picture of the main problem. For example, if you are anxious, do you experience chest pain, shortness of breath, trembling, sweating, and feelings of dread that are common in panic attacks, or is your anxiety unaccompanied by physical symptoms? If you are depressed, are you unable to function because of low energy, diminished appetite with weight loss, insomnia, suicidal preoccupation, or do you accomplish your daily activities even though you're chronically unhappy?

There are a number of different kinds of anxiety, mood, and psychotic disorders that are distinguished by the associated symptoms, not the main problem. It is important, therefore, to carefully assess the presence or absence of various associated symptoms in order to determine which psychiatric disorder is present. Effective treatments for the same chief complaint may differ when the chief complaint is accompanied by different associated symptoms. Part III describes the major psychiatric syndromes and the treatments helpful for each.

Determining the nature of psychiatric symptoms and whether there was a syndrome present was of paramount importance in a twenty-one-year-old woman who came to see me. She had had significant conflict with her boyfriend and assaulted him. When the police arrived, she was quite agitated and could not be calmed down, and they brought her to the emergency room. She had been drinking some alcohol, and the decision was made to admit her to the psychiatric unit. On the unit she complained of mood swings, and her moods appeared to shift rapidly on the ward from irritability, to tearfulness, and to relative calm. She was diagnosed with bipolar disorder and placed on Depakote. Over several days her mood swings appeared to even out, and she was discharged.

I carefully questioned her about her mood swings when we first met. There were no alterations in sleep, appetite, energy level, or changes in her thoughts or speech as are seen in bipolar disorder. Her mood was relatively stable when she was getting along with her boyfriend. When they argued, however, she would become very angry. It appeared to me that her "mood swings" appeared to be caused primarily by arguments with her boyfriend. I went over this with her in some detail and came to the conclusion that she probably did not have bipolar disorder. Upon sharing this with her, she felt that everything she learned about the illness did not really apply to her. Although she clearly had variability in her mood, we understood that these variations were more accurately seen as reactions to external stress. We agreed that she needed counseling with her boyfriend, which she engaged in. She gradually tapered off the Depakote and had no further need for medication.

Another woman who had never been on medication was referred to me by a clinician for evaluation of bipolar disorder. This woman had gone to the clinician with her husband because of chronic marital difficulties. Her husband complained that she periodically became quite withdrawn, had no energy, and didn't provide very good care for their children. At other times she would be quite energetic, enthusiastic, though irritable at times, but exercise poor judgment in financial matters and in regard to her children. For example, she decided spontaneously during one school vacation to go down to Florida for a week. She charged it all to a credit card, even though they couldn't afford to take such an expensive vacation. The ups and downs of his wife's mood were very troubling to her husband, and he was considering separation.

I questioned her about her symptoms during our first meeting. She had periods of depression lasting weeks and at times months that were accompanied by low energy, tearfulness, feelings of helplessness and hopelessness, and excessive sleep. She also had periods lasting as long as a few weeks, in which she needed less sleep, her activity level increased, her thoughts speeded up, she talked more, nonstop at times, and would often use alcohol inappropriately.

This woman clearly had bipolar disorder. Placing her on medication significantly ameliorated her ups and downs and allowed her to function far more effectively as a parent and in her marriage.

With both of these women, as with anyone who is considering medication, it is important to use medication not just for the "chemical imbalance" or the diagnostic label that may be all too easily applied. Rather, it is important to sort out whether or not a specific psychiatric syndrome actually exists.

Educate yourself about the different syndromes and make sure that the one you choose fits your symptoms as closely as possible. For example, if you have mood swings and wonder whether you have bipolar disorder, seek information from your doctor, books at a library or bookstore, through the Internet, and through organizations such as the American Psychiatric Association or the National Alliance for the Mentally Ill. Part III describes the symptoms of different psychiatric disorders.

Don't believe everything you hear or read, however, for there is a great deal of misinformation in the media. Go over what you have learned with your doctor. At a minimum you should decide with your doctor exactly which psychiatric syndrome you both believe is present as you consider the possible usefulness of medication. Even if neither one of you can be fully certain, and this is frequently true because of the difficulties that we discussed in the first section, you should at least be in agreement as to what you are doing together. Keep an open mind regarding things that aren't fully clear, and always be ready to revise your thinking.

Assess the Effects of Symptoms on Your Life   The presence of a psychiatric syndrome should not in and of itself determine whether you take medication. It is also important to consider the amount of distress your symptoms cause you, the degree of impairment of your functioning, and the effects of your difficulties on others.

For example, a man I once saw complained of unhappiness that had troubled him for many years. He very much wanted to try Prozac. Although he found that his mood slightly improved, he noticed marked sexual dysfunction. He decided that he would rather stay off antidepressants and avoid the sexual dysfunction, in part because his depression was mild and did not impair his ability to lead his life. He began to exercise regularly, decreased his work week to four and a half days a week from six, and spent more time with his wife in leisure activities. These changes helped his depression more directly without impairing his sexual functioning, and he decided to stay off antidepressants.

It is also important to determine whether the syndrome bothers you or whether it bothers other people. Many people with mild depression find that they note minimal benefit from antidepressants, while those around them may notice a significant improvement. While I do not believe that you should take medication merely to satisfy other people, it is important to weigh their observations carefully so that you can make the best judgment for yourself.

Taking medications because other people see the benefit is a major issue when children cause disruption in school. The disruptive child often leads to the four *P*'s: the *principal* calls the *parent,* who calls the *pediatrician,* who calls in the *prescription.* Learning disabilities, stresses in life, normal rambunctiousness, and classroom expectations of docile children can also contribute to the perception of a child as disruptive, difficult, and in need of medications. These issues can be lost in the rush to medication if the focus is only on the effects of the child's disruptiveness and not on the need to make a full assessment.

If your symptoms are severe, you may want medication to alleviate your distress right away. Although this is reasonable, don't let the intensity of your symptoms and your need for immediate relief override your willingness to consider other treatment alternatives.

3. Assess the Factors That Shape Psychiatric Syndromes

Current Influences   There are several areas in your day-to-day life that influence the presence and severity of any psychiatric syndrome that you may be experiencing and will shape the treatment you choose.

Life Stresses   Sometimes the problems in life are only too clear. Your distress may directly follow illness, the death of someone close to you, the breakup of a relationship, sudden unemployment, or the departure of children from home. Other times, the reasons may not be obvious. For example, maybe you've become depressed over what appears to be a relatively small event. It may not be immediately apparent that this small event reminds you of earlier difficulties in life. Panic attacks often appear to come out of the blue with no apparent cause. Upon careful review, however, the issues that led to the intense anxiety often emerge.

There are three basic areas of life that often cause difficulty: your current relationships, your work, and issues related to your stage of life. A breakup of a six-month relationship may overwhelm you initially. The most appropriate treatment may be psychotherapy to help you put your loss into perspective so that you can move on. On the other hand, if you have just lost your spouse of forty years, you may need medication to prevent a serious depression as you adjust to life alone after so many years together. Being fired from work may be enormously distressing and cause anxiety and depression for which medication may be useful. You may also benefit from group therapy to explore difficulties you may have relating positively with others. As age-related issues evolve—developing a lasting intimate relationship in your twenties, a career in your thirties, health changes in your forties, and the departure of your children as they grow into adulthood—depression and anxiety often occur.

Coping Skills   We each have our own unique coping style with which we manage the ups and downs of life. Ideally we engage in activities that are constructive when things are difficult, such as seeking support from friends and family, engaging in new activities, exercising regularly, eating sensibly, and avoiding the excessive use of alcohol and other drugs.

Some people have learned specific skills to help them manage their psychiatric symptoms. For example, many people with attention deficit disorder use appointment books, a scheduled routine, and support from other people who organize them at work. Many people with anxiety have learned relaxation techniques and know the importance of avoiding caffeine and engaging in regular exercise.

If you lack coping skills, you can learn some. People with a wide variety of psychiatric disorders can be helped with a number of simple day-to-day techniques that can significantly diminish the impairment and distress caused by their disorder. It is important for you and your physician to identify these coping skills so your improvement can proceed as quickly as possible and treatment can be as effective as possible. For example, relaxation techniques to help with anxiety can significantly enhance whatever medications and therapy you choose for yourself.

Physical Complaints and Medical Problems Physical conditions and medical problems affect the assessment and treatment of your psychiatric problem in five ways.

First, some physical problems may initially manifest themselves as psychiatric symptoms. For example, anxiety or depression may be the first symptom you experience if you have a thyroid disorder. A lack of energy or depression may be from colon cancer. It is important to determine that you do not have a physical illness causing your psychiatric problems. The specific physical conditions that can give rise to psychiatric problems are noted in part III.

Second, you may be taking medications or undergoing treatment that can cause psychiatric symptoms. For example, some cardiac and antihypertension medications cause depression. Some antiasthmatic medications can cause anxiety and worsen psychotic thinking. The medications that can cause psychiatric problems will be described in more detail in part III.

Third, physical problems can obscure psychiatric difficulties. For example, you may experience depression if you have Parkinson's disease, rheumatoid arthritis, chronic back pain from back injuries, or heart problems. The depression may go undiagnosed or be attributed to the disorder itself and never become a focus of treatment. As a result you may be more depressed and experience needless impairment in your day-to-day functioning.

Fourth, medical conditions can complicate the treatment of any psychiatric disorder. For example, certain antidepressants can be dangerous if you have heart problems or blood pressure abnormalities.

Finally, the form of treatment recommended for relief of psychiatric problems must take into account the physical problems you may have and any treatment you are undergoing. While regular exercise may be important to your recovery if you are thirty, it may not be possible if you are eighty and have heart problems or an unsteady gait.

Use of Drugs There are several ways in which substance use and dependence can influence a psychiatric disorder, its assessment, and recommended treatment.

First, substance use may *cause* whatever psychiatric problem you have. For example, excessive alcohol use can cause anxiety, depression, and insomnia. Achieving abstinence through involvement with groups such as Alcoholics Anonymous and other psychoeducational methods may be sufficient to improve psychiatric symptoms, although you may need some psychotherapy to help you begin to lead an effective and satisfying life without substances.

Sometimes people turn to drugs and alcohol because they seem, on the surface, to alleviate distress. For example, if you have chronic anxiety, you may become dependent on alcohol, thinking it minimizes your anxiety. It can be difficult to stop drinking unless you get some help for your anxiety. As alcohol exacerbates anxiety, effective treatment requires targeting both anxiety and the use of alcohol.

Sometimes both disorders are present, and both can be considered primary. For example, some people use marijuana at the time they experience the gradual onset of the disorganized thinking of schizophrenia. Although marijuana may generate euphoria, it can also disorganize a person's thinking. Treatment often needs to be directed both at the substance use as well as the thought disorder of schizophrenia.

Any treatment recommendations will vary significantly depending on the presence or absence of any substance abuse and its relationship to a psychiatric problem.

If you are using alcohol, marijuana, or any other drugs, it is vitally important to get some help to stop your use and address your psychiatric problems as well. There are far more productive ways to manage the distress you feel, ways that will help you to lead a satisfying and meaningful life. Millions of people have found that giving up alcohol and drugs was an important step in getting their lives back on track. Value your mind and body enough to make the best effort you can to get better.

Past Issues   Your past circumstances need to be taken into account in order to accurately assess and treat any psychiatric problem.

Previous Psychiatric Problems   Previous episodes of distress can help determine treatment for your current difficulties. You may get a head start on addressing your current difficulties by reviewing what you learned about the cause of your previous problems and what helped you. For example, if psychotherapy was insufficient for depression that emerged after the breakup of a relationship and you needed antidepressants to get better, it may make sense to start antidepressants at the first sign of depression, without waiting until your functioning is significantly impaired.

Previous Psychiatric Treatment   It is extremely important to review any previous treatment. If medication has been effective before for similar symptoms, the same medication may be helpful again. If certain medications or treatments haven't worked before, it makes little sense to try them again.

Sometimes previous treatments weren't effective because the treatments themselves weren't carried out adequately. For example, the potential value of an antidepressant is unknown if you took it for only a few days, because antidepressants take weeks to work.

Childhood Events   Some childhood experiences cause psychiatric problems later in life. Sexual abuse, physical abuse, and emotional neglect due to parental substance abuse, illness, or death contribute to anxiety and depression in adults. Some experiences are so severe that posttraumatic stress disorder develops in childhood and people form their identities and adult functioning around them.

Your early childhood experience may also shape the way you manage problems as an adult. For example, if you covered up feelings of anger, sadness, or anxiety as a child, you may find that you do the same thing as an adult in your relationships with adults, at work, or with your children. You may have difficulty asserting yourself and helping to change a situation at work that makes you angry because you never learned to express anger appropriately as a child. This may contribute to depression as an adult because you feel helpless in unsatisfying situations.

Finally, your childhood experiences can influence the form of treatment with which you feel most comfortable. If you were sexually abused by a man, you may feel more comfortable with a woman therapist. If you have been harmed significantly by others, you may not want to engage in group therapy because of your fear of being attacked or criticized by others. It might make sense to consider individual therapy until you are feeling more confident about addressing interpersonal issues effectively in a group format.

Other Family Members with Psychiatric Problems   As we previously discussed, there is no clear genetic cause for any psychiatric disorder. Nevertheless, many disorders do appear more common in some families. It is important to assess whether siblings, parents and their siblings, grandparents, and sometimes even more distant relatives have had similar or different psychiatric problems. This assessment can offer insights that may illuminate your diagnosis.

It is also important to understand what treatment has been effective for your relatives. While psychiatric disorders are heterogeneous in nature, there may be biological similarities among family members that lead them to respond well to the same medication. Even if you may not know exactly whether your brother has an anxiety disorder or depressive disorder, the fact that he responded to Prozac may provide a clue as to what medicine could be helpful for you.

4. Make a *Complete* Diagnosis

We discussed the difficulties with making a diagnosis in part I. Nevertheless, you need to come to some understanding about the difficulties you are having in order to figure out how to help yourself most effectively. The conclusions you reach will affect the treatment you choose. For example, if you've suddenly begun to experience panic attacks and you feel that nothing in your life causes them, you are more likely to look for medication as a solution. On the other hand, if you connect the panic attacks with the feeling of being out of control ever since your father died of a sudden heart attack, you will probably be more open to psychotherapy and relaxation techniques. If you see schizophrenia strictly as a brain disease, then medication can seem like the only sensible treatment. If you see it as an illness that strongly affects you as a person, however, you are more likely to see the additional value provided by psychotherapy and rehabilitation to help you cope successfully with the illness.

Assess the Etiology, Pathogenesis, and Syndrome   Use all the information you can gather about the etiology, pathogenesis, and syndrome. For example, if you are feeling sad and hopeless with tearfulness and insomnia, it's likely you will decide that you have depression (the syndrome). You've been somewhat depressed all your life, and you believe you may have a biological/genetic vulnerability to depression because your mother, aunt, and grandmother have also experienced depression (the etiology). You wonder if your depression is due in part to your parents' divorce when you were a child, but believe it's mostly due to your recent separation from your spouse (the pathogenesis).

Perhaps your seven-year-old boy is hyperactive and disruptive at school and his teacher suggests that he needs evaluation for medication. After learning about attention deficit/hyperactivity disorder (ADHD) from your doctor and some books from a bookstore, you decide that he does have ADHD. You know your son has always been very active, but he's worse since he began first grade. You feel that the etiology may be biological in nature, but the recent worsening in his symptoms (pathogenesis) is really due to the restrictiveness of full-time school.

Assess the Biological, Social, and Psychological Realms of Your Life
Your diagnosis should include consideration of the three areas of life that shape psychiatric problems: the biological (your brain), the psychological (your mind), and the social (your life). Consider each one separately as you try to understand what is contributing to your problems.

Could you have two disorders? It can be confusing if you have symptoms that suggest two disorders. For example, perhaps you experience hallucinations and delusions, as well as symptoms characteristic of manic episodes. Do you have bipolar disorder with psychotic thinking or schizophrenia with manic episodes? The diagnostic label often given to such people is schizoaffective disorder ("schizo" for psychotic thinking, "affective" for mood disturbance of either mania or depression), but no one really knows whether certain difficulties are best understood as a disorder of thought or mood.

There is substantial debate over how to understand multiple syndromes in the same person. The current practice in the field of psychiatry is to isolate each syndrome with its own separate diagnosis. This often makes no sense. For example, some people with chronic psychotic thinking and depression also experience panic attacks. Three diagnoses could be applied: schizophrenia, depression, and panic disorder. It seems unrealistic to think they have *three* illnesses, however, each with its own separate etiology, pathogenesis, and syndrome. Only a good understanding of the underlying biology and psychology, which we do not yet possess, can help us to sort this out, so there is no satisfactory solution at present.

On the other hand, isolating each syndrome ensures that each problem becomes a focus of treatment. This is clearly a good thing. If you feel that you have symptoms of two or more disorders, say anorexia and depression, make sure you don't lose sight of either one. Try to sort out the etiology and pathogenesis as best you can, keeping in mind that your focus is on your treatment, not a sterile exercise in psychobiology.

Keep an Open Mind   As you make your diagnosis, be open to new information. Be prepared to change your mind as you gather more information and begin treatment. Maybe you'll come to believe that your depression isn't "biological" at all but instead is due to emotional deprivation during childhood. Maybe you'll come to believe that your son doesn't have ADHD, that he really is just rambunctious, and that the school needs education about how to manage high-energy boys.

Come to an Agreement with Your Doctor about Your Diagnosis   It's most beneficial if you agree with your psychiatrist about your full diagnosis, that is, sharing what you believe is the syndrome of symptoms, the cause of your illness, and what has made it worsen to the point that it now needs treatment. You may have some ideas about your difficulties and what would be most helpful based on something that you recently read or heard about. Discuss what you have learned with your physician. Although your doctor or psychiatrist may have one view of what the problem is, you may have another. For example, you may feel that your problems are primarily due to your current situation while the doctor may think you have more long-standing difficulties. You won't get much help if you begin therapy with the idea that your problems will be solved in a few weeks while your doctor thinks it will take months or even years.

5. Know Your Treatment Preferences

Express Your Treatment Preferences   They matter! It is important for you to communicate to your doctor what kind of treatment you would like. Although many primary care physicians are most comfortable prescribing medication, say you want to talk to a therapist if that's what you believe would help you the most.

On the other hand, you may have done some reading or have heard about a specific medication that you think may be helpful for you, and be quite clear that you want to try it. It is important that you bring this up so that the physician doesn't give you medicine that you think is only second-best. If the two of you disagree about what would be best for you, make sure that you understand the reasons for the disagreement so that you can come to the best decision together.

Assess Your Motivation   The success of any treatment depends on how willing you are to go along with it. Although psychotherapy and relaxation techniques can help many people with anxiety, they won't be effective for you if you don't do them. If your doctor is recommending medication, but you don't want to take it because of your concern about side effects or because you don't think you need it, you won't get much benefit if your ambivalence leads you to take it inconsistently.

Consider How You Will Pay for Treatment   These days the funding of psychiatric treatment is in flux. Managed care companies, insurance companies, pharmaceutical companies, and the medical profession are all vying to get your dollars.

It is wise to inform yourself about what the costs of any treatment will be. This may mean a detailed discussion with your doctor about how soon any treatment, such as psychotherapy or medication, can begin to provide you benefits, whether that treatment will need to be continued indefinitely, and how much it will cost you if your insurance company doesn't pay.

Many people are shocked by the high cost of medications for their disorders. Many people are unable to pay the high cost of newer medications like olanzapine, Effexor, and Depakote. Although some of the older medications such as Elavil, Thorazine, and lithium are significantly cheaper, they tend to cause side effects that are more troubling.

Make sure that you can afford medication that you and your doctor think can be of help. It is very distressing to have to stop medication that is effective merely because of cost. It can also be difficult to change medications. For example, changing an antidepressant commonly involves significant ups and downs in a person's mood as one medication wears off and the other one begins to kick in. Try to select an affordable medication at the beginning of treatment.

Consider the Negative Aspects of Any Treatment   Any treatment that you choose may have a downside. Besides ineffectiveness and cost, medications commonly cause side effects. Psychotherapy can be time-consuming and expensive. Behavioral techniques and short-term psychotherapy can be helpful in the short run, but the benefits may wane over time. You will need to weigh the pros and cons of the problems associated with any treatment. It is a good idea to explore this ahead of time to avoid wasting your time, money, and effort with a treatment that you are unwilling to complete.

6. Create Your Treatment Plan

Consider All Treatments   It is essential that you consider all options, not just medications, before deciding on which treatment, or combination of treatments, is best for you. Educate yourself about what each treatment involves. Although some treatments may appear vague or complicated at first, you may get enormous benefit from them. For example, many people are skeptical when I describe the importance of relaxation techniques in minimizing their anxiety. The techniques sound cumbersome, ineffective, and perhaps even silly. However, people quickly notice that they are able to relax more effectively when they practice these exercises regularly. It is important that you consider alternative treatments with more than just a shake of the head.

Compare Treatments   Compare the treatments with the benefits that you hope to derive from medication. Although it may seem that taking a pill is the simplest alternative, often this is not so. For example, antidepressants for depression can seem very straightforward. People who jump right into them, pay a couple of hundred dollars a month, and then find their sexual lives severely curtailed begin to rethink the usefulness of medication and consider alternatives. Do yourself a favor and make your assessment *before* you've spent your time and energy on something that isn't going to help.

Don't Rush to Medication   Most people are in significant distress when they first show up and go on medication. It can be hard to consider other forms of treatment during the initial visit. However, even if medication is effective for you, keep other treatments in mind. For example, a woman came to see me for long-standing symptoms of depression that had worsened recently when she and her husband discussed separation. She clearly needed medication, which helped her feel somewhat better within a few weeks. However, she felt that her depression was truly better only after she began couples therapy with her husband to address the areas of conflict between them.

You need to take extra precautions if you are considering medication and you are not an adult white male. The next chapter focuses on why.

CHAPTER 4

People for Whom Psychiatric Drugs Pose Extra Risk

Psychiatric research in this country has concentrated on white male adults for reasons that are largely political and financial, not medical. Many important aspects of the psychiatric treatment of children, women, the elderly, and people of varied ethnic backgrounds have not been systematically investigated. This lack of research on other populations has led the medical and psychiatric profession to make treatment recommendations for these populations by extrapolating findings made by studying the adult white male.

Unfortunately, these extrapolations do not take into account the differences in the biological makeup of members of these groups. There are important issues unique to each group, and any member of these groups should take extra caution in the use of medication.

Children

Children are vulnerable. Because of their smaller size, limited cognitive skills, and dependence on others, adults protect them from harm and exploitation in myriad ways. These issues are relevant to the prescription of psychiatric medications to children.

As a parent, you have the legal authority to decide whether your child should receive any medical treatment. Although you will likely discuss the issue of medication with your child, the decision is essentially yours. If you are a parent trying to decide about the usefulness of medication for your child, you have more to weigh than if you were deciding just for yourself. There are four major areas of concern.

Your Support How you view your child's difficulties will have an enormous impact on how he or she understands the symptoms and copes with them. While you may feel angry and frustrated by certain behaviors or lack of improvement, it is important to be as supportive as possible. Educate yourself by learning as much as you can about the symptoms and possible treatments. This can help you understand your child's difficulties within a framework based on the two of you working together to master the problems as best you can, rather than on your feelings about your child's problems.

Ethics   The major ethical issue is to determine exactly whom you are trying to help. Few children are able to articulate that they feel some internal distress and want medication. The issue of whether or not to prescribe medication generally arises because of a child's difficulty functioning in some area of life. If you or an outside observer notices some impairment in your child, you must first decide whether the behavior is abnormal or merely disruptive to those who notice it.

As there is no objective measure to prove or disprove the presence or absence of any psychiatric disorder, this can be a difficult assessment. For example, if your child's teacher thinks your child has attention deficit disorder and may need medication, it is important to get a complete picture of the child's experience in the classroom. You need to decide whether your child is behaving in a manner that is out of the normal range or whether the school has an especially low tolerance for children who are active and energetic with a tendency to be rambunctious. Even if it turns out that he does have attention deficit disorder, some school programs are able to manage a child with attention deficit disorder without the use of medication through implementation of a strong behavioral plan. If your school does not have this capability, you must ask yourself whether you are medicating your child for the child's symptoms or the limitations of the school.

This is not an idle question. Millions of children now receive Ritalin to help them function better in school. Critics of schools and the psychiatric profession believe, however, that while many children derive substantial benefit from medication, some of these children are taking medication to help the schools, not the children. They feel that the medication makes children docile enough to tolerate a system that discriminates against energetic children who aren't quiet in large groups and who don't like to sit at desks for hours every day.

Following the guidelines set forth in chapter 3 should help you feel confident that the medication is truly for your child's benefit.

Evaluation of the Child   The baseline assessment for children is similar to the one outlined in chapter 3 for adults. There are several areas that need special mention, however.

Diagnostic Evaluation   Obviously it will be important to perform a full psychiatric evaluation of your child should he or she be experiencing symptoms of distress. The purpose of the evaluation is to determine the presence or absence of any specific psychiatric syndrome, in spite of our current inability to do so with precision.

Your child deserves a complete evaluation by a knowledgeable practitioner. Many pediatricians do not have the training and experience necessary to distinguish between disorders that may have some common symptoms but in fact require very different treatment, such as attention deficit disorder, learning disabilities, oppositional disorder, and conduct disorder. If your child's problems are significant enough that they are causing him or her distress and you are considering medication, he or she deserves an evaluation by a professional trained to perform one. Medical doctors with graduate training in child psychiatry are most qualified to perform this evaluation—child psychiatrists, behavioral pediatricians, and child neurologists with special expertise in childhood behavioral problems.

Life Stresses   As much as adults, children are affected by things going on around them. Many children do not verbalize their thoughts and feelings about changes that occur in their lives, so it can be easy to assume that they are handling things well. However, changes in your home life, the physical health of your child and other members of your family, the child's functioning at school, or relationships with peers will assuredly affect your child. Each of these areas should be investigated as part of the evaluation. Contact with your child's teacher at school is important both during the evaluation process and after treatment has begun.

Your use of alcohol or drugs affects your child, even though it may not be readily apparent to you. It is worthwhile to discuss your use of alcohol or drugs with the mental health professional who is evaluating your child to assess whether your use is contributing to your child's distress.

Physical Exam   There should be a physical examination of your child if there are symptoms disruptive enough to call for the administration of medication. A physical exam should include baseline temperature, pulse, blood pressure, height, and weight. A pregnancy test should be considered for any girl who might be pregnant, because medications may have adverse effects on the developing fetus.

Laboratory Tests   Laboratory tests frequently recommended as part of a comprehensive pediatric examination or premedication workup include the following:[1]

1. Complete blood count
2. Urinalysis
3. Blood urea nitrogen
4. Serum electrolyte levels
5. Liver function tests
6. Serum lead level determination
7. Thyroid function test (if lithium is prescribed)
8. Kidney function test (if lithium is prescribed)
9. Electrocardiogram (EKG—if tricyclic antidepressants are prescribed)
10. Electroencephalogram (EEG—if child is at risk for seizures)

Rating Scales   Once the presence of a psychiatric disorder has been suspected and consideration has been given to the use of medication, it may be useful to perform an objective assessment of the severity of symptoms with the use of a specific rating scale. Rating scales are a series of questions designed to determine the presence or absence of the signs and symptoms in different disorders. Rating scales can be self-report, filled out by the child; an informant report, filled out by you or a teacher; or a professional report, filled out by a psychiatrist, social worker, or pediatrician. Examples of scales include the Connors Teacher Rating Scale and Parent Rating Scale, which are commonly used to assist in the diagnosis of ADHD.

After medication is prescribed, the scale is repeated to determine whether there has been improvement. Although rating scales are somewhat objective, there is the subjective element of any rater's assessment of the individual questions. As a result, the rating scale itself should not be held in higher regard than assessments by the school, teacher, you, or your child, but it can be a useful aid.

Target Symptoms   As discussed in chapter 16, it is important to determine whether there is a target symptom that may improve with medication. Although fire setting, lying, stealing, and refusal to do homework may be very troubling behaviors, they are not amenable to specific medication. On the other hand, if a symptom such as stealing is part of a depressive syndrome, in which a child steals to "fill up" with some concrete object what he feels is lacking inside, then direct treatment of the depression with medication may help to modify the stealing behavior. Nevertheless, the target symptom of the medication would not be stealing, it would be the symptoms of the depression, such as sadness, lack of energy, poor sleep, poor appetite, and lack of motivation.

Treatment Issues   The prime treatments for children in distress are psychotherapy and behavioral interventions. Medications should be used as one part of a total treatment program, not alone.

Alliance   Although you are the decision maker about medication, bring your child into the decision-making process as an important partner. Forming an alliance with your child around the symptoms and treatment stimulates interest in seeing the treatment succeed. It can also start the process of self-observation, so that a child monitors his or her own behavior with the goal of improving.

Forming a good treatment alliance with teenagers is especially important. Most teenagers want to be independent and resent any perceived threat to their autonomy. Many will actively resist any treatment that they feel is forced on them. Educating them about the nature of their problems and listening to their treatment wishes can help to secure their cooperation for treatment that may be initially unappealing but ultimately beneficial.

Physiology of Children   The brain continues to develop throughout childhood, adolescence, and adulthood. For example, some neuroanatomical pathways in the brain are not completed until the adult years. This may explain why symptoms of many psychiatric disorders are somewhat different in children and adults. It may also be why some psychiatric disorders such as schizophrenia and bipolar disorder are relatively rare in prepubertal children and have their onset usually in the late teens and early twenties. As a result of these differences, medications may have different effects in children.

Because of their smaller size, children may need smaller doses of medication than adults. However, children tend to require larger doses of medication *per pound of body weight* in order to achieve the same blood levels and therapeutic efficacy as adults. This is because the liver is proportionally larger in children. As a result, medication is more rapidly metabolized by the liver and excreted by the kidneys.

Safety   Besides knowing whether medication may help your child, you need to know whether medication may harm your child. You are well advised to be cautious about this issue. A number of psychiatric medications can indeed be dangerous for your child. Although the rate of mortality is extremely low with the vast majority of psychiatric drugs, some people have died who have taken desipramine, valproate, and clozapine.

You need to educate yourself about all the potential side effects that your child may experience from any medication he or she takes. Some of the side effects may not be immediately obvious. For example, the use of methylphenidate can impair a child's growth and height. Lithium use for many years can impair kidney function. Obviously if a child is on lithium for bipolar disorder beginning at the age of twelve or fourteen, there are potentially many decades of use. The effects of lithium on kidney function when it is begun in the teenage years and continued for twenty, thirty, or forty years have not been definitively evaluated and determined to be safe.

Besides side effects, you also want to know whether medication may change your child's personality. A child's personality is shaped by physical characteristics, temperament, behavior, moods, thoughts, sense of humor, intelligence, interpersonal relationships, and other things. Ideally, of course, medication should work only on those aspects of the psychiatric syndrome that are troubling. For example, a child who was otherwise well and then became depressed would take medication and the symptoms of depression would improve.

Medication sometimes affects more than the narrow psychiatric syndrome and may change a child's personality in ways that permit better functioning. For example, your daughter may be painfully shy. Antianxiety medication may help her interact more easily with other people. This will allow her to get out more, be more confident in school, and establish and maintain friendships more easily. Your child with ADHD may find that overtalkativeness and physical rambunctiousness is so extreme that it turns other kids off. Medication can sometimes tone down the hyperactivity and impulsivity, aiding the ability to make and keep positive relationships with others.

Medications can affect personality in ways that can have negative consequences as well, however. SSRIs such as Paxil, Luvox, Prozac, and Zoloft can inhibit a person's sexual drive and the ability to become aroused and achieve orgasm. How medication-induced alterations in sexual development in children and teenagers might affect their sexual adjustment as teenagers, and as adults, is unclear.

As the guardian of your child's total health, and not just the administrator of medication, do not ignore your own concerns about the effects of medication on your child's personality. Make them part of a conversation between you, your doctor, and the child.

Lack of Research   Most medications have not been approved by the FDA for use in children. You should be aware that many doctors prescribe these medications anyway, based primarily on clinical experience. These medicines may be helpful to your child, but you should be aware that the research supporting their use is lacking.

Drug Holidays   Because children are growing in so many different ways and the safety of most psychiatric medications for use over the long term has not been established, most clinicians feel it is advisable to minimize the use of medication by using the smallest dose for the shortest period of time. For example, if a teenager becomes depressed in response to the loss of an important relationship, antidepressants may be helpful until the teen has regained his or her former level of functioning, but can then be stopped. On the other hand, children who experience psychotic disorders or bipolar disorder may need to take medication continuously in order to prevent worsening of their symptoms. The wisdom of a drug holiday is best determined by considering the issues raised in stopping a medication, discussed in chapter 16.

Women

The improvement in opportunities for women over the last few decades should not blind us to the oppression women have experienced in the past and continue to experience now. The medical and psychiatric professions have contributed many sorry chapters to this story. These include denying entrance to women to medical schools until the 1960s, preventing midwives from practicing obstetrics in order to preserve this lucrative area of business for obstetricians, and blocking efforts at finding safe and effective contraception. The psychiatric profession denied the frequency of sexual abuse and the devastation it caused until the 1980s, and has persistently described women's psychological development as deficient, based largely on theories derived from the study of men.

One terrible period in the treatment of women by the psychiatric profession occurred in the fifties and sixties. This was a time when women were supposed to be satisfied with a very constricted role in life. Many women were upset at the restrictions placed on their hopes and dreams. Many became distressed, anxious, or depressed. Millions were given medications to blunt their distress, medications that turned out to be addictive. The underlying social message was that there was something the matter with women and they needed to be fixed with medication. In fact, of course, the feelings of distress that these women experienced were entirely reasonable and should not have been blunted with medication. Rather than acknowledge the legitimacy of women's distress and help them to change things in society so that they were not so oppressed, psychiatry, wittingly or not, was one of the oppressive forces that women experienced during these years.

Because of the greater presence of women in positions of power in society and medicine, some of the more overt oppression of women has receded. Nevertheless, there is still cause for concern with regard to the treatment of women by the psychiatric profession.

For one thing, the frequency of anxiety and depression is much higher in women than it is for men. Their use of psychiatric medications for these two disorders is also much higher. Even accounting for the higher prevalence of psychiatric disorders in women, however, they are still given medication more frequently than men are. For example, Elizabeth Ettore, a psychiatrist who has written widely on the psychopharmacological treatment of women, studied one hundred men and women who had used psychiatric drugs for a period of nine years. Ninety percent took habit-forming benzodiazepines either on their own or in combination with other psychiatric drugs. Many patients grew concerned about the duration of their drug use and asked their doctors to help them stop. Male patients were twice as likely to receive support from their doctors in their desire to stop. One-third of women users were told that there was no alternative to their drug use, while only 6 percent of men heard this message.[2]

Another cause for concern is that factors unique to women have often been used as justification for excluding women from drug research.[3] The onset of menarche at puberty, the hormonal changes that occur throughout the menstrual cycle, and the dramatic shifts in hormone levels at menopause all cause significant changes in a woman's physiology. Females also experience different rates of drug absorption, distribution throughout the body, metabolism, and excretion. How these changes affect women has not been adequately understood by the psychiatric and medical profession.

Another complication is the use of hormone therapy for menopause and contraception. Hormone pills may be very effective for the specific indications for which they are used, namely to minimize the effects of menopause and to prevent pregnancy, but they have other far-reaching effects on women's physiology. The effects of hormone replacement therapy on psychiatric disorders, and on the way that medications are handled and how they may influence the effectiveness of psychiatric medications, are largely unknown.

This lack of knowledge can be very significant on a practical basis. For example, many women notice that they experience more anxiety, depression, or irritability a few days prior to the onset of their menstrual period. If this occurs when they are on medication, it is difficult to know whether it is due to the hormone changes themselves, to the ineffectiveness of the medication, or to alterations in the way the body reacts to the medication. Adequate research into the differences in the way that medications are handled by the body throughout the menstrual cycle could help to provide an accurate assessment that would be useful to guide treatment.

In the absence of this research, it is difficult to make sensible recommendations. It is especially important, therefore, to closely monitor your symptoms and responses to medication. It may be useful to chart the intensity of your symptoms if they wax and wane in relation to your menstrual cycle.

Medication During Pregnancy   Pregnancy is an important event in a woman's life. Anxiety, depression, and other psychiatric problems can dramatically shift with the knowledge that you are pregnant and with the physiological changes that occur in your body.

Pregnancy will affect your physiological status in a number of ways. For example, the volume of distribution for a drug is larger, effectively decreasing the amount of drug available to the brain at any given dose. Other changes include a decrease in gastrointestinal motility and an increased rate of breakdown of many drugs.[4] Hormonal shifts during pregnancy may intensify these effects, all of which can significantly alter the level of drug in the body. For example, doses of tricyclic antidepressants required to minimize depressive symptoms may increase as much as 60 percent during the second half of pregnancy.[5] If you decide to take medication during pregnancy, consider getting regular checks of blood levels of the medication to ensure that you are getting an adequate amount.

Most drug research studies have specifically excluded pregnant women following the realization in the 1960s that abnormal limb formations were caused by the use of thalidomide during pregnancy. Because of the lack of research, the use of any psychiatric medication during pregnancy has not been determined to be safe by the U.S. Food and Drug Administration (FDA). As a result the FDA has not approved any drug for use during pregnancy. Although this makes a great deal of sense ethically, we are left with little knowledge upon which to base decisions.

Most of the information we have has been derived from anecdotal reports of women who were taking medications during pregnancy and either did or did not have problems. Unfortunately, this method does not serve as a valid guide because it is difficult to distinguish the spontaneous occurrence of a birth defect from one that is caused by psychiatric medication.

You need to consider the effects on your health and the health of your child in determining whether medication should be taken during pregnancy. You should weigh the risks and benefits of being both on *and* off the medication.

Your Health   There are several possible benefits to the use of medication during pregnancy. First, medication may control your symptoms so they don't worsen to the point where you would jeopardize your physical health or your ability to manage the physical and mental stress of labor and the decisions that sometimes need to be made in the midst of labor. For example, many women with bipolar disorder and schizophrenia stay on medication to prevent an exacerbation of symptoms that would impair eating, sleeping, and judgment about issues related to the pregnancy. Second, medication may help you to feel calmer and thereby minimize the physiological consequences of stress. Third, continuation of medication throughout pregnancy may prevent postpartum psychiatric episodes. Finally, you may be better able to relate to and care for your infant if your psychiatric symptoms are under control with medication.[6] The risk to your health of being on medication is essentially the same whether or not you are pregnant.

Going off medication puts you at risk for a return of your symptoms. This may cause you significant distress. On the positive side, you will not experience any side effects.

The Health of the Fetus   If you are pregnant, of course you are concerned about the effects of medication on the fetus. There are several ways in which a medication may adversely affect a fetus. The most obvious one occurs when a medication causes a birth defect, an effect called teratogenesis. Lithium can cause an abnormally formed heart in the fetuses of a very small percentage of women who take it during the first trimester of pregnancy. Benzodiazepines can cause a cleft palate. A description of the teratogenic effects of each medication is listed in part IV.

Any medication may cause the same side effects in the fetus as it does in the mother. These include movement disorders caused by antipsychotics, and an increased heart rate and lower blood pressure from some antidepressants. These would be undetectable in the fetus but could possibly be detrimental.

There may be effects on the child after birth. For example, antipsychotic medication can cause poor muscle coordination for many months after birth in some infants. This can impair the ability to nurse effectively.

There may be withdrawal effects after birth when the child is no longer exposed to the medication. For example, the abrupt withdrawal of tricyclic medications that are used for depression and anxiety can cause a flulike syndrome that includes symptoms of nausea and stomach cramps. This may complicate the course of the first few days of an infant's life if the mother took such a drug throughout pregnancy.

There may be harmful effects on a fetus that do not manifest themselves until long after birth. For example, the use of diethylstilbestrol by women who were pregnant in the 1950s and '60s has caused vaginal cancer in their female offspring in adulthood.

Finally, a medication may cause the brain to grow differently in ways that we are not able to measure at this time. For example, the alterations in brain chemistry caused by antidepressants may affect the growth patterns of individual brain cells. These may cause changes in a person's cognition or emotions that are too subtle for us to pinpoint at this time.

There are some possible benefits to your child if you stay on medication. First, significant stress in the mother can impair the growth of the fetus. Your child will benefit if you are happy and relaxed. Second, you need to be able to make good decisions about your diet, sleep, and activities during pregnancy, labor, and delivery. Your child will not do well if you are too depressed to eat during pregnancy, too fearful to decide whether you need an emergency caesarean section during labor, or too disorganized to push during the contractions heralding delivery.

There is a lot to consider in weighing the risks and benefits to you and your child if you take or don't take medication. There is no quick and easy way to decide what you should do. Discussion with your obstetrician, psychiatrist, and partner is essential to ensure that all issues are considered.

If you are able to manage your symptoms with alternative psychiatric treatments, then serious consideration should be given to going off medication. For example, many people using antidepressants like Paxil, Tofranil, Prozac, and Zoloft are able to stop their medication without significant difficulty. People using benzodiazepines, such as Xanax or Klonopin, are often able to stop their use with a combination of psychotherapy, relaxation techniques, and changes in their life directed toward reducing stress.

Medication Use during Breast Feeding   Medications are passed in breast milk, though in smaller concentrations than through the placenta during pregnancy, and can have direct effects on a child. You need to weigh the risks and benefits of medication to you and your infant as outlined above for use during pregnancy.

The Elderly

Psychiatric medications are frequently used by those over sixty-five years of age. Not only do the elderly experience anxiety, depression, psychotic disorders, and bipolar disorder, but they may also suffer from Alzheimer's disease and related cognitive difficulties. Many psychiatric medications can provide enormous benefit to the elderly: old age does not preclude the use of psychiatric medications. However, there are three issues pertinent to the issue of psychiatric drugs for the elderly that need to be taken into account. If you are over sixty-five, or are caring for an elderly person, it is important that you consider these issues to be sure that the kind and amount of medication are appropriate and beneficial.

Physiological Differences   The elderly are more sensitive to the effects of medications than those under sixty-five. There is enhancement of some brain enzymes with aging and there is increased sensitivity of receptors in several neurotransmitter systems.[7]

Drugs in elderly people tend to reach higher levels and last longer than in younger patients. There are two reasons for this. First, there is an increase in body fat composition and decreased muscle mass. Many drugs that are stored in fat tissue will be more widely distributed in the body and will take longer for the body to metabolize and excrete. Water-soluble drugs that are not stored in fat tissue, such as lithium, are distributed throughout a much smaller volume in the body and thus can reach higher tissue concentrations. Second, the liver enzymes that break down drugs decline with age, so that an elderly person takes longer to metabolize psychiatric drugs.

Side Effects   Age-related changes in other body systems also make the elderly more sensitive to the side effects of many medications. For example, changes in the receptors of blood vessels make them much more vulnerable to experiencing low blood pressure from medications that are not particularly troublesome to younger people. The age-related decrease in bowel motility makes them more vulnerable to constipation from medications that have this tendency. Symptoms of prostatic enlargement may be significantly worsened by a wide variety of psychiatric medications. Gait and balance can be more easily affected by medications that would not be troubling to a younger person.

The increased sensitivity to impaired coordination and lower blood pressure renders the elderly at greater risk for experiencing complications from these side effects. They fall more and, as a result, have an elevated risk of hip fractures.[8]

Other Medical Problems   The elderly are also more likely to experience other medical problems with the heart, liver, kidney, and other organ systems.

Many elderly people are on a wide variety of other medications because of these medical problems. These other medications can interact with psychiatric medications such that either one or both are increased or decreased in the body. The medications may also combine to contribute to side effects that would not be experienced in either one of them alone. For example, delirium can be caused by the addition of some psychiatric drugs to certain medical drugs when either one alone wouldn't cause significant difficulty.

Kidney and liver problems can lead to decreased metabolism of psychiatric drugs. This can increase the potency of a single dose when compared to someone without those medical problems.

Because of these differences, the maxim "Start low and go slow" is a good guide for the prescription of any psychiatric drug to people over the age of sixty-five. Exercise, relaxation techniques, establishment of a good social support system, and psychotherapy are important alternatives to consider in place of, or as an adjunct to, psychiatric medications.

Non-Caucasians

If you are a member of an ethnic minority living in the United States, you are undoubtedly aware that members of ethnic minorities have historically been unable to access good quality medical care on a routine basis. Unfortunately, the medical and psychiatric professions continue to ignore the unique needs of non-Caucasians. Bigotry and discrimination against different ethnic groups by the white majority are at the root of this problem.

Because of the widespread manifestations of bigotry prevalent in our society, problems specific to the delivery of health care also affect your ability to obtain high-quality psychiatric care. These include the low numbers of minority psychiatrists, language barriers, ignorance about cultural practices that may shape your difficulties and influence your treatment preferences, and the lack of research into health problems that disproportionately affect minorities.

There are many issues that should make you cautious if you are considering medications. First, the symptoms, incidence, and prevalence of different psychiatric disorders vary among different ethnic groups. For example, seeing visions and hearing the voices of family members who have recently died are part of the normal grieving process among some Hispanic groups, while they might be considered a psychotic disorder among Caucasians. Members of different cultures can experience different symptoms of depression, such as physical problems more than overt sadness. Syndromes of unusual behavior and experiences common to other cultures but not well studied by the psychiatric profession, such as *rootwork* in European and African descendants in the southern United States, *colera* among Latinos, *latah* among Indonesians, and *pibloqtoq* among Eskimos may lead to misdiagnosis and inappropriate treatment if your psychiatrist is unfamiliar with your cultural background.

Differences in *pharmacokinetics,* the way that drugs are absorbed, distributed, stored, metabolized, and excreted, will affect your response to treatment with medication. These differences are most pronounced in the metabolic breakdown of medications, a process that permits and facilitates excretion. For example, alcohol, clonazepam, and phenelzine are metabolized quickly or slowly depending on the presence or absence of a certain enzyme process called acetylation.[9] Members of some ethnic groups possess this process, while members of other ethnic groups do not.

Differences in *pharmacodynamics,* the effect a drug has on your body, will also affect your response to medications. For example, African Americans have been found to be more sensitive to the effects of benzodiazepines. As a result of both pharmacokinetic and pharmacodynamic differences, you may need a higher or lower dose of a medication than that demonstrated to be of benefit to a study population consisting largely of whites.

Members of different ethnic groups may be more sensitive to certain side effects of medications. For example, African Americans may be at higher risk for developing tardive dyskinesia[10] and some Hispanic groups experience more side effects from tricyclic antidepressants than do Caucasians.

Finally, ethnic minorities are not uniform. Different ethnic groups are composed of people from widely different cultures and areas of origin (Asians from China are quite different from those Japan). Intermarrying among different ethnic groups makes the evaluation of these issues even more complex.

Unfortunately, while a few differences are well documented, there is very little systematic research documenting how members of different ethnic groups can best use psychiatric medications. As a result, there are no specific guidelines about how to use any specific drug for any ethnic minority.

There are several principles that can help you get the most out of medication, however. First, it is vitally important that your psychiatrist be familiar with your ethnic heritage and cultural practices. If this is not the case, do your best to explain your symptoms, your understanding of your difficulties, and your expectations for treatment in the context of your background. Enlist friends or family members to assist you if you are having difficulty communicating. Don't be afraid to take time to do this.

Make sure you come to an understanding about your difficulties with your psychiatrist. If you don't understand what the psychiatrist believes is the problem or agree with the treatment, resolve the conflict *before* you start treatment.

If you agree that medication makes sense, discuss with your psychiatrist whether there are any known variations in the way medications might affect members of your ethnic background.

Educate yourself *well* about common side effects before you start medication. If you experience other side effects, consider whether they may be due to your biological makeup. If so, further use of the drug may be unwise.

Once you start medication, observe the physical and psychological effects carefully. If you notice no therapeutic benefits or side effects, it may be that you metabolize the drug more quickly than is customary in Caucasians. If side effects are more intense than expected, it may be that you metabolize the drug more slowly and it is building up in your system. In either case, adjust the dosage in response to the signals from *your body,* not a dosage scheme derived from studies on people different from you.

CHAPTER 5

Alternative Treatments for Psychiatric Problems

Medication is most helpful when it is used in conjunction with other things you do to help yourself. Try to get the most out of any medication you take by augmenting it with other sensible aids. Some things you can do on your own, while others require the expertise of others. Specific aids for each disorder will be described in part III.

Diet

Diet affects your physical health. Deficiencies of vitamins and minerals cause illnesses. The best-known example is the development of scurvy among British sailors during their long voyages at sea. The addition of limes to their diet prevented the disease. The important ingredient in the limes was later determined to be ascorbic acid, vitamin C. Other vitamin deficiencies can cause blindness, rickets, pellagra, anemia, beriberi, and dementia. A lack of iodine can lead to hypothyroidism.

A great deal has been written about the effect of diet on your mental health. Diets that are low in fat, low in carbohydrates, high in carbohydrates, low in protein, high in protein, and rich in certain vitamins and minerals, and those that avoid certain kinds of foods such as dairy products and meat have all been touted as aids to attain emotional well-being.

Various supplements in dietary components have been suggested as the cause or cure for various psychiatric disorders. For example, the ingestion of large amounts of B vitamins has been promoted as an aid for depression. Although people who are depressed sometimes have low levels of B vitamins because of their poor dietary intake, there is insufficient evidence to demonstrate that B vitamin deficiencies cause depression, or that ingestion of large amounts can cure it. Most other claims promoting the specific benefits of these specialized diets also lack a valid foundation. They are generally pioneered by one person and backed up with anecdotes, not rigorous scientific research. They generally fall from favor when people aren't helped all that much and the next fad comes along.

A varied diet of foods from different food groups, low on fats and sugars, eaten two to four times a day is sufficient if you do not have any other significant health problems. If you do, then it is important to alter your diet no matter what psychiatric problems you are experiencing. For example, people with diabetes need to minimize their sugar intake in order to avoid hypoglycemic reactions. People with high blood pressure and certain kinds of heart problems generally do better if they maintain diets that are low in salt.

It's also important to maintain an appropriate level of caloric intake. Symptoms of many psychiatric disorders can intensify somewhat if you eat only one meal a day, or if you are not eating enough. For example, palpitations, tremor, sweating, restlessness, and irritability from anxiety can be more troublesome if you eat only a single meal at dinnertime.

If you feel that nutrition is a way to maintain a certain balance in your life, then by all means continue your dietary regimen, as long as it is not so extreme that you get significant metabolic disruptions.

Exercise

Regular exercise is important for everybody regardless of whether they have psychiatric problems. Although none of us needs to become a marathon runner or look like Arnold Schwarzenegger, regular physical activity can go a long way toward promoting emotional well-being. It helps us feel more energetic and vibrant both during the exercise itself and afterwards. It is an active way of participating in the world and promotes feelings of strength, competence, and self-esteem. The health benefits of exercise include greater muscle strength and lower blood pressure and, in combination with an appropriate diet, can reduce obesity. Exercise can help some psychiatric disorders in specific ways, which will be detailed in part III.

Psychotherapy

Almost everything has been described as psychotherapy from orthodox psychoanalysis in which a person lies on a couch for several days a week for many years to shorter forms of once weekly psychotherapy, group therapy, activity therapy, and adventure-based therapy. We sometimes call our daily activities "driving" therapy, "garden" therapy, and even "work" therapy. Psychiatrists tend to have a narrower definition of psychotherapy and see it as a series of meetings between a therapist and a client in which they work together to help the client to overcome a psychological problem. There are several forms of psychotherapy that can be of enormous benefit to people with different psychiatric problems.

Unfortunately many insurance companies limit the amount of money that they will pay for any form of psychotherapy. They discriminate against people with psychological problems and the treatments they will cover and hide behind a maze of double talk and regulations that will prevent you from getting the treatment you need. As a result you may not be able to engage in any beneficial form of therapy except meeting a therapist a few times to go over your problems and discuss ways of managing them.

Don't be bullied by insurance companies and HMOs to restrict your treatment to the use of medications when psychotherapy can be far more effective and result in long lasting changes. Persistence with an insurance company can pay off. Under threats to complain to a state regulating industry, they may agree to fund appropriate treatment.

Consider paying for psychotherapy out of your own pocket. Although this may seem like a large expense, consider what you are paying for discretionary spending such as smoking, clothes, restaurants, and entertainment. Most people can afford psychotherapy if they put their minds to it.

Behavioral   Behavioral therapy focuses specifically on your behavior and seeks to change it through a series of exercises. There are several kinds of specific behavioral techniques that may help you.

Systematic Desensitization   This is a process in which you and your therapist establish a hierarchy of situations ranging from those that you handle easily to those that are most difficult. You practice the easiest ones first. When fully comfortable with the initial situation, you progress to the next situation in the hierarchy. You practice at each stage in the hierarchy until the difficulty is mastered before moving to the next stage. Systematic desensitization is a slow process in which the problem is gradually mastered step by step. If you become overwhelmed at any step, you scale back the difficulty of each task by breaking it up into smaller increments and increasing the frequency of practice.

Flooding   This is essentially the opposite sequence. One imagines the most difficult experience possible and seeks it out. The experience is purposely overwhelming. With regular practice however, similar experiences in life become much more tolerable. For example, if you panic in crowds and stores, three to four times a week you go to the most crowded large space you can find, such as a downtown shopping district or a mall. Regular practice gives you the confidence to go to a less crowded place as well, and makes it relatively easy by comparison. Many therapists accompany their clients to begin flooding and gradually reduce their involvement as proficiency is gained.

Relaxation Techniques   Relaxation techniques are mental and physical exercises to induce a state of calm and relaxation. The goal of a relaxation technique is to achieve that sense of relaxation in a calm situation and gradually gain proficiency in achieving that same state of calmness and relaxation in anxiety-provoking situations.

There are many different forms of relaxation techniques. *Relaxation tapes* provide soothing sounds such as the waves of the ocean. These are often a good way to begin learning how to relax. In *progressive muscular relaxation* a person slowly clenches and relaxes each of the body's muscle groups, in sequence, one after the other. Each clenching and unclenching should be gradual and take roughly ten to fifteen seconds. As the exercise proceeds, most people notice that they are physically much calmer. In using the *breathing technique* one sits quietly and comfortably breathing slowly in and out and saying "in . . . out . . . in . . . out . . ." with each breath. As thoughts come to your mind, you let them pass through and refocus your attention on your breathing. With *meditation,* one develops a sense of relaxation by concentrating on a word or phrase while simultaneously letting the body relax deeply. Attention is paid not so much to breathing or to the muscles, but rather to the word itself. Focusing on the word itself helps you to maintain a state of relaxation by overriding any thoughts that do come to mind. In *self-hypnosis,* you learn to imagine yourself in a calm place and embroider it with as many details as possible. Regular practice at hypnosis then allows you to recall this image and the sense of relaxation it brings when you are feeling distressed. It is best learned by working with somebody who is an expert at hypnosis and can teach it to you.

Cognitive Therapy   Cognition is the mental process of thinking and knowing. Aaron Beck, a professor of psychiatry at the University of Pennsylvania School of Medicine, has written a number of books exploring the element of cognition in both anxiety and depression. Although he acknowledges that there are many root causes for these disorders, he has written widely about his research demonstrating that these disorders are maintained in part by mistaken or dysfunctional cognitive appraisal of a situation. For example, one type of dysfunctional thinking is called "catastrophic thinking," which occurs when people lose their perspective on a situation and dwell on the worst possible outcome.

He developed cognitive therapy to help people correct their dysfunctional appraisal of situations. Cognitive therapy is short-term, problem-oriented, and primarily educational. Some techniques commonly used in cognitive therapy include homework between sessions and role-playing in the session itself.

Psychodynamic Psychotherapy   Psychodynamic psychotherapy shares with psychoanalysis the belief that much of your psychological distress is due to unconscious conflicts about people and events in the past. The process of therapy involves meeting with a therapist once or twice a week.

Psychodynamic psychotherapy has profoundly helped many people. It can be slow going at first, and you may need months of treatment to notice substantial benefits. Full resolution of old conflicts can take years.

Interpersonal Therapy   This form of therapy was pioneered by psychiatrist Gerald Klerman. You meet with a therapist weekly, usually for no more than a few months. You focus on your current relationships with others and how they contribute to your distress. You work on one or two current problems, rather than unconscious feelings, with the goal of coping better with interpersonal situations.

Group Therapy   While the treatments listed above generally involve a therapist and an individual, there are advantages to treatment in a group setting led by a
therapist. Groups commonly meet weekly and focus on issues common to the
group members. These issues could include disorders such as depression or anxiety, or life problems such as cancer or divorce. Sometimes groups are made up of
people in similar situations, such as single adults, teenagers at school, or women
who have been sexually abused. Group therapy is an enormously powerful tool
that can significantly aid in your recovery from psychiatric problems.

Many people avoid group therapy because they dislike having to share their
problems with strangers. Although some initial hesitancy is reasonable, it is unfortunate when the normal reticence to share private experiences with others interferes with the use of such a powerful aid.

Self-Help Groups

The first self-help group was started by two people struggling with alcoholism.
Their work led to the creation of Alcoholics Anonymous, or AA, which has helped
millions of people in many countries achieve and maintain sobriety and abstinence
from alcohol. The principles that have made AA so useful for so many people have
been extended to a wide variety of self-help groups that focus on overeating, gam-
bling, or compulsive sexual behavior.

These principles include the belief that the disorder itself is something that
you are unable to manage on your own. Second, meeting and discussing your difficulties with other people opens up ideas as to how best to combat the problem. Finally, helping other people by sharing your experience allows you to solidify your
ability to master your difficulties.

There are several advantages to self-help groups. They are free. You will probably derive considerable emotional support by meeting regularly with people who
have similar problems. Also, self-help groups empower you to make changes in
your own life without looking to somebody else to make them for you.

A Crisis Plan

You may benefit from developing a crisis plan if your symptoms sometimes overwhelm your ability to lead your life. Mary Ellen Copeland has written about the
value of developing a crisis plan. Her recommendations are contained in her work
entitled *Wellness Recovery Action Plan* (WRAP).[1] One purpose of a WRAP is to
help you address any worsening of your symptoms as soon as possible in an effort
to avoid any further decompensation. The other purpose is to outline your wishes
for care should you be unable to advocate on your own behalf.

She recommends writing down your plan in a loose-leaf notebook, so it can be
improved as you learn more about what is helpful for your illness. She divides the
plan into five parts.

The first part is a daily maintenance list of things you do for yourself every day to keep yourself feeling good. These include eating sensibly, exercising, relaxation techniques, contact with a partner and friends, work, and engaging in fun activities. Extra activities might include getting a massage, meeting with a mental health professional, spending time with pets, doing laundry and housework, planning vacations, and planning other activities.

The second part involves making a list of "triggers," external events or circumstances that may produce symptoms. Although the reaction to these events may be normal, your symptoms may get worse if you don't respond to them. Triggers include anniversary dates of losses or trauma, conflict with family, friends, or people at work; physical illness; being criticized; stress; or even a lack of sleep. Write a specific plan you will follow if one of your triggers occurs. For example, if the trigger is conflict with your family, your plan may be to perform some deep breathing exercises, call a friend to talk about the situation, and talk about it with your therapist.

The third part is a list of early warning signs that signal the need for further action to prevent your symptoms from getting worse. Some early warning signs include increased anxiety, irritability, craving drugs or alcohol, lack of motivation, isolating yourself, feeling unconnected to your body, and not keeping appointments. Make a plan you will follow should these early warning signs occur. These plans may include doing things on the daily maintenance list, seeking an early appointment with a mental health professional, and spending additional time with family and friends.

The fourth part is a description of symptoms that occur when things are breaking down or getting worse. Such things may be irrational responses to events, withdrawal from your usual activities, excessive sleeping, thoughts of self-harm, and risk-taking behaviors. Again, make a plan you will follow if these symptoms occur.

The last part describes a plan to follow if you need others to make decisions for you. It describes your symptoms, people who can help you during a crisis, medications, other treatments that may help you or that you want to avoid, treatment facilities where you prefer to be treated, and things that other people can do for you.

Hospitalization

Psychiatric hospitals have a terrifying reputation because of dehumanizing abuses that occurred in the past. Thankfully, vast improvements have been made in most psychiatric wards and hospitals in the quality of care that people receive and the efforts to ensure your rights and dignity. Hospitalization is used far less frequently now than in the past because outpatient treatments are much more effective, but there are still times when hospitalization is the most appropriate treatment alternative.

The most common reason that leads people to go to a psychiatric hospital at this time has to do with issues of safety. If you are depressed and suicidal, too paranoid to eat sensibly, or your teenager is behaving unsafely, a hospital can provide a contained environment that will allow treatment to proceed in a safe setting.

The other major reason for hospitalization is to receive treatment that cannot be performed outside the hospital. For example, if you have schizophrenia, you may want to go into the hospital to start clozapine because of the severity of the initial side effects. If you are elderly and have medical problems, you may benefit from hospitalization to intensively monitor your physical condition as you add psychiatric medications.

Residential Treatment

Some people live in a therapeutic community that focuses on helping them to manage their psychological problems in the hope that they will be able to function more effectively when they return to the community. For example, if you have schizophrenia, you may find it helpful to live in an environment with staff who help you with your day-to-day life because the intense disorganization of your thinking may impair your ability to do so. You may move on from residential housing after a few months or a year or two, although some people require residential treatment for extended times. If you are struggling to overcome addiction to alcohol or drugs, you may need residential treatment beyond the one- to four-week period generally needed for detoxification. Stays range from months to years. During this time you can use the structure of the residential setting to help you maintain abstinence, learn your warning signs for when you are vulnerable to drinking or using drugs again, and learn other ways of coping with your difficulties besides using drugs.

Teenagers, and sometimes even younger children, go to residential facilities when their behavior becomes unsafe and their caregivers are not able to help them maintain their safety. Residential living for behaviorally disordered children and adolescents generally focuses on teaching effective ways of managing their emotions before they act out in dangerous ways, helping them further their education, and teaching them skills that will enable them to return to home as soon as possible.

Psychosocial Rehabilitation

Psychosocial rehabilitation focuses on improving your hygiene, social skills, vocational skills, anger management, money management, travel skills, and other concrete tasks in life. Psychosocial rehabilitation treatments include one-on-one teaching, role-playing, real life practice, job training at a site with a job coach, and group therapy focused on developing productive ways of managing self-destructive urges.

For example, vocational training is especially helpful if your psychiatric problems impaired your schooling and ability to obtain and hold a job. Sometimes the content of the training at a specific task is necessary. You may need help learning how to conduct yourself during an interview and when you start your job. One person with schizophrenia felt that he could not work and came to my office for help one day instead of going to work. His concern was that there was a man standing closely behind him at the job site. Because of his paranoia he felt very uncomfortable about someone so close to him. With the assistance of his job coach, his working arrangement was changed so that there was no one standing behind him. More comfortable, he was able to maintain the job for many years thereafter.

Sometimes anxiety and fearfulness about starting work or doing something in the community are managed best by role-playing or even practicing the skills in the community with a case manager, therapist, or rehabilitative counselor, rather than by increasing medication or trying a medication change. For example, many children with attention deficit/hyperactivity disorder (ADHD) can benefit from medication. However, many also benefit from a strong behavioral program to help them manage their impulsivity and intense feelings in appropriate ways. Adults with ADHD can often benefit from working with a therapist to develop strategies for circumventing and coping effectively with their deficits.

PART III

Psychiatric Syndromes and Their Treatment

CHAPTER 6

Anxiety

Whether we call it "nerves," "the willies," or "the jitters," we all experience anxiety when something threatens our health, job, marriage, or other important aspects of our lives. Although the experience of anxiety is uncomfortable, it is actually a good thing. It signals us to prepare for future challenges, whether we are to meet with the Internal Revenue Service, study for exams, or ask our boss for a raise.

When anxiety is prolonged beyond the situation that caused it or is more intense than warranted, however, it is no longer beneficial or normal. It is intensely distressing and can be disabling. It can overwhelm your body with sensations, prevent you from doing what you want, and compel you to do what you don't want.

Anxiety is common. Twenty-five percent of the U.S. population, more than sixty million people, will experience a syndrome of anxiety over the course of their lives. Women experience anxiety syndromes at twice the rate of men.

The etiology is probably multifaceted. There appears to be a biological component, as it runs in families. The pathogenesis is complex as well. It is likely that predisposing factors like biology and trauma alter the nervous system so that a person is more likely to experience anxiety in stressful situations. When a person experiences anxiety, their reaction may make them more or less likely to experience it again in the future.

Symptoms

Anxiety can affect four different areas of your life. Anxious *thoughts* can be normal or pathological, depending on the intensity and frequency with which they occur. For example, it's normal to keep a watchful eye over your health, but a consuming fear that every unusual bodily sensation is a sign of a fatal illness is a sign that anxiety has become excessive. The physical *sensations* of anxiety can range from a mild inner feeling of restlessness to intense agitation with palpitations, shortness of breath, sweating, dizziness, nausea, numbness and tingling in the extremities, and chest pain. The main *emotion* present in anxiety is fearfulness. This is merely unpleasant when mild, but can be overwhelming if it is full-blown panic. Your *activity* is generally affected if you are anxious. Maybe it's merely trembling hands, the urge to bite your nails or twirl your hair, but sometimes anxiety is so severe it is difficult to sit still. You may experience insomnia. You may avoid certain places or engage in rituals like handwashing to allay your anxiety.

Treatment Options for Anxiety

There are a number of things you can do to help anxiety. These other aids are generally far more helpful for you in the long run than any medication, but only if you pursue them conscientiously.

Diet   A proper diet can improve anxiety. It is important to eat balanced meals (with some protein and carbohydrates such as grains and vegetables) three to four times a day and avoid the ingestion of products high in sugar.

   The reason for this is somewhat complex but is important to understand. The body needs energy to run. This energy is produced by the conversion of food to glucose, or blood sugar. When your blood sugar is low, the adrenal gland (a small gland next to the kidney) releases the hormone adrenaline. Besides increasing blood sugar, however, adrenaline also causes many of the physical effects of anxiety: increased heart rate, palpitations, sweating, goosebumps, and an inner feeling of restlessness.

   Your diet affects the level of glucose in your blood, and, therefore, how much adrenaline you produce. Fasting for more than four hours depletes glucose, causing an increase in adrenaline and the symptoms of anxiety. Eating foods high in sugar, such as candy or sodas, initially cause an elevation in blood sugar. This is quickly followed by a rebound to low blood sugar, however, which increases adrenaline and the symptoms of anxiety.

Drugs   Stopping *caffeine* can decrease the intensity of your anxiety immediately. Stopping *tobacco* use can make you more anxious at first, though you will feel better in the long run. It may make sense to hold off on attempts to quit smoking until you get some control over your anxiety. You should stop any *alcohol* use, however. If you continue to drink alcohol in spite of attempts to stop, seek treatment to help your efforts.

Exercise   Regular exercise can be especially important for people experiencing anxiety. Besides the invigoration exercise produces, it causes the release of adrenaline, which helps the body perform the exercise itself. After the exercise is over, however, the body decreases the production of adrenaline, so you feel less anxious. Also, regular exercise helps you become accustomed to a body that is more energetic, with an elevated heart rate and palpitations, and sweating. This can help you to tolerate the feelings of anxiety when they do occur.

Relaxation Techniques   Relaxation techniques are exercises that you perform to feel calmer. The advice to "take a deep breath" is actually describing a relaxation technique. Relaxation techniques include relaxation tapes, deep breathing exercises, muscle relaxation exercises, meditation, self-hypnosis, and biofeedback. Your ability to relax will improve if you practice relaxation techniques several times daily in calm situations. As your ability to relax improves, you will be increasingly able to maintain a calm feeling in situations that previously led you to be anxious. Most people are unable to learn relaxation techniques without the guidance of a manual or therapist. Fortunately many books describe the use of relaxation techniques, and most therapists are familiar with their use.

Psychotherapy   Psychotherapy was the mainstay of treatment for anxiety until the current fad for drugs. Group and individual behavioral, cognitive, interpersonal, and psychodynamic psychotherapy significantly improve and often cure the symptoms of anxiety. Which therapy would be best for you depends on the precise nature of your symptoms and will be discussed under the syndromes of anxiety described below.

Medications   The number of medications used in the treatment of anxiety is vast. Bromide, chloral hydrate, paraldehyde, urethane, and sulfonal were used in the 1800s. Barbiturates like phenobarbital, a derivative of barbituric acid, were introduced in the early 1900s. The 1950s saw the introduction of drugs from many different chemical classes: meprobamate (Miltown), methaqualone (Quaalude), ethchlorvynol (Placidyl), and glutethimide (Doriden). These drugs are rarely used now because they cause sedation, are addictive, and are frequently lethal in overdose attempts.

Many new drugs have been created that are currently more popular. In general, the drugs used currently are more effective, tend to cause less sedation, and are less lethal if taken in an overdose. They are not without their problems, however. Which one you choose will depend on the type, duration, and severity of your symptoms, your use of other treatments, and your attitudes about medication (discussed in chapter 16). The group names are derived from their chemical structure, their action in the brain, or the effect produced. Different pharmaceutical companies create their own unique drugs from a basic chemical structure or action in order to capture a piece of the market for a particular class of drugs, which accounts for why some groups have so many individual drugs.

Medications Used in Anxiety

Benzodiazepines
   Alprazolam (Xanax)
   Chlordiazepoxide (Librium)
   Clonazepam (Klonopin)

continued

Medications Used in Anxiety (continued)

    Clorazepate (Tranxene)

    Diazepam (Valium)

    Lorazepam (Ativan)

    Oxazepam (Serax)

Selective serotonin reuptake inhibitors (SSRIs)

    Citalopram (Celexa)

    Escitalopram (Lexapro)

    Fluoxetine (Prozac)

    Fluvoxamine (Luvox)

    Paroxetine (Paxil)

    Sertraline (Zoloft)

Tricyclic antidepressants (TCAs)

    Amitriptyline (Elavil)

    Clomipramine (Anafranil)

    Desipramine (Norpramin)

    Doxepin (Sinequan)

    Imipramine (Tofranil)

    Nortriptyline (Pamelor)

    Protriptyline (Vivactil)

    Trimipramine (Surmontil)

Monoamine oxidase inhibitors (MAOIs)

    Isocarboxazid (Marplan)

    Phenelzine (Nardil)

    Selegiline (Eldepryl)

    Tranylcypromine (Parnate)

Beta-blockers

    Propranolol (Inderal)

Antihistamines

    Hydroxyzine (Atarax, Vistaril)

Antipsychotics

    Standard antipsychotics

        Chlorpromazine (Thorazine)

        Fluphenazine (Prolixin)

        Haloperidol (Haldol)

        Loxapine (Loxitane)

        Mesoridazine (Serentil)

Molindone (Moban)
Perphenazine (Trilafon)
Thioridazine (Mellaril)
Trifluoperazine (Stelazine)
Thiothixene (Navane)
Atypical antipsychotics
Olanzapine (Zyprexa)
Risperidone (Risperdal)
Quetiapine (Seroquel)
Miscellaneous
Buspirone (Buspar)
Duloxetine (Cymbalta)
Gabapentin (Neurontin)
Trazodone (Desyrel)
Venlafaxine (Effexor)
Herbal remedies
Chamomile
Hops
Kava
Lemon
Passion flower
Valerian

Benzodiazepines   Named for their chemical structure, benzodiazepines are frequently used for the acute symptoms of anxiety because they are very effective and work within an hour. They can be used intermittently, an attribute that some people find attractive. Immediate side effects include sedation, poor physical coordination, and memory impairment. Daily use for months can dull your emotions, impair cognitive skills, and contribute to depression. There is some anecdotal evidence that they may cause brain shrinkage after years of use. Most troubling of all is that they are habit-forming. If used daily for more than four weeks, you can experience rebound anxiety when a dose wears off as part of a withdrawal syndrome. This can lead you to think that your anxiety is returning and you need the medication, when really you are just treating a withdrawal syndrome. This pernicious cycle has ensnared millions of people in the United States into a daily cycle of anxiety, benzo dose, relief, and then rising anxiety until the next dose. (I previously wrote a book about this problem called *The Benzo Blues*.) Don't let this happen to you. Even if benzos help you initially, learn and use alternative methods of managing anxiety as quickly as you can so you can get off them.

Selective Serotonin Reuptake Inhibitors (SSRIs) Named for their action in the brain and initially marketed for depression, SSRIs have proved to be enormously helpful for people with different syndromes of anxiety. They need to be taken every day and generally take some weeks to become effective, so they are not useful for acute anxiety. Their day-to-day side effects are minimal in most people, although some people experience fatigue and a few become agitated. Most people notice decreased sexual drive and impaired sexual response, side effects that can cause considerable distress.

Tricyclic Antidepressants (TCAs) Named for their chemical structure, TCAs are effective for some forms of anxiety. They need to be taken every day and generally take some weeks to work, so they are not effective for acute anxiety. They have been supplanted by other drugs, notably the SSRIs, because of their tendency to cause weight gain, dry mouth, constipation, sweating, and light-headedness due to low blood pressure.

Monoamine Oxidase Inhibitors (MAOIs) Named for their action in the brain, MAOIs are also very effective. They too must be taken every day, and they take weeks to become effective. Common side effects include weight gain, dry mouth, insomnia, impaired sexual response, and light-headedness due to low blood pressure. Their most troubling side effect is the potential to cause a stroke if you ingest adrenaline or adrenaline-like substances. MAOIs can be used only with a fairly strict diet that avoids foods or medicines that contain adrenaline or adrenaline-like substances. These include cough and cold medicines, and a variety of food products such as aged cheese and processed meats. (A full list of the dietary restrictions is listed in part IV.) As a result, MAOIs need to be used with extra caution. At low doses, many people are able to use selegiline without rigorous adherence to the diet. Low doses are often not effective for depression, however.

Beta-Blockers Named for their ability to block the action of adrenaline on beta receptors in cells of the heart, lung, and other muscles, these medications should, in theory, be very helpful to minimize the symptoms of anxiety. Although a single dose can calm performance anxiety, they are not effective for other kinds of anxiety.

Antihistamines This group of medications reduces the excessive mucus secretions in respiratory infections and allergies. They also make people tired, however, and are sometimes used to decrease anxiety because of this sedative quality. They start working within thirty minutes. They can be taken intermittently and are not habit-forming. Their effects are mild.

Antipsychotics These medications are generally used to treat the hallucinations, delusions, and disorganized thinking in schizophrenia and bipolar disorder, and, if present, in depression. They can be helpful when severe anxiety overwhelms your ability to think clearly. They work within an hour or two, are not habit-forming, and can be used intermittently. Their side effects can be quite unpleasant, however, including sedation, emotional blunting, and weight gain. Use for more than a year can lead to tardive dyskinesia, a disorder that consists of constant, rhythmical, involuntary movements of muscles of the body, most commonly the tongue, face, hands, and feet. These side effects limit the use of antipsychotics to people who experience disabling anxiety and for whom other medications have provided no relief.

Miscellaneous   Buspirone is generally used in chronic anxiety. Daily doses for weeks are required for effectiveness. Common side effects include nausea, dizziness, and drowsiness, although most people are not significantly bothered by any side effects. Although research demonstrates some effectiveness, Buspirone is used infrequently because it has not proven helpful for most people with anxiety.

Duloxetine and venlafaxine are similar to the SSRIs in that they block the reuptake of serotonin. However, they also block the reuptake of norepinephrine. Although less commonly used than the SSRIs, these medicines are equally effective.

Trazodone was initially marketed as an antidepressant. Its usefulness in depression is limited because of the marked sedation people experience, but some people find the sedative quality helpful in reducing their anxiety.

Gabapentin has been used to prevent seizures in some people. It causes pronounced sedation, and some people have noticed a decrease in their level of anxiety. Most people notice sedation as the only side effect.

Many herbal remedies are used for anxiety. They may be helpful for people who have only mild symptoms of anxiety, as their effects are quite subtle. Valerian and kava are the strongest of those listed. Kava should not be used for more than a few months because it can lead to liver problems. Valerian acts in a manner similar to benzodiazepines, although there is no documented evidence so far that it is habit-forming.

Syndromes of Anxiety and Their Treatment

Your body and mind contain complex structures to alert you to danger and respond to it effectively. There are many ways for these systems and structures to malfunction. As a result, there are many different syndromes of anxiety, each with its own unique etiology, pathogenesis, and constellation of symptoms. Each syndrome requires a different approach.

Biological Causes of Anxiety   It is important to rule out any medical causes of anxiety. *Thyroid disorders, hypoglycemia, Cushing's disease,* and *pheochromocytoma,* a rare tumor of the adrenal gland, can cause symptoms similar to anxiety. You should consider a medical exam if your anxiety does not have an obvious cause.

Many drugs cause anxiety. Work with your doctor to avoid theophylline preparations used for asthma. Avoid decongestants like pseudoephedrine (Sudafed) and phenylephrine, as they invariably make people more anxious. The recreational drug that worsens anxiety the most is caffeine. Don't forget that caffeine is in sodas and chocolate, not just coffee and tea. Although you may feel calmer when you first drink alcohol, it causes a rebound anxiety when it wears off that may last for some days. The act of smoking may be a habit that relaxes you, but the nicotine in tobacco worsens anxiety. Cocaine, hallucinogenics, and amphetamines can make people acutely anxious during the period of intoxication.

Anxiety in a Crisis   Sudden events like the death of a family member, physical illness, being fired, or involvement in a natural disaster can distress you and over-whelm your ability to cope. You may develop symptoms of anxiety, even though you've never had them before. Symptoms are generally limited to anxious thoughts and a feeling of apprehension, although you may be agitated and unable to sleep.

If your natural supports are insufficient to help you regain your equilibrium, psychotherapy is the treatment most likely to be of help. It can help you to express your feelings about the event so that you are able to make productive changes that allow you to move on in your life.

Benzodiazepines can be quite helpful in crises like these. They start working within thirty minutes, and the side effects of impaired memory and muscle coordination are usually negligible. They can also help you get to sleep. They are habit-forming if taken longer than four weeks, though, so try to limit your use.

Anxiety that arises as a result of a crisis may persist long after the crisis is over. If it does, you can help yourself the most if you maintain a good diet, eliminate caffeine and alcohol, and exercise regularly. You should definitely see a therapist to help you sort out your reaction to what happened and why you've become stuck. SSRIs or TCAs may help you feel less anxious, though they can take weeks to become effective.

Panic Disorder   The syndrome of panic disorder consists of "panic attacks," the sudden onset of intense fearfulness accompanied by palpitations, shortness of breath, sweating, chest pain, nausea, and fears of dying or having a heart attack. Panic attacks can occur in a variety of situations and psychiatric disorders but most commonly occur in people who suffer from anxiety. The attacks themselves last from a few minutes to a few hours and are extremely unpleasant and intensely dis-tressing. The worry about having another attack can be as disabling as the attacks themselves, especially if your worrying leads you to stay home and avoid anything that may precipitate an attack.

If you have panic disorder, you will benefit from eating a proper diet, eliminat-ing caffeine and other drugs, exercising regularly, and practicing relaxation tech-niques. Psychotherapy can help you work on issues in your current life and past experiences that contribute to your anxiety. You may see a therapist for just a few sessions to help you during your current difficulties, or work for months or years on the underlying issues that led to your anxiety in the first place.

The treatment of panic disorder with medications can be divided into an acute and maintenance phase. Benzodiazepines provide the fastest and most effective relief. They are a poor choice for extended treatment, however, because of their addictive qualities and the heightened level of general anxiousness experienced with chronic use. SSRIs and TCAs take some weeks to become effective, but once this period is over, they generally provide lasting relief without daily anxiety. MAOIs are effective long-term, but their side effects are more troubling. Antipsychotics, antihistamines, beta-blockers, buspirone, and trazodone are generally ineffective for panic disorder.

Although some people rely on medications for years, the constant worry about having another attack takes its toll. It's hard to enjoy life and vigorously pursue all that it has to offer if you are constantly monitoring your level of anxiety and shaping what you do depending on how anxious it makes you feel. Psychotherapy and relaxation techniques may require more effort than medications, but they provide genuine long-lasting relief from anxiety so that you make your life as meaningful and satisfying as possible.

Phobias   A phobia is an intense fear of objects such as animals or insects, environmental situations such as storms or water, or situations such as crowded or open spaces.

A single phobia, such as a fear of dogs, is generally best treated with behavioral therapy. The feared object isn't around enough to make treatment with medication useful or sensible.

Social phobia, which is a fear of embarrassment in social or performance situations, is experienced by 10 to 20 percent of the population. Behavioral psychotherapy aimed at helping you maintain calm in increasingly public situations is the most beneficial treatment. SSRIs and TCAs aid many people. Beta-blockers can help you feel calm for a specific event but will not work when taken on a daily basis.

Agoraphobia is a fear of being unable to escape from a crowded place. It often accompanies panic disorder, although some people experience agoraphobia without ever having a panic attack.

Benzos can make it easier to leave home. Having a pill in your pocket can fortify your courage to face the world. However, it is easy to become dependent on them. You then wind up spending enormous amounts of your mental energy assessing your current level of anxiety, how anxious you will be in the next two hours, and how anxious you'll be if you take a dose, a double dose, or skip it altogether. Anxiety, reinforced by the chronic use of benzos, can become a compass telling you where you can go and what you can do. Life gradually becomes a chore as you give up more and more of your activities. Try not to fall into the trap of chronic benzos just because they seem to help you at first.

SSRIs and TCAs help many people with agoraphobia. MAOIs can be helpful, too, but their side effects are more troubling. The side effects of antipsychotics make them a poor choice for phobias. The other medications are ineffective.

Posttraumatic Stress Disorder (PTSD)   PTSD occurs after a traumatic experience that is potentially life-threatening. Symptoms include reexperiencing the event through intrusive recollections, nightmares, flashbacks, avoidance of people and situations similar to the events of the trauma, and persistent symptoms of increased arousal such as insomnia, hypervigilance, and an exaggerated startle response.

A sensible diet, the elimination of caffeine, alcohol, and drugs of abuse, regular exercise, and relaxation techniques can help you to gain some measure of control over the symptoms of PTSD. You may find psychotherapy helps to free you from the influence of the trauma in your life, though this work can be painful, difficult, and time-consuming.

There are no medications to "cure" PTSD, but they can minimize the intensity of some of the symptoms. SSRIs can lessen the intensity of anxiety, flashbacks, and improve sleep. TCAs and MAOIs can do the same thing but tend to cause more side effects. Benzos can minimize the anxiety and improve sleep, but are habit-forming and tend to lose their effectiveness after some months. You will go through a period of intense anxiety due to withdrawal effects if you stop them after months or years of use, so avoid their use for longer than four weeks. Antipsychotics in small doses can be helpful if your symptoms are truly overwhelming and other medications and treatments have proved inadequate. The other drugs listed above are usually ineffective.

Generalized Anxiety Disorder   The major feature of this syndrome is excessive anxiety and worry about a number of activities and events in your life. You may find it difficult to control the worry and may notice chronic restlessness, easy fatiguability, difficulty concentrating, irritability, muscle tension, or insomnia.

A sensible diet, the elimination of caffeine, alcohol, and drugs of abuse, regular exercise, and relaxation techniques can help you feel somewhat more relaxed on a day-to-day basis. Psychotherapy may help you directly address the issues in your life that lead you to be anxious.

SSRIs and TCAs provide some benefit on a long-lasting basis and are probably the best first choice. Benzodiazepines are often used for this syndrome. They offer the most relief initially, but carry the problems associated with addiction: ineffectiveness over time with a rebound in symptoms if they are tapered off or stopped. Buspirone helps some people, but its effects are so mild most people experience minimal relief. Small doses of Trazodone can help but may make you tired. The side effects of antipsychotics make them a poor choice. The other medications are ineffective.

Obsessive-Compulsive Disorder (OCD)   The syndrome of OCD is extremely distressing. When severe, it can impair work, relationships, and any semblance of a normal life. Obsessions, persistent intrusive thoughts, are invariably present. Common obsessions include persistent fear of contamination by germs and repeated doubts about such things as turning off the stove. Compulsions are repetitive behaviors or mental acts performed to reduce anxiety about some dreaded event or situation. Handwashing and checking rituals are common.

Although behavior therapy provides some people with partial relief, the most effective treatment is medication. Fluvoxamine (an SSRI) and clomipramine (a TCA) were the first two medications that research proved could be beneficial. Other SSRIs and TCAs have subsequently been shown to provide significant aid as well. Other medications and treatments generally provide no benefit.

CHAPTER 7

Attention Deficit/Hyperactivity Disorder

Attention deficit/hyperactivity disorder (ADHD) is the name given to a persistent pattern of inattention, hyperactivity, and impulsivity. The problems are generally first noted in childhood, especially if there is excessive activity. These behaviors can be enormously distressing to you and those around you. In childhood, they may have impaired your learning, disrupted classrooms, alienated teachers and friends, and frustrated family members. In adulthood, they may impair your employment and intimate relationships. You may feel that there is something wrong with you or that the world is an unfriendly place, but in either case, you may find it difficult to find satisfaction in your life.

There has been a great deal of controversy in recent years about the existence of ADHD and the wisdom of using medication. At one end are those who believe that ADHD is a biological disorder best treated with medication. On the other end are those who believe that these behaviors are normal. These people tend to believe that the main difficulty is a society that finds exuberance disruptive and that medication is inappropriate. A third group believes that these behaviors are abnormal but are due to stress, not abnormal biology, and that psychotherapy is the treatment of choice. Adherents of each group have published books and articles and appeared on radio and television to promote their viewpoints.

There is some validity to each position. Differences in brain scan imaging have been demonstrated in some children who have been labeled with ADHD, suggesting a biological or genetic etiology. Some children given the label of ADHD *are* more active than others, disruptive even, but their "symptoms" resolve in a more accepting environment. The behaviors seen in children with ADHD can also be seen in some children with stressful life experiences, such as parental abuse, neglect, alcohol use, and divorce. These behaviors improve when children begin to cope effectively with these situations, either because life changes or because psychotherapy helps them learn productive ways of managing their bottled-up feelings.

As the physiology of normal brains is not well understood, and we don't know what differences may be present in the brains of people who exhibit these tendencies, there is no definitive way to resolve the debate to everyone's satisfaction at this time.

Diagnosis

The syndrome of ADHD consists of a variety of behaviors that demonstrate hyper-activity, inattentiveness, and impulsivity. Manifestations of hyperactivity include difficulty staying seated, feeling as if there was an engine inside of you that won't slow down, being constantly on the go, and having difficulty relaxing during leisure activities. Inattention is demonstrated by being easily distracted, making frequent mistakes in work, daydreaming, difficulty starting and finishing tasks, difficulty listening in conversations, losing things necessary for tasks, and being forgetful in daily activities. Impulsivity can be seen by saying things without thinking of their consequences, interrupting people, being impatient while wait-ing, buying impulsively, and switching from task to task in a haphazard fashion. Some people with ADHD are irritable and find themselves in frequent arguments. Many people with ADHD abuse alcohol, caffeine, and other drugs to alter their mood and thinking.

It's important to recognize that many people with these behaviors display a number of very positive characteristics as well. They are often creative and ener-getic. They may be able to "hyperfocus" on tasks that greatly interest them. They are often personable, funny, and quite likable.

We all display some of these behaviors at times, and they can all be seen in "normal people." The difference between those with ADHD and others is a matter of degree. Children can manifest these behaviors in understimulating environ-ments or if there is a chaotic and disorganized home life.

These behaviors are also seen in other psychiatric syndromes. Learning dis-abilities can impair comprehension and performance in school and masquerade as ADHD, especially if a child reacts to the failure by excessive motor activity. Children who are oppositional by nature may have difficulty functioning in school in a manner that looks like ADHD. Hyperactivity, excessive speech, dis-tractible thinking, and irritability are often seen in bipolar disorder, and the two can be difficult to tease apart. Some people have both syndromes. People with anxiety or posttraumatic stress disorder can be chronically restless, al-ways on the go, easily distractible, impulsive, and irritable. Excessive use of caffeine or the use of marijuana, cocaine, or alcohol can also cause some of these symptoms.

There is no blood test or brain scan that can definitively determine whether someone has ADHD. Sophisticated neuropsychological testing, performed by psychologists, involves a series of mental exercises probing your visual, auditory, and verbal skills, memory, learning style, and organizational ability. Such testing can demonstrate the presence of thinking patterns that are abnormal and that may play a role in the behaviors of ADHD. Questionnaires that ask about these behav-iors can suggest ADHD.

You should seriously consider neuropsychological testing to document your thinking style and how it affects your behavior. Even if you don't have ADHD, you may uncover some cognitive weaknesses that can be helped by training and tutoring. Consultation with a psychiatrist can help you sort out whether symptoms are due to another psychiatric syndrome. If you are evaluating your child, consultation should be with a child psychiatrist, as most pediatricians and family practitioners do not have the training to distinguish between different psychiatric syndromes and are not familiar with the range of treatments appropriate for each disorder.

Treatment

There are three treatment options you can pursue if you decide that you have ADHD after educating yourself about the disorder, obtaining neuropsychological testing, and consulting with a psychiatrist.

Shape the Environment   Search for a good "fit" with the environment. Children with ADHD will probably not do as well in a large class in which the teacher expects everyone to remain seated throughout the day. A small class that allows a lot of physical movement led by a teacher who values exuberance and creativity can make a world of difference to your child's academic growth and emotional well-being. Helpful modifications in school can include taking untimed tests, sitting next to the teacher, receiving individualized homework assignments, and receiving permission to leave the classroom when overstimulated. Adults with ADHD tend to perform better in an environment with a clear structure although it can feel restrictive. New challenges can bring out the best in both children and adults.

Shape the Behaviors   Shape your behavior to take into account the difficulties caused by ADHD. Use lists, written reminders, appointment books, schedules, and modern technology to help you start and finish tasks. Develop routines so that your internal disorganization interferes with your life as little as possible and your natural creative abilities can flourish. Write down a weekly schedule of all activities. This includes work, exercise, errands, appointments, and entertainment and anything else you do regularly. By following this routine regularly, accomplishing these tasks becomes a habit you follow with little mental effort.

If your child has ADHD, structure will help organize behavior. Use lists, written reminders, alarm clocks, and computers to assist in organizing and accomplishing tasks. Develop a behavior plan in which there are clear expectations for behavior, with rewards for success built in. Try to be as positive as you can in your feedback— many children with ADHD respond best to praise.

Consider Medication   Many people have misgivings about medication in general, and especially for ADHD. Following the assessment outline provided in chapter 3 should help you come to a decision about which medication is the right one for you. If you decide to try it, observing the guidelines for medication use described in chapter 16 should ensure that you use it safely and derive the greatest benefit.

Stimulants   This class of medications, named for their effect on a person's level of alertness, often appears to have a calming effect on people with ADHD. On the surface, this is somewhat paradoxical—how does a "stimulant" calm people down? Stimulants do not work any differently in the brains of people with ADHD, however. They help both "normals" and those with ADHD by improving concentration and permitting a person to behave in a more focused way. A person with ADHD can seem calmer, because the hyperactivity, impulsivity, and distractibility are toned down by the greater degree of concentration.

Stimulants are helpful for many behaviors associated with ADHD. They are the medications most frequently prescribed because they are usually well tolerated with a minimum of side effects. Many who have tried the other classes of medications believe that stimulants provide the most powerful effect.

They work within an hour, but their effects generally last only two to four hours. As a result, they need to be taken several times a day. Long-acting, sustained-release preparations are available and last four to eight hours, although many people believe they are not as effective as the standard preparations. You may find a combination of the standard and sustained-release forms provides the most benefit. You may prefer to take the same dose every day or tailor your dose to the day's activities, often taking less during weekends and vacations.

Most people notice few day-to-day side effects. There is a mild appetite-suppressant effect, but weight loss in an otherwise healthy person is minimal. It can be difficult to get to sleep if a dose is taken too close to bedtime.

Stimulants can worsen the tics seen in Tourette's disorder and can cause them on their own. Most professionals believe that the presence of Tourette's in the patient or the patient's family precludes the use of stimulants, and that stimulants should be stopped if tics appear.

Children may experience slight growth retardation. Periodic holidays from the medications, such as occur over the summer, can minimize this.

Stimulants can be abused for the euphoria they sometimes induce. Dextroamphetamine probably causes the strongest effect, then methylphenidate, and there is a minimal effect with pemoline. Anyone who wants to stay awake, concentrate more effectively, and feel energized will find them to be helpful. Students and truck drivers are the two groups most likely to abuse them. Sniffing methylphenidate has become popular among some high school students. People who abuse other drugs, such as cocaine, speed, and heroin, may "spice" up their use of these other drugs with stimulants. There is little reason to fear that they will be abused if they are prescribed sensibly to people with ADHD. There is no documented evidence that they lead children or adolescents to abuse other drugs.

Medications Used in Attention Deficit/Hyperactivity Disorder

Stimulants
  Dextroamphetamine (Dexedrine)
  Dextroamphetamine and L-amphetamine (Adderall)
  Methamphetamine (Desoxyn)
  Methylphenidate (Concerta, Focalin, Metadate, Ritalin)
  Pemoline (Cylert)

Miscellaneous
  Atomoxetine (Strattera)

Antidepressants
  Tricyclics
    Desipramine (Norpramin)
    Imipramine (Tofranil)
    Nortriptyline (Aventyl, Pamelor)
  Bupropion (Wellbutrin)
  Fluoxetine (Prozac)

Antihypertensives
  Clonidine (Catapres)
  Guanfacine (Tenex)

Antipsychotics
  Standard Antipsychotics
    Phenothiazines
      Chlorpromazine (Thorazine)
      Thioridazine (Mellaril)
      Trifluoperazine (Stelazine)
    Haloperidol (Haldol)
  Atypical Antipsychotics
    Aripiprazole (Abilify)
    Olanzapine (Zyprexa)
    Quetiapine (Seroquel)
    Risperidone (Risperdal)
    Ziprasidone (Geodon)

Stimulants can worsen and even cause psychotic thinking and manic episodes. Extra vigilance should be taken if they are prescribed to someone with these symptoms.

They carry a small risk of seizures. It can be reasonable to try stimulants in people with seizure disorders as long as there is simultaneous use of antiseizure medications and seizure frequency is followed carefully.

Miscellaneous   Atomoxetine exerts the same basic therapeutic effect as stimulants. It improves attention span, excessive motor activity, and impulsivity. However, it works quite differently from the stimulants. It is taken every day, usually at bedtime, and gradually affects functioning after two to four weeks of use. Advantages include a continuous beneficial effect rather than the waxing and waning seen with stimulants. Once-daily dosing is sufficient. It does not produce euphoria, so it is not abused. Some people do not find it as effective as stimulants. Rarely, it can cause suicidal thoughts or liver failure.

Antidepressants   This class of medications is generally used in the treatment of depression, but they are often useful in the treatment of ADHD. All antidepressants can increase the frequency of seizures in people who have a seizure disorder.

Tricyclics   Named for their three-ringed structure, these medications are taken once or twice a day and can take weeks to take effect. Many people notice an improvement in their symptoms, but most feel that stimulants provide a more robust effect.

Common side effects include fatigue, dry mouth, constipation, weight gain, sweating, and low blood pressure.

Rare side effects include the risk of irregular heart rhythms. At least six prepubertal children who have taken tricyclics have died, five on desipramine. Although desipramine was not definitively proved to cause the deaths, it was strongly suspected.

Bupropion   This is taken two or three times a day and generally takes some weeks to show effectiveness. It can cause anxiety, headaches, insomnia, and tremor. It carries a higher risk of seizures than other antidepressants when taken at high doses.

Fluoxetine   Some people find that their concentration and attention span improve with fluoxetine. Fluoxetine is taken once a day and generally takes some weeks to show effectiveness. Day-to-day side effects are minimal, although some people experience nausea, insomnia, and agitation for the first week or so. Many people notice a decrease in sexual desire and impairment of their sexual response, which doesn't go away.

Antihypertensives Generally used to treat hypertension in adults, clonidine and guanfacine have also been shown to help some people with ADHD. They are most useful to modulate mood and activity level in children who are hyperactive and explosive. They have little effect on attention, but can be used in people with a personal or family history of tics. They are perhaps most useful as an augmentation to stimulants. The main side effect is sedation.

Antipsychotics This class of medications is most helpful in combating the hallucinations and delusions often seen in schizophrenia and bipolar disorder. They are also used to control aggressive behavior in Alzheimer's disease. They are often termed "major tranquilizers," because they markedly reduce agitation.

   They have been used with some positive effect in people with ADHD, although stimulants are clearly superior. They also have a wide variety of side effects that make them unsuitable in the routine treatment of ADHD: sedation, blunted emotions, stiffness, restlessness, tremor, and tardive dyskinesia, a neurological disorder in which there are constant rhythmical, involuntary movements of the mouth, tongue, hands, trunk, and feet.

How to Start I usually recommend a trial of stimulants first. They are the most frequently effective and are generally well tolerated with a minimum of day-to-day side effects. Additionally, the onset of effectiveness is usually seen within hours or days. My personal experience is that most people find methylphenidate the most effective, so I generally start with that. If stimulants are effective, and they usually are, the next task is to optimize the dosing regimen. Because of the short duration of action, it can take several adjustments to arrive at the dosing schedule that works best for you.

   Your dosing regimen should maximize the effects of the stimulant over the course of the day. For many people, this means using the sustained-release preparations. You may find a combination of the sustained-release and the standard forms most beneficial. Many people take the largest dose when they need to be at their best. This is usually in the morning when work first begins. Students with night classes often take the largest dose in the evening. Many people cut back on their dose during leisure activities on weekends or vacations.

   Atomoxetine is a reasonable first choice as well, although it may not be as effective in some people. Some people find a combination of atomoxetine and a small dose of a stimulant is most effective for them.

   If stimulants and atomoxetine are ineffective, it is reasonable to try antidepressants, with the exception of desipramine in children. The difference in side effects leads some people to choose one antidepressant over the other. A combination of stimulants with one of the antidepressants is reasonable. Clonidine or guanfacine can be added to decrease motoric hyperactivity.

Antipsychotics should be used only if behavior is unsafe and there are no alternatives. Atypical antipsychotics are preferable because of the lower incidence of side effects (see chapter 14 for a full description of different antipsychotics).

CHAPTER 8

Bipolar Disorder and Mood Swings

Bipolar disorder, formerly called manic-depressive disorder, is characterized by wide swings in mood. Most of the time you will probably experience *euthymia,* when your mood, thoughts, energy, and outlook are normal. During manic periods, however, you may feel euphoria, with your mind full of ideas about how wonderful you are and all the great things you will do. Your thinking may go so fast that other people can't keep up with you. You may talk rapidly without stopping, have boundless energy and sleep little. The effects of mania may seem beneficial if symptoms are mild. Your thinking, energy, and enthusiasm may lead you to start projects and carry them through more effectively than if you weren't manic. In fact, many people begin successful businesses driven by manic thinking. More often, however, judgment is significantly impaired by manic thinking, disrupting relationships, work environments, and financial well-being. As much as you may enjoy feeling manic, you may feel ashamed by your behavior during a manic episode when it is over.

At times you may experience depression. When depressed, your thoughts are slowed, you have no energy, you have no plans, and you may feel hopeless about the future. Depression in bipolar disorder sometimes occurs after a manic period is over, regardless of whether there is anything in your life that distresses you. Other times it may occur in response to an external event, but the intensity of the depression is more intense than is warranted. Suicide is a real risk if you are depressed and have bipolar disorder.

Bipolar disorder occurs equally in men and women in about 1.5 percent of the population. Your risk of developing bipolar disorder is increased tenfold if your parents or siblings have it. You may first develop symptoms in your teens, although pronounced symptoms are more likely to emerge in your twenties. Some people don't develop pronounced symptoms until their forties. More than 90 percent of individuals who have one manic episode go on to develop another. On average, four episodes occur in a ten-year period. The interval between episodes decreases with age in some individuals. Most people return to their usual ability to function in between episodes, but about 25 percent will continue to demonstrate mood variability and difficulties in work and relationships.

There is no accepted etiology or pathogenesis for bipolar disorder. Most clinicians believe that the disorder is genetic in origin, but no specific genetic defects or linkages have been determined. Although stress may play a role in the precipitation of any individual episode of mania or depression, it is not thought to cause the disorder itself.

Symptoms

The symptoms of bipolar disorder vary depending on the mood. There is a characteristic group of symptoms present during mania, and a different group present in depression.

Symptoms during Mania   Your mood will probably be euphoric, happy, and enthusiastic when you are manic, maybe even "too good." As the episode continues, you may notice that the euphoria turns into irritability. This may lead you to argue and even fight with others.

Increased energy   You will almost certainly feel increased energy. You may feel boundless energy and enjoy all the things you are able to do.

Pressured Speech   You will probably talk at a more rapid pace than usual. You may feel unable to stop talking to the point that other people have to interrupt you.

Racing Thoughts   Your thoughts will speed up. They may go so fast that you are unable to process them and be unable to communicate them to others. They may jump rapidly from subject to subject, a phenomenon called *flight of ideas.*

Sleep Alteration   You will probably sleep less without feeling tired. When symptoms are pronounced, people can go many days without sleep.

Dietary Changes   You may notice that you are hungrier and eat more, or that you have no appetite and eat less. Whichever it is, it is likely that you will lose weight.

Increased Sexual Drive   You will probably notice an increased sexual drive, and may act sexually in ways you later regret.

Inflated Self-Esteem   You may have grandiose ideas about yourself and your abilities. Although there may be some validity to these ideas at the beginning of an episode, manic thinking can embellish them to the point that they are untrue.

Impaired Insight and Judgment   You may lose your ability to accurately perceive what is happening to you and the consequences of your actions.

Increased Activity   You may develop and carry out cleaning, hobbies, activities, and plans at work far more energetically than when you are not manic. If your judgment becomes significantly impaired, you may ignore the consequences of what you are doing, and engage in inappropriate sexual behavior, spending sprees, and fights with others.

Psychotic Thoughts You may hear voices (hallucinations). You may experience delusional beliefs, which tend to have a grandiose theme, such as the belief that you are rich, powerful, important, or have special powers. Psychotic symptoms occur in a minority of people who experience mania.

Symptoms during Depression You will invariably have a *depressed mood,* and feel sad, empty, discouraged, and hopeless as part of your experience of depression. You may be more irritable than sad, but an underlying unhappiness is present. You may cry uncontrollably many times a day for no apparent reason.

Diminished Enjoyment of Life You may lose your interest in activities, hobbies, work, and even relationships if you are depressed. This loss of interest may seem reasonable, but is usually part of the depressive syndrome, not an accurate assessment of your life. Psychiatrists refer to this as *anhedonia,* or an absence of pleasure.

Feelings of Helplessness, Hopelessness, and Worthlessness You may feel that your problems are insurmountable and that you are inadequate to manage them. When severe, these feelings can so shape your perspective of yourself that you believe you are a terrible person who has acted wrongly.

Diminished Energy You may feel tired and without energy all day.

Activity Level Changes Your movements and even your speech may be significantly reduced and slowed down, as if you were moving in slow motion. Alternatively, you may feel agitated and unable to sit still, even wringing your hands continuously.

Sleep Alteration You may experience insomnia, which is common with depression. Some people have difficulty falling asleep, others toss and turn, and others wake up after a couple of hours and can't get back to sleep. Less likely, you may sleep excessively.

Dietary Changes You may notice that food doesn't taste as good. Your appetite may be diminished. If you eat less, you may lose significant amounts of weight. Less commonly, you may eat more than usual and even gain weight.

Impaired Ability to Think Depression can impair your concentration, memory, and ability to make decisions.

Psychotic Thoughts You may hear voices (hallucinations) that berate you for supposed failings. You may experience delusional beliefs, which tend to have a negative, nihilistic quality to them, such as the belief that your body is malfunctioning in some way.

Suicidal Thoughts   Depression can be so severe that you may think your only way out is to die. As depression worsens, you may develop a specific plan to kill yourself. Suicidal thoughts are a sign you need professional help.

Treatment Options in Bipolar Disorder

The treatment of bipolar disorder has two phases. One goal is the *restoration* of a normal mood during an acute exacerbation of either mania or depression. Equally important is the *maintenance* of a normal mood, by preventing recurrences of either mania or depression.

Treatment of Acute Mania   Mania may require an emergency evaluation by your psychiatrist or a visit to a hospital emergency room if you don't have a psychiatrist. It can be a medical emergency if the symptoms impair your perception of reality and judgment to the point that your safety or that of others is jeopardized. Hospitalization is generally sensible, especially if it's your first episode and you don't know which medications work for you. Mania can lead to death if poor nutrition, insomnia, and physical exertion are extreme. In the most severe circumstances, electroconvulsive therapy (ECT) may be needed to calm your physical agitation and prevent collapse.

There are several things to do to lessen mild manic symptoms, however. Remove any influences that may worsen your symptoms, such as caffeine, cocaine, amphetamines, or other recreational drugs. Decrease the stimulation in your life by staying home with one or two people who help you maintain a quiet atmosphere. Don't go to parties, malls, movies, or any activity that may be exciting. Engage in quiet activities that will calm you down, such as listening to quiet music. Avoid conflict with others. Avoid strenuous physical exercise. Sleep as much as possible, as sleep itself can decrease the intensity of a manic episode.

Medications   These supportive measures are not curative, however, and the most important treatment for you is medication. It generally takes some weeks to bring an episode of mania under control. It may take months if medication is not taken faithfully. Three kinds of medication have proved beneficial.

Mood Stabilizers   Mood stabilizers are invariably used as soon as possible in an acute episode, in part because they are also used to prevent future episodes. They generally take one to two weeks to exert their effects, however. Lithium and carbamazepine are frequently effective. Valproate is probably the most helpful in an acute episode, because it causes sedation when first begun, a side effect that is actually helpful during acute mania. Oxcarbazepine is similar to carbamazepine and shows promise as a mood stabilizer. The atypical antipsychotics olanzapine, risperidone, and quetiapine can be helpful in acute mania. Olanzapine and risperidone can also

Medications Used in Mania

Mood Stabilizers
  Carbamazepine (Tegretol)
  Gabapentin (Neurontin)
  Lamotrigine (Lamictal)
  Lithium (Eskalith, Lithobid, Lithonate)
  Oxcarbazepine (Trileptal)
  Topiramate (Topamax)
  Valproate (Depakene, Depakote)

Benzodiazepines
  Alprazolam (Xanax)
  Chlordiazepoxide (Librium)
  Clonazepam (Klonopin)
  Clorazepate (Tranxene)
  Diazepam (Valium)
  Lorazepam (Ativan)
  Oxazepam (Serax)

Antipsychotics
  Standard Antipsychotics
    Phenothiazines
      Chlorpromazine (Thorazine)
      Fluphenazine (Prolixin)
      Mesoridazine (Serentil)
      Perphenazine (Trilafon)
      Thioridazine (Mellaril)
      Trifluoperazine (Stelazine)
    Haloperidol (Haldol)
    Loxapine (Loxitane)
    Molindone (Moban)
    Thiothixene (Navane)
  Atypical antipsychotics
    Aripiprazole (Abilify)
    Clozapine (Clozaril)
    Olanzapine (Zyprexa)
    Quetiapine (Seroquel)
    Risperidone (Risperdal)
    Ziprasidone (Geodon)

Alternative remedies
  Omega 3 fatty acids

help prevent future manic episodes. Lamotrigine appears to be helpful for preventing depression without causing mania. Gabapentin and topitramate have not been proven to provide significant benefit in large-scale studies, but some patients find them helpful.

Benzodiazepines   Immediate calming is generally noted with benzodiazepines. Their effects are moderate, however, and are not sufficient treatment by themselves. Clonazepam and lorazepam are most frequently used in the treatment of mania, although all benzodiazepines provide the same benefit.

Antipsychotics   The powerful effects of antipsychotics, generally used in schizophrenia, may be needed to calm the tremendous physical and mental excitement that manifests itself in a manic episode. Antipsychotics are invariably necessary when psychotic symptoms are present. Risperidone, olanzapine, and quetiapine usually cause the fewest side effects, but they may not be as effective as the others. Chlorpromazine and thioridazine cause the most sedation but can also cause low blood pressure, so are generally avoided these days. Clozapine is rarely used in mania because it can cause a fatal blood reaction. The rest can all cause uncomfortable muscle spasms, restlessness, and tremor. Of these, haloperidol is the most widely used, often with adjunctive medication to minimize the muscular side effects.

Alternative Remedies   Omega 3 fatty acids (O3FA) may be helpful for people with bipolar disorder. O3FA are chemicals involved in the intricate biochemistry of all cells in the body, including neurons, the cells that make up the brain. Examples of O3FA include eicosapentanoic acid and docosahexanoic acid, commonly found in salmon and other fish and available as concentrates. They are beneficial for some types of heart problems. They may also slow down communication between neurons.

In one study, investigators gave large doses of O3FA to people with bipolar disorder.[1] Many people appeared to derive significant benefit from O3FA, although they also took other medications. Although this report is not sufficient evidence for everyone who has bipolar disorder to start taking O3FA, these compounds may provide another aid in the treatment of bipolar disorder if further investigation confirms their usefulness. As with any drug, however, there are side effects. There may be mild effects on blood clotting, and many people note an unpleasant fishy taste. Reports of other side effects may follow if use becomes more widespread.

Prevention of Mania   Once the acute episode has been brought under control, the goal becomes the prevention of future episodes.

Mood stabilizers are the cornerstone of treatment because of their demonstrated effectiveness in reducing the frequency and severity of future episodes. You have about a 60 percent chance of experiencing a positive effect from a mood stabilizer. People respond most frequently to lithium and valproate. Fewer appear to respond to carbamazepine, while the effectiveness of gabapentin and lamotrigine is unproved. Some people need two, or even three, mood stabilizers to gain control over their symptoms.

The side effects of the mood stabilizers can be troubling. Lithium often causes increased appetite with weight gain, tremor, increased thirst and frequent urination, and can impair thyroid and kidney function when taken for many years. Valproate can cause fatigue when first started and increased appetite with weight gain. People often notice some mild hair loss after two to three months on valproate, though it generally grows back without difficulty. Rarely, valproate and carbamazepine can cause potentially serious blood disorders. All three require regular blood work to measure levels in your body and ensure that you are not having a toxic reaction. Lamotrigine can cause a rash and liver failure.

In spite of the difficulties associated with the use of mood stabilizers, however, it is essential that you work to determine a regimen that works for you and *stick with it*. There are three reasons for this. First, it is important to reduce further disruptions in your life. You have a 90 percent chance of having a second manic episode if you've already had one, and mood stabilizers substantially reduce the likelihood that you will have another. Second, there is some evidence that reducing the frequency and severity of episodes may actually reduce the severity of the illness over time. Third, stopping an effective mood stabilizer may render it less effective in the future. For example, if you stop lithium after a two-year period of being free of symptoms and you then become manic, it may be ineffective when you restart it.

Unfortunately, mood stabilizers may not be sufficient. You may have only a partial response, and you may not respond at all. The addition of a benzodiazepine may be all you need if you obtain partial control with a mood stabilizer, allowing you to avoid the long-term side effects of antipsychotics. They are most useful in helping you sleep adequately, although some people use them to maintain a stable mood during the day.

Antipsychotics are the class of medications most likely to help you if mood stabilizers are ineffective. Olanzapine and risperidone are often effective as mood stabilizers. Other atypical antipsychotics may also be helpful. Atypical antipsychotics often cause significant weight gain and can cause diabetes and elevations in cholesterol and triglycerides. Standard antipsychotics are less likely to cause weight gain but are much more likely to cause tardive dyskinesia, a syndrome of involuntary muscle movements, generally affecting the mouth, face, hands, and feet. Clozapine, an atypical antipsychotic, can be helpful in bipolar disorder. However, it has a number of serious side effects, which make it appropriate only for people who have exhausted all other remedies.

Treatment of Depression   The treatment of depression in bipolar disorder is largely the same as outlined in chapter 9. That information will not be repeated here, but it is worth your while to be familiar with it. There is one important additional fact, however: all antidepressants can cause manic episodes. It is preferable to try to avoid antidepressants if possible. Sometimes the symptoms of depression are mild and relatively short-lived. It may be better to tolerate a few days, or even a week or two, of unhappiness rather than resort to drugs that may cause more problems.

Often, however, the depression in a person with bipolar disorder has an autonomous quality that may be a direct biological effect of the illness, not a reaction to troubling events in life. Antidepressants may be the best aid at such times. Many people with bipolar disorder respond relatively quickly to antidepressants.

There are two important guidelines you should follow if you decide to use antidepressants. First, never use an antidepressant without a mood stabilizer to provide protection against having a manic episode. Second, it is generally better to stop the antidepressant when you feel better, because you will probably remain in a good mood once you have improved. Although mood stabilizers may provide some protection, it is useful to minimize your risk of another episode as much as possible.

You may find that you become depressed if you stop your antidepressant. If this is the case, it may make sense for you to remain on the antidepressant except when you experience symptoms of mania.

Prevention of Depression　　Although depression may be part of your illness, you may also experience depression for all the reasons anyone else does, too. It is important to take proper care of yourself to minimize the feelings of depression that arise in response to issues in your life. As described in chapter 9, maintaining a proper diet, eliminating drugs that can exacerbate depression, exercising regularly, and working on issues in life that lead you to be depressed can be of significant help.

Bipolar Disorder Syndromes and Their Treatment

The abnormal mood swings characteristic of bipolar disorder have been recognized for centuries. Because of our lack of understanding of the etiology and pathogenesis of abnormal mood swings, however, the specific syndrome has been, and continues to be, in some dispute. This is in part because there is no laboratory test that accurately diagnoses the presence or absence of bipolar disorder.

In the last twenty years, there has been increasing recognition that there are several distinct syndromes in which the symptoms of bipolar disorder are present. They differ primarily in the severity and duration of the symptoms. Because of the absence of a solid understanding of abnormal mood swings, however, your symptoms may not fit neatly into one of the four syndromes described here. There is a great deal of research investigating the nature of moods, however, and the best we can do at this point is to hope our ability to diagnose abnormal mood swings more specifically will improve.

The treatment of bipolar disorder is complex. No specific decision tree or guideline can steer you through and guarantee a successful outcome because so much depends on your response to different medications. The best advice is to make each decision about medication knowledgeably and carefully. Record your response to medications and the side effects you experience so that you are able to develop increasingly accurate information about which drugs, or combinations of drugs, are helpful at different stages of your illness.

Biological Causes of Mood Variations Possible causes of mania include multiple sclerosis, Cushing's disease, and hyperthyroidism. These are invariably diagnosed long before you have manic symptoms. Steroids, stimulants, and antidepressants can cause a full-blown manic episode. Cocaine and speed cause manic symptoms during periods of intoxication.

Thyroid disorders, anemia, cancer, Alzheimer's disease, and Epstein-Barr virus infections can lead to depression. Many rare medical conditions can also cause depression, so you should consider a physical examination and appropriate laboratory work if your symptoms do not quickly improve with whatever treatment you choose. Obviously you need treatment for any medical disorder you may have. Ideally, your depression will resolve when you obtain treatment for your medical problem, although you may require treatment with antidepressants indefinitely if you have Alzheimer's or Parkinson's disease. Many prescription and recreational drugs can also contribute to depression. Coordinate the treatment for your medical problems with your primary care doctor and psychiatrist if you take medication that can cause depression. Try to stop recreational drugs that can worsen your mood once the euphoria has worn off.

Bipolar I This label is given to the classic syndrome of mood swings recognized for centuries. Manic symptoms usually begin gradually and worsen steadily. They last for at least two weeks, but can go on for months if no treatment is begun. Psychotic symptoms are occasionally present. A mild, brief period of depression usually follows the period of mania. You may notice symptoms of depression and mania at the same time, sometimes called a "mixed" episode. You may notice that the manic episodes occur at the same time of year, often the fall or spring. Teenagers with the Bipolar I syndrome commonly experience mood irritability as their primary symptom rather than euphoria.

The restoration and maintenance of a normal mood needs to be an ongoing focus in Bipolar I. If you are lucky, a single mood stabilizer will prevent all but the most transient of symptoms. Benzodiazepines and antipsychotics may be necessary during exacerbations of mania. It may take two or three episodes to sort out which specific drugs in these classes will be the most helpful and cause you the fewest side effects. Antidepressants may be necessary briefly but are rarely needed for a prolonged period of time.

Avoiding caffeine and recreational drugs, maintaining adequate sleep, and minimizing stress in your life may help you avoid exacerbations of mania.

If you have more than four episodes a year of either mania or depression, a condition sometimes called "rapid-cycling," your symptoms will probably not respond as well to medications as if you have only one or two a year. If this is the case, you will probably need to be on a combination of mood stabilizers. You may need to take antipsychotics both during acute exacerbations and to maintain a normal mood.

Bipolar II   This label is applied if you primarily experience episodes of depression, which may last for many months. The symptoms of mania are brief and may be so mild that you merely feel "normal."

You will probably find the extended depressions the most troubling aspect of this illness. Many people stay on antidepressants indefinitely to minimize the depression. This is reasonable, but you should also stay on a mood stabilizer to prevent a "switch" into mania.

Cyclothymia   This disorder is characterized by mood swings in which the symptoms are milder and tend to last briefer periods of time than in Bipolar I.

Symptoms of cyclothymia often respond to a lower dose of a mood stabilizer than is commonly used in Bipolar I. Antipsychotics and benzodiazepines are generally unnecessary. Antidepressants may be helpful, but their use puts you at risk of a manic episode if you do not use a mood stabilizer.

You may want to tolerate the swings in mood without medication. You may enjoy the highs, find the lows only minimally troubling, and wish to avoid doctors, medication, and side effects. Sometimes, however, cyclothymia progresses to bipolar disorder. You are taking a risk of a manic episode if you avoid medication.

Mood Swings   Some people, particularly those who have experienced traumatic experiences in childhood, such as sexual or physical abuse, experience pronounced mood swings. Although some clinicians and patients refer to these mood swings as "bipolar disorder" and may equate the "ups" with mania, there are several important differences. First, they rarely last more than a few hours, often occurring several times over the course of the day. Second, the ups and downs are generally associated with a specific event, such as a conversation with a family member or boss, and do not have the autonomous quality of a genuine manic episode, in which a person is impervious to the opinions and actions of others and the events around them. Third, mood-stabilizing drugs, so useful for genuine bipolar disorder, provide minimal benefit. Finally, antidepressants often provide substantial benefit without causing a manic episode, whereas they invariably precipitate a manic episode in people with genuine bipolar disorder.

CHAPTER 9

Depression

Although we have all been sad because of experiences in life, depression goes beyond the demoralization produced by difficult circumstances. It is a much deeper level of distress. It infects our sense of who we are and what we feel capable of doing. It alters our view of the world and our place in it. We feel hopeless about our life and unable to improve it. Any action seems hard and pointless.

Depression is common. More than 20 percent of the U.S. population, fifty million people, experience depression over the course of their lives, with 10 percent depressed at any given time. Women develop depression at twice the rate of men. The probability that a person will experience depression is increased with premature parental loss, a neglect of emotional needs in childhood, traumatic experiences in childhood, a lack of social supports, and recent life stresses. There appears to be a genetic component to depression as well.

The effects can be devastating. Many people feel unhappy for years, unable to enjoy even the simplest pleasures in life. Some are so troubled that they are unable to work, maintain friends and family relationships, or engage in any activity beyond what is necessary for survival. Some require hospitalization just to stay alive. Sadly, some commit suicide out of despair.

What is especially troubling about depression is that many people never seek or receive adequate treatment. The depression itself can sap the energy and motivation needed to seek help. The social stigma against "mental illness" can stop people from getting help as well.

Don't let this happen if you are depressed. It is vital that you know that you can feel better! Don't give in to despair. The despair you feel is actually a sly tool of the illness working against you, not an accurate view of yourself or the world. Many forms of treatment can be enormously helpful for you and your depression. If you feel too hopeless to pursue treatment on your own, enlist a family member to help you get the help you need.

Symptoms

A syndrome of depression occurs when the feeling of depression persists over time and is accompanied by other symptoms. These symptoms affect your feelings, thoughts, and behaviors.

Depressed Mood   You will probably feel sad, empty, discouraged, and hopeless as part of your experience of depression. You may be more irritable than sad, but an underlying unhappiness is present. You may cry uncontrollably.

Diminished Enjoyment of Life   You may have lost your interest in activities, hobbies, work, and even relationships if you are depressed. This loss of interest may *seem* reasonable, but is usually part of the depressive syndrome, not an accurate assessment of your life. This is *anhedonia,* an absence of pleasure.

Feelings of Helplessness, Hopelessness, and Worthlessness   You may feel that your problems are insurmountable and that you are inadequate to manage them. When severe, these feelings can so shape your perspective of yourself that you believe you are a terrible person who has acted wrongly.

Diminished Energy   You may feel tired and without energy all day.

Activity Level Changes   Your movements and even your speech may be slowed down, as if you were moving in slow motion. Alternatively, you may feel agitated and unable to sit still, even wringing your hands continuously.

Sleep Alteration   You may experience insomnia. Some people have difficulty falling asleep, others toss and turn, and others wake up after a couple of hours and can't get back to sleep. Less likely, you may sleep excessively.

Dietary Changes   You may notice that food doesn't taste as good. Your appetite may be diminished. If you eat less, you may lose significant amounts of weight. Less commonly, you may eat more than usual and even gain weight.

Impaired Ability to Think   Depression can impair your concentration, memory, and ability to make decisions.

Psychotic Thoughts   You may hear voices (hallucinations) that berate you for supposed failings. You may experience delusional beliefs, which tend to have a negative quality to them, such as the belief that your body is malfunctioning.

Suicidal Thoughts   Depression can be so severe that you may think your only way out is to die. As depression worsens, you may develop a specific plan to kill yourself. Suicidal thoughts are a sign you need professional help.

Treatment Options for Depression

You will get the most out of whatever medication you choose if you combine it with other aids.

Diet   If you are so depressed that you have had significant weight loss, you may have difficulty motivating yourself and getting things back on track because you are so tired and run-down physically. You need to maintain a diet that provides adequate caloric intake and contains enough variety to ensure that you are getting the nutrients you need. Avoid sugar sweets between meals as they can lead to low energy after the sugar "high" wears off.

Drugs   You will help your depression if you eliminate alcohol, caffeine (it can impair sleep at night and lead to a lack of energy when it wears off), and nicotine (it impairs your breathing and your taste for food).

Exercise   Regular exercise can be very beneficial if you are depressed. It can improve your energy during the day as well as your sleep at night. The physical feelings of increased energy, elevated heart rate, and powerful exertion help you to feel competent and strong in at least one area of your life, especially when other areas may be in some disarray. Maintaining the discipline to perform regular exercise helps to counteract the paralyzed helplessness that you may feel.

Light Therapy   Many people notice that their mood is somewhat more down in the winter months and improves in the spring and summer. This has been called seasonal affective disorder, or SAD. Researchers have investigated the possibility that exposing yourself to certain kinds of light for periods of time during the day can bring about a mild improvement in mood in some people. Light therapy is insufficient for people with significant depression.

Psychotherapy   Different kinds of psychotherapy, described in chapter 5, can be very helpful if experiences in your life contribute to your depression. Discussing current issues as well as difficult experiences in your past can help you develop a more positive perspective about yourself and the world.

Group therapy may be helpful to offset your sense of isolation and lack of support, and challenge your pessimistic outlook on life. Strongly consider group therapy if your depression is due to the death of a loved one or the presence of a family member who abuses alcohol, issues around which group therapy can provide enormous relief.

If you feel too depressed to talk, you may benefit from vigorous treatment with medication before you try to tackle problems in therapy.

Hospitalization   If you are profoundly depressed or even suicidal, hospitalization can be enormously helpful. The care that you get in the hospital can ensure that you eat adequately, exercise regularly, attend to your medical problems, and work intensively on the problems that lead you to be depressed.

Hospitalization should be seriously considered if you have thoughts of suicide or have tried to hurt yourself. It can be very difficult to see that things may look better for you in the future when your perspective on your problems is so distorted. It is important that you get the support you need during your period of greatest vulnerability so that you do not harm yourself.

Electroconvulsive Therapy   Severe depression can be treated successfully with electroconvulsive therapy (ECT). ECT was widely used in the 1950s and '60s, when it fell out of favor because of its abuse by the psychiatric profession. It has undergone a resurgence of popularity in recent years, as hospitalizations have gotten shorter and people look to the quick improvement it can provide. Although ECT is effective, it causes pronounced memory problems and its effects are transitory. Although the process of ECT is no longer as barbaric as the image of Jack Nicholson being shocked in *One Flew over the Cuckoo's Nest,* it is dehumanizing. I do not recommend ECT unless it's a life-threatening emergency, when it may be the only sensible choice for people who are so ill that they aren't eating food and are refusing medication.

Medications   The categories into which medications are placed are derived from their chemical structure, chemical effects, or effects on your behavior. There is no classification scheme that neatly characterizes all the medications used for depression. All improve the symptoms of depression in most people, but none work for everyone. There is no "best" drug, although people sometimes respond better to one than another. There is no accepted protocol for determining which drug should be chosen. The choice of an individual drug is based on your responsiveness to the drug, your willingness to live with its side effects, and your physician's concerns that the drug might exacerbate an existing medical problem.

Selective Serotonin Reuptake Inhibitors (SSRIs)   Named for their action in the brain, SSRIs have proved to be enormously helpful for depression. They need to be taken every day and take some weeks to become effective. Their side effects are minimal in most people, although some people experience fatigue and a few become agitated. Most people notice decreased sexual drive and impaired sexual response, side effects that can cause considerable distress.

The drugs in this class have slight differences. Paroxetine also helps with anxiety and often causes mild sedation. Sertraline tends to cause increased energy. Fluoxetine remains in your system for many weeks after you stop taking it, which can complicate a switch to another medication. Fluvoxamine has been researched and prescribed mostly for obsessive-compulsive disorder, so there is less experience with its use in depression than the other SSRIs. Citalopram and escitalopram do not appear to have the problems of the others, and either makes a good first choice. Symbyax is a combination of fluoxetine and olanzapine, an atypical antipsychotic. This is generally a poor choice because a dosage adjustment of one medication requires changing doses of the other medication even when that is not desired.

SSRIs may cause a general soothing of anger and irritability over day-to-day events. This is an effect separate from depression. Although you may like this, it is not clear that this is a good thing. Getting angry or irritated about annoying issues may be unpleasant, but it can also spur you on to do something

Medications Used in Depression

Selective serotonin reuptake inhibitors (SSRIs)
Citalopram (Celexa)
Escitalopram (Lexapro)
Fluoxetine (Prozac, Sarafem, Symbyax)
Fluvoxamine (Luvox)
Paroxetine (Paxil)
Sertraline (Zoloft)

Tricyclic antidepressants (TCAs)
Amitriptyline (Elavil)
Amoxapine (Asendin)
Clomipramine (Anafranil)
Desipramine (Norpramin)
Doxepin (Sinequan)
Imipramine (Tofranil)
Nortriptyline (Aventyl, Pamelor)
Protriptyline (Vivactil)
Trimipramine (Surmontil)

Monoamine oxidase inhibitors (MAOIs)
Isocarboxazid (Marplan)
Phenelzine (Nardil)
Seligiline (Eldepryl)
Tranylcypromine (Parnate)

Heterocyclic antidepressants
Nefazodone (Serzone)
Trazodone (Desyrel)

Stimulants
Methylphenidate (Ritalin)

Miscellaneous
Bupropion (Wellbutrin)
Duloxetine (Cymbalta)
Maprotiline (Ludiomil)
Mirtazapine (Remeron)
Venlafaxine (Effexor)

Alternative medicines
Ginkgo
S-adenosylmethionine (SAMe)
St. John's wort

about them. Many people stay on SSRIs primarily for this effect. Although there is no obvious harm to this, many of us feel troubled about this national experiment with tranquilization.

Tricyclic Antidepressants (TCAs)   Named for their chemical structure, TCAs are the "gold standard" for treatment of depression because of their effectiveness. They need to be taken every day and take some weeks to work. They have been supplanted by other drugs, notably the SSRIs, because of their tendency to cause weight gain, dry mouth, constipation, sweating, and low blood pressure.

Desipramine and nortriptyline are the two most commonly prescribed TCAs because they tend to cause the fewest side effects. Desipramine sometimes increases energy, while nortriptyline often causes mild fatigue, effects that can be useful if you are either agitated or have no energy. Amitriptyline is frequently used to aid sleep because it causes the most sedation.

Monamine Oxidase Inhibitors (MAOIs)   Named for their action in the brain, MAOIs are also very effective. They too must be taken every day and take weeks to become effective. Common side effects include weight gain, dry mouth, insomnia, impaired sexual response, and low blood pressure. Their most troubling side effect is the potential to cause a stroke if you ingest adrenaline or adrenaline-like substances. MAOIs can be used only with a fairly strict diet that avoids foods or medicines that contain adrenaline or adrenaline-like substances. (A full list of the dietary restrictions is found in part IV.) As a result, MAOIs need to be used with extra caution. At low doses, many people are able to use selegiline without rigorous adherence to the diet. Low doses are often ineffective for depression, however.

Heterocyclics   Named for their ringed chemical structure, these medications can be effective for depression. The most troubling side effect is sedation, which often prevents maintenance of an adequate dose. Some psychiatrists believe that these medicines are somewhat less effective than those described above.

Stimulants   Named for the effect they produce, stimulants are most commonly used in the treatment of attention deficit disorder. They have been abused in the past by people who enjoy their ability to produce a burst of physical and mental energy. As a result, they are used infrequently for depression because so many other alternatives exist. Nevertheless, they can be effective antidepressants. Methylphenidate is the stimulant commonly employed. Although people notice improved energy right away, improvement in depression may take some weeks.

Miscellaneous   The four medications in this group have different chemical structures and act in different ways in the brain. Each must be taken daily and requires two to four weeks to become effective.

Alternative Medicines   St. John's wort can be helpful for depression. There are reports that ginkgo may be helpful in some people. S-adenosylmethionine is a substance produced by the body involved in the biochemistry of cellular processes. There are a number of studies which suggest that it may be useful in the treatment of depression, although studies necessary to gain FDA approval have not been undertaken. It appears to have few side effects, although rigorous evaluation of its potential for side effects has not been performed. It can be quite expensive and it may be ineffective if it is poorly manufactured.

Syndromes of Depression and Their Treatment

Thyroid disorders, anemia, cancer, Alzheimer's disease, and Epstein-Barr virus infections can lead to depression, so you should consider a physical examination and appropriate laboratory work before starting treatment. Ideally, your depression will resolve when you obtain treatment for your medical problem, although you may require treatment with antidepressants indefinitely if you have Alzheimer's or Parkinson's disease.

Some antihypertensive medications and recreational drugs can also contribute to depression. Coordinate the treatment for your medical problems with your primary care doctor and psychiatrist if you take medication that can cause depression. Try to stop recreational drugs that can worsen your mood.

Psychiatrists have created many classification schemes over the years to aid in sorting out which treatments are most effective for depression. These schemes have described depression in such terms as unipolar, bipolar, endogenous, reactive, atypical, postpartum, involutional, psychotic, seasonal, and others. The specific terms are derived primarily from how depression is understood. The descriptive terms keep changing because advances in our understanding of depression keep undercutting the validity of whatever scheme is in vogue. We will develop accurate terms only when we truly understand the etiology and pathogenesis of depression in the biological, psychological, and social realms.

Whatever diagnostic terms are used, however, there are two main syndromes of depression: *acute* and *chronic*. They can both occur by themselves or with other syndromes. For example, people with bipolar disorder experience acute depression, but the symptoms are indistinguishable from people with acute depressions who do *not* have bipolar disorder. Many people with schizophrenia experience a chronic unhappiness that isn't all that different from people with chronic depression who do not have schizophrenia.

Chronic Depression If you've been depressed for years, psychiatrists in the 1990s would call this *dysthymia,* a word derived from the Greek, meaning "abnormal mind" but commonly taken to mean depression. Chronic depression may wax and wane in severity but is present to some degree almost all the time, perhaps even starting in childhood. This form of depression may have become such a part of your outlook on life that you are perhaps unaware you could feel differently.

Chronic depression has a pernicious effect on your life that can be surprisingly subtle. It may be hard for you to see that you are, in fact, depressed because your negative outlook has been such a big part of you for so long. You may not even realize that it is depression which makes you find your relationships with others unfulfilling, your work as a burden to be borne, and the obstacles of life insurmountable.

Acute Depression   This form of depression generally occurs more abruptly, often following the death of a loved one, a physical injury or illness, or an unwanted change in your family or work. You are vulnerable to developing acute depression if you suffer from chronic depression or bipolar disorder. The symptoms of acute depression are generally more severe than in the milder chronic depression (which is why psychiatrists often call this *major depression*).

Acute depression calls for immediate intensive treatment to prevent a slide into such a state that hospitalization is necessary to maintain your nutrition and self care and to prevent suicide.

How to Start   Several antidepressants are "first-line" treatments, that is, they are the most likely to help you with the fewest side effects. I usually recommend a trial of an SSRI because these medications are the most frequently effective and the most easily tolerated. Unfortunately, they frequently inhibit sexual desire and impair sexual responsiveness, effects that intensify at higher doses. You may not care about this when you first start medication if you are focused mostly on the relief you hope to derive, but as you improve, this may become more important to you. After a couple of weeks paroxetine tends to make people tired after a dose, so this may be a useful one to try first if you experience insomnia. Some people try venlafaxine first, but blood pressure can rise and needs to be closely monitored. Bupropion is a reasonable drug to start with, although it can cause anxiety and insomnia. Additionally, the dose needs to be carefully monitored in order to prevent seizures.

TCAs were the mainstays of treatment until the SSRIs came out in the late 1980s. They are very effective, especially in cases of severe depression, but commonly cause weight gain, constipation, light-headedness from low blood pressure, and dry mouth, side effects that are unpleasant enough to make most people choose an alternative. TCAs are sometimes used first in severe depression in spite of their side effects because of some evidence that they are the most effective. Nortriptyline tends to make people drowsy after they take a dose, so may be the best choice if you experience insomnia.

You may respond best to MAOIs or SSRIs if you have "atypical" symptoms, such as excessive sleep and increased weight gain.

Some antidepressants are generally used only if trials of other antidepressants have failed. These "second-line" drugs include the MAOIs and stimulants. You may find stimulants helpful if you are elderly and suffer from a lack of energy as part of your depression. Trazodone, nefazodone, and mirtazapine tend to cause significant sedation. Although this can be helpful for insomnia, the sedation tends to last into the next day. Maprotiline has a greater tendency to cause seizures than other antidepressants.

Three additional tips: 1) You will generally improve only with the addition of an antipsychotic if you experience hallucinations or delusional thinking. 2) Benzodiazepines can relieve the intense agitation that may accompany your depression. 3) Extra caution needs to be taken in the treatment of depression if you have bipolar disorder in order to prevent the occurrence of a manic episode. The use of antidepressants in bipolar disorder is discussed in chapter 8.

Monitoring the Effectiveness of Your Antidepressant   Although you may notice some effects right away, an antidepressant generally takes some weeks to become fully effective. You should observe any physical or psychological changes as you evaluate its effectiveness and be on the lookout for side effects.

If the Medication Is Effective   If you're fortunate, and many people are, the drug you choose will be helpful without side effects that are significantly troubling to you. However, you may experience unpleasant side effects with any antidepressant. It is important to sort out whether a particular side effect is transitory or will continue as long as you take the medication.

If the side effect is one that will continue, there are three options. First, you can lower the dose. Unfortunately, the dose at which the side effect disappears may not alleviate depression. Second, you can consider adjunctive treatment. For example, yohimbine can improve the diminished sexual desire caused by SSRIs. (Adjunctive treatments to minimize side effects are described in chapter 19.) Third, you can change to a different antidepressant. If the side effect is one that is common to all drugs in that class, such as dry mouth and weight gain from TCAs, it may make sense to change to a different class.

You may want to go off the medication after you've been feeling better for a while. Most people do best if they stay on the medication until the situation that led to the depression has resolved. If you have had more than one bout of depression, however, research has shown that you are likely to suffer additional depressive episodes in the future. Recurrent bouts of depression are probably best treated by staying on the medication indefinitely.

If the Medication Is Not Effective   If you stopped the trial prematurely because of a side effect, it is reasonable to change to a different antidepressant. Depending on the problem you experienced, you may want to choose a new medication in the same class or a different one.

You may remain depressed even after an adequate trial of a high enough dose for a long enough time. This generally means the highest dose recommended by the manufacturer for a minimum of two to three weeks. You should probably obtain a blood level if you take a TCA to ensure that you have an adequate amount in your system. (Therapeutic blood levels have not been determined for other antidepressants.) It is reasonable to change to a different antidepressant if you remain depressed after an adequate trial, because you may respond positively to a different one.

If you have tried several antidepressants without benefit, consider *augmentation.* Augmentation with lithium or thyroid supplementation has helped some people. Augmentation strategies include using two antidepressants of different classes at the same time. A combination of a TCA and an SSRI has helped many people. Some combinations of antidepressants should not be taken because they can cause severe side effects. For example MAO inhibitors should not be combined with TCAs or SSRIs because of the potential for life-threatening reactions. Two SSRIs should not be taken at the same time because of the possibility that a person may experience the "serotonin syndrome," symptoms of which include fever, muscular rigidity, instability in blood pressure and pulse, and changes in mental functioning that can be so severe as to progress to delirium and coma.

If You Experience Suicidal Thoughts or Behavior   Suicidal thoughts frequently occur in people with depression. Very infrequently (less than 1%), people who take antidepressants find that they begin to experience suicidal thoughts when they've never had them before. Sometimes people who've had some suicidal thoughts find that they become more frequent or more intense. How or why this occurs is not entirely clear. It may be a specific reaction to the drugs in some people. It may be that the drugs give people more energy and motivation to do things, fueling hopelessness rather than hope, resulting in more intense suicidal thoughts.

Whatever the cause, you need to contact your provider if you experience suicidal thoughts, especially if they are getting more intense or more frequent. You need to make sure you can keep yourself safe until you regain your perspective that life is worth living and can be good for you. You may need to change medications or change other aspects of your treatment to feel better. These decisions are best made in consultation with your provider—don't decide that the antidepressant isn't working and stop it on your own.

If You Don't Feel Better   There are three things to keep in mind if you continue to feel depressed in spite of using antidepressants. First, is your *complete* diagnosis of depression correct? For example, are there medical problems that are contributing to your depression and need treatment? Is your distress better understood as unhappiness over your life situation rather than depression? Discuss this issue with your doctor.

Second, are there other treatments that might help you? For example, do you need to go to Alcoholics Anonymous and get some help stopping your alcohol use? Should you engage in therapy to address issues that are troubling you, such as couples therapy with your spouse to work on communication problems?

Finally, and most important, don't give up! Depression is an insidious condition that changes your perspective and makes you think you can't lead an enjoyable life. This isn't true—but it will take effort on your part to use the tools we have to make your life better.

CHAPTER 10

Developmental Disorders

Developmental disorders are characterized by severe impairments in several areas of functioning noticeable in the first few years of life. Social interaction skills are invariably impaired and often accompanied by poor communication skills, stereotyped behaviors, and mental retardation. While some people with developmental disorders are able to achieve independent functioning as adults, many require assistance from others to maintain their hygiene, nutrition, clothing, and shelter.

Diagnosis

The *Diagnostic and Statistical Manual* (DSM-IV), the standard diagnostic manual for psychiatrists, recognizes five subtypes of pervasive developmental disorders (PDD). In *autistic disorder,* the main deficit is impaired social interaction and communication. There is a reduced repertoire of activity and interests, a rigid adherence to specific nonfunctional routines or rituals, and motor mannerisms such as flapping of the hands. It is most common in males. There is severe impairment in social interaction in *Asperger's disorder,* but there are no delays in cognitive functioning, age-appropriate self-help skills, and curiosity about the environment. Language is not delayed, but there may be alterations in the rate and rhythm of speech. There can be excessive involvement and preoccupation with odd interests. The label of *childhood disintegrative disorder* is given to children who develop normally for the first few years but then lose their ability to communicate and interact appropriately with others. They also show repetitive patterns of motor behavior. *Rett's disorder* occurs exclusively in females. It is characterized by a few months to a year or two of normal development followed by slowed head growth, a loss of hand skills with subsequent development of repetitive handwashing or hand-wringing, a gradual loss of interest in the social environment, impaired gait and trunk movements, and a severe impairment in language development. Some children have a combination of deficits that do not fit precisely into one of these four and are given the label of *pervasive developmental disorder not otherwise specified.*

There are a variety of abnormal behaviors that may distress the individual or the caregivers. There is generally a marked impairment in interpersonal relatedness, which interferes with day-to-day functioning. There may be self-injurious behavior such as hand-biting or head-banging. There may be excessive motor activity, restlessness, and insomnia. There may be inattentiveness and distractibility. There may be irritability and aggressive behavior toward others. There may be non-goal-directed repetitive motor behavior, such as posturing with fingers. There may be an excessive preoccupation with inanimate objects such as string. Marked distress and disruptive behavior may follow any deviation from a rigid routine.

The etiology of these disorders is presumed to be biological. The theory in the middle of the twentieth century that autism was due to cold, rejecting parents has been thoroughly disproved. The pathogenesis is also unknown. In particular, there is little understanding of how and why there are such marked impairments following periods of normal functioning.

It is important to screen for any medical conditions that may cause such profound difficulties. Brain scans, complete blood work, and evaluation by a pediatrician and a neurologist can ensure that treatable medical causes are not overlooked.

Treatment

If you are the parent or guardian of a child with a developmental disorder, it can be a lifelong effort to ensure that he or she does as well as possible. New strategies are required as the child reaches school age, puberty, and young adulthood.

The main goal of treatment is to help your child achieve as much independent functioning as possible. Take advantage of any educational opportunities in your area. Schools may fund placement at residential programs that offer intensive learning environments. Occupational, speech, and language therapy are important. It is useful for family members to learn as much about the disorder as they can and to seek emotional support informally or through support groups.

Psychologists can create programs to teach behaviors that are increasingly appropriate and independent. Detailed behavior programs can often be effective in ameliorating aggressive behavior toward others or self-injurious behaviors like hand-biting, although short-term management with medication may be needed.

Medications   A wide variety of medications have been tried for developmental disorders, but none effect dramatic improvement. They can, however, sometimes diminish some of the core symptoms and aggressive or self-injurious behavior. These improvements may enhance the effectiveness of other interventions. The choice of which medication to use depends, therefore, on the target symptom. Some medications can improve more than one symptom. In general, very low doses are used at first, and the dose raised gradually while closely monitoring target symptoms.

Antipsychotics   This group of drugs is named for the ability to reduce psychotic hallucinations, delusions, and disorganized thinking. Psychotic symptoms are not usually present in developmental disorders. However, antipsychotics can reduce agitation, aggression, rage, impulsivity, hyperactivity, and withdrawal.

Medications for Developmental Disorders

Antipsychotics
 Standard antipsychotics
  Phenothiazines
    Chlorpromazine (Thorazine)
    Thioridazine (Mellaril)
    Trifluoperazine (Stelazine)
  Haloperidol (Haldol)
Atypical antipsychotics
 Aripiprazole (Abilify)
 Olanzapine (Zyprexa)
 Quetiapine (Seroquel)
 Risperidone (Risperdal)
 Ziprasidone (Geodon)

Antihypertensives
 Clonidine (Catapres)
 Guanfacine (Tenex)

Beta-blockers
 Nadolol (Corgard)
 Propranolol (Inderal)

Mood stabilizers
 Carbamazepine (Tegretol)
 Lamotrigine (Lamictal)
 Lithium (Eskalith, Lithobid, Lithonate)
 Valproate (Depakote)

Selective serotonin reuptake inhibitors
 Citalopram (Celexa)
 Escitalopram (Lexapro)
 Fluoxetine (Prozac, Sarafem, Symbyax)
 Fluvoxamine (Luvox)
 Paroxetine (Paxil)
 Sertraline (Zoloft)

Stimulants
 Dextroamphetamine (Dexedrine)
 Methylphenidate (Concerta, Focalin, Metadate, Ritalin)

Miscellaneous
 Buspirone (Buspar)
 Gabapentin (Neurontin)
 Naltrexone (ReVia, Trexan)

Following the first use of chlorpromazine in the 1950s, many antipsychotic drugs have been marketed. Standard antipsychotics, released before 1985, block the neurotransmitter dopamine. They generally begin to work within a matter of days, although some effects may be noticeable one to two hours after just one dose.

Standard antipsychotics cause a variety of unpleasant day-to-day side effects. They cause emotional blunting, fatigue, weight gain, sexual dysfunction, and dry mouth. Muscular side effects are often the most unpleasant and include decreased muscle movements, rigidity, tremor, muscle spasms, and restlessness.

They also cause tardive dyskinesia, a disorder of abnormal, involuntary, constant, rhythmical muscle movements. The movements usually affect the tongue, mouth, hands, fingers, trunk, and toes. The symptoms of tardive dyskinesia can persist even if the medication is stopped. There is no cure for tardive dyskinesia, although vitamin E can sometimes reduce the severity of the symptoms. There is a 10 to 30 percent chance of developing tardive dyskinesia after using a standard antipsychotic for more than one year.

A number of antipsychotic drugs have been marketed in the last decade. These "atypical" antipsychotics exert effects on neurotransmitters other than dopamine, which may account for several differences from standard antipsychotics. First, they cause fewer muscular side effects. Second, there is a much lower rate of tardive dyskinesia. Finally, some people find them more effective than standard antipsychotics.

All atypical antipsychotics can cause substantial weight gain (an increase of 10 to 20% of your current body weight in the first couple of months), diabetes, and elevations of cholesterol or triglycerides (another form of fat in the blood). People with a family history of diabetes are at a higher risk for developing these complications. These serious complications are associated with high blood pressure, heart attacks, strokes, and gallbladder problems. It's not clear if high doses are more likely to cause these problems than low doses. It's not clear if atypical antipsychotics cause these changes in metabolism directly or whether the changes result from weight gain. In either case, it is important to monitor your weight and be tested regularly for the presence of high cholesterol and diabetes. Careful dieting and exercise can minimize weight gain and even permit weight loss in people who have gained weight.

There are significant differences among atypical antipsychotics. Aripiprazole appears to be the least likely to cause weight gain, high cholesterol, and diabetes. However, approximately 25 percent of people who take it experience agitation, insomnia, and a worsening of their symptoms. Ziprasidone is the most likely of the atypical antipsychotics to cause an abnormal heart condition called QTc prolongation (see chapter 19). This condition is infrequent, even with ziprasidone (less than 1%), but is potentially serious. Ziprasidone must be taken twice a day because the body metabolizes it quickly. This is a problem if you have difficulty taking medication regularly. It should be taken with meals to enhance absorption by the intestines—taken without food causes roughly 50 percent less absorption. Risperidone tends to cause stiffness and restlessness at dosages above 6 mg a day. Although many people improve on doses lower than 6 mg a day, many people need more. Quetiapine causes pronounced sedation. Olanzapine appears to cause the most pronounced weight gain and problems with cholesterol and diabetes.

Antihypertensives Generally used to treat hypertension in adults, clonidine and guanfacine have also been shown to help some people with developmental disorders. They are most useful to modulate mood and activity level in children who are hyperactive and explosive. The main side effect is sedation.

Beta-Blockers Named for their ability to block the action of adrenaline on beta receptors in cells of the heart, lung, and other muscles, these medications minimize aggressive behavior in some people. Their lack of side effects makes them attractive, although they cannot be used in certain heart conditions, asthma, hyperthyroidism, or diabetes. Their effects are generally modest at best.

Mood Stabilizers Named for their general effect in the treatment of bipolar disorder, these drugs generally take one to two weeks to exert their effects. Carbamazepine, lithium, and valproate are used most frequently. Oxcarbazepine is similar to carbamazepine and shows promise as a mood stabilizer. Lamotrigine appears to be helpful for preventing depression without causing mania.

The side effects of the mood stabilizers can be troubling. Lithium often causes increased appetite with weight gain, tremor, and increased thirst and frequent urination, and can impair thyroid and kidney function when taken for many years. Valproate can cause fatigue when first started and increased appetite with weight gain. People often notice some mild hair loss after two to three months on valproate, though it generally grows back without difficulty. Rarely, valproate and carbamazepine can cause potentially serious blood disorders. All three require regular blood work to measure levels in your body and ensure that you are not having a toxic reaction. Lamotrigine can cause a rash and liver failure.

Selective Serotonin Reuptake Inhibitors (SSRIs) Named for their action in the brain, these medications are generally used for depression and anxiety. They do not alter the basic course of a developmental disorder. They may decrease repetitive behaviors, aggression, and self-mutilatory behavior. They carry the risk, however, of causing agitation or psychotic symptoms to emerge.

Stimulants Named for their general effect on a person's level of alertness, this class of medications is primarily used in the treatment of attention deficit disorder, although it is also used in narcolepsy, and sometimes in depression. Stimulants can sometimes improve hyperactivity, rage, and impulsivity in developmental disorders. They may increase internal preoccupation and withdrawal, however.

Miscellaneous A few other medications have been tried with limited success. Their value has not been demonstrated in the scientific literature, although some individuals may derive some benefit. Buspirone, generally used in anxiety, may reduce agitation and explosive outbursts in some individuals. Gabapentin reduces anxiety and agitation in some people. Naltrexone has been tried in the treatment of developmental disorders with mixed results. It may cause a modest improvement in activity level and attention, but is used primarily for self-injurious behavior, such as head-banging or hand-biting.

CHAPTER 11

Drug Dependence

Dependence on psychoactive drugs is of epidemic proportions in the United States and around the world. Tens of millions of people use alcohol, opiates, marijuana, cocaine, and amphetamines on a daily basis. The use of these drugs disrupts the lives of people who use them and those around them. It impairs friendships and functioning at work. It is responsible for the loss of lives in traffic accidents and crime. It impairs physical and emotional health and costs billions of dollars in health-related injuries, illnesses, and rehabilitation.

Many different treatments have been tried over the last few decades to help people who are dependent on drugs. The first, most successful, and most popular is Alcoholics Anonymous (AA). It is now a worldwide organization of self-help groups involving millions of people who meet regularly to help them avoid alcohol. Many self-help groups have modeled themselves on AA to help with various problems—Narcotics Anonymous, Overeaters Anonymous, and Gamblers Anonymous. Other treatments used to treat drug dependence include individual and group psychotherapy, residential treatment, and medication.

If you are dependent on drugs, you are probably aware of the negative effects of your use of drugs even if you are unable to stop. You have probably considered stopping your use and may have already made many attempts to do so. You may have already tried AA or counseling. You may have considered medication with the hope that it can provide some aid in your struggle to stay sober.

Treatment with medication is best undertaken as part of a comprehensive plan to achieve and maintain sobriety. This plan varies, depending on which drug you use. There are no medications that have helped reduce the craving or use of cocaine, hallucinogens, or marijuana. Some medications may be useful to help you end your dependence on alcohol, nicotine, and opiates.

Alcohol

People with the syndrome of alcohol dependence range from those who have a couple of drinks every day to those who regularly consume large amounts to the point of intoxication, and experience adverse consequences to their health, relationships, and employment. Definitions of alcoholism, alcohol abuse, and alcohol dependence emphasize different aspects of a person's experience with alcohol. Some focus on the frequency and duration of use. Others note the impairment of health or functioning. DSM-IV, the American Psychiatric Association's standard diagnostic manual, requires both.

There appears to be a genetic component in the etiology of alcohol use, although one's development, upbringing, and environment also play a role. The pathogenesis is complex as well.

However excessive drinking is defined, stopping your alcohol use can be a difficult task. The alcohol itself and the life you lead are intertwined in many ways, and abstinence will require major changes in how you spend your leisure time, your methods of relaxation, and your relationships. There are several aspects to your recovery.

If you possess strong will power and determination, you may be able to stop your alcohol use on your own. If you drink daily, you will probably go through a period of physical withdrawal, with symptoms of restlessness, tremor, anxiety, and insomnia. Many people find it hard to stop on their own and find the support of AA and therapy helpful.

If your use has been heavy, however, you should not try to stop drinking abruptly on your own. In addition to the unpleasant effects listed above, you may experience high blood pressure, rapid pulse, seizures, delirium tremens ("DTs"), hallucinations, and other physical changes. These changes can be dangerous and even lead to death, so medical care is essential. Benzodiazepines are often used during detoxification in order to prevent these serious complications.

Some people are unable to achieve or maintain sobriety even with the help of therapy and AA. You may require hospitalization or residential treatment to prevent you from obtaining alcohol and to give you the intensive support you need to make it through each day.

Once you have attained sobriety, the task is to maintain it. Many people go through repeated relapses. If you relapse, don't castigate yourself. Try to understand what led to the relapse so that you are better able to prevent it in the future. AA and counseling can be enormously beneficial in this regard.

Medications   A variety of medications have been tried in an effort to help people maintain sobriety.

Disulfiram   This alcohol-sensitizing agent changes the way alcohol is metabolized by the body. If you drink after taking it, acetaldehyde collects in your system as a breakdown product and produces a toxic reaction with symptoms of elevated pulse, low blood pressure, nausea, vomiting, and headaches. In a severe reaction, there can be respiratory and cardiac impairments that lead to death. The intensity of the effects is proportional to the amount of disulfiram and alcohol ingested. The basic idea is that you will avoid alcohol under the threat of these unpleasant reactions.

Disulfiram is rarely used in the treatment of alcohol dependence for practical reasons. It does not change your motivation, so if you want to drink, you just stop

---

Medications for Alcohol Dependence

Primary drugs

    Acamprosate (Campral)

    Disulfiram (Antabuse)

    Naltrexone (ReVia, Trexan)

    Benzodiazepines

        Alprazolam (Xanax)

        Chlordiazepoxide (Librium)

        Clonazepam (Klonopin)

        Clorazepate (Tranxene)

        Diazepam (Valium)

        Lorazepam (Ativan)

        Oxazepam (Serax)

Secondary drugs

    Antidepressants

    Mood stabilizers

---

taking it. If you use alcohol anyway, it is dangerous. If you are strongly motivated to stop your use, disulfiram provides no additional help. It is primarily helpful for people who are in a residential setting like a hospital or halfway house who want to maintain sobriety, lack the will power to do so, have the disulfiram administered by staff, and don't drink while they are on it.

Acamprosate   This anticraving agent affects GABA receptors in the brain and has been shown to decrease the frequency of relapse in people who have achieved abstinence.

Naltrexone   This anticraving agent blocks opioid receptors in the brain. Some people who are actively involved in counseling and take naltrexone are less likely to relapse.

    Many clinicians who work with people dependent on alcohol are skeptical of naltrexone and acamprosate. After an extended period of dependence on alcohol, maintaining sobriety is a task that requires an ongoing commitment to lifestyle changes that have nothing to do with the effects of a medication. Scientific studies and further use of naltrexone over the next few years will clarify its effectiveness.

Benzodiazepines   Named for their chemical structure, this class of medications is generally used in the treatment of anxiety. It is helpful for the acute withdrawal symptoms of alcohol. Some people stay on benzodiazepines past this period, believing they help to maintain sobriety. If you are anxious enough to feel the need for medication after you have withdrawn from alcohol, however, then you need to consider the possibility that you have an anxiety disorder. If you do, then you should vigorously pursue treatment for it, as abstinence is difficult to maintain in the face of intense anxiety.

Benzodiazepines are habit-forming. Cessation after more than four weeks of use produces a characteristic withdrawal syndrome. If you take them for extended periods, you will find that you continue to experience anxiety each time a dose wears off, a mini-withdrawal. Many people find that benzodiazepines are very difficult to stop once they have become dependent on them, a problem that has ensnared millions of people in the United States and many more worldwide. The substitution of benzodiazepines for alcohol merely replaces one addictive substance for another. Abstinence from habit-forming medications should be your goal.

Antidepressants   If you feel depressed, you may wonder whether antidepressants will help you to stop drinking. (See chapter 9 for a complete list of antidepressants.) Antidepressants do not change your craving or response to alcohol. However, you may be depressed even apart from your alcohol use. If so, you may derive benefit from treatment of your depression. This treatment may include antidepressants, although many people derive enormous benefit from other treatments as well. If you are depressed, you may find an antidepressant boosts your motivation so that you are more interested and willing to endure the difficulties in achieving and maintaining abstinence.

Mood Stabilizers   Used in the treatment of bipolar disorder to minimize wide mood swings (see chapter 8), there is no evidence that mood stabilizers reduce drinking in people *without* bipolar disorder. Some people with bipolar disorder find a reduced craving for alcohol when they take a mood stabilizer. It is not clear why this is true. Some people have speculated that the alcohol itself soothes the intense mood swings of bipolar disorder. The craving for alcohol is thus reduced when the mood swings are adequately treated with appropriate medication.

Nicotine

Thirty percent of the U.S. population smokes cigarettes and a small percentage in addition to that use pipes, cigars, and smokeless tobacco. Regular use of tobacco causes heart disease, lung cancer, mouth cancer, emphysema, and bronchitis, and causes several hundred thousand deaths each year. Dependence on tobacco is partly due to the presence of nicotine, which produces slight changes in awareness and attention that some people find pleasing. Nicotine produces physical dependence. If smoking is abruptly stopped, the withdrawal from nicotine can cause depression, insomnia, irritability, restlessness, anxiety, difficulty concentrating, decreased heart rate, a craving for cigarettes, and increased appetite with weight gain. The symptoms can begin within hours.

It is difficult to stop smoking after years of use. Most people make multiple attempts before they are successful.

Many treatments have been tried to aid the effort to stop smoking. Hypnosis and behavior modification have helped some people. Use of nicotine gum or patches decreases the nicotine withdrawal symptoms, but the craving for cigarettes remains.

Recent studies have demonstrated that the antidepressant bupropion (Wellbutrin, Zyban) appears to help some people stop smoking. Whether the effects will persist long after the drug is stopped is unclear. Other antidepressants have not been shown to provide significant benefit.

Opiates

Opiates are drugs derived from the juice of the poppy plant, such as opium, codeine, and morphine. Synthetic opioids include heroin, hydrocodone (Vicodin), meperidine (Demerol), oxycodone (Percodan), and propoxyphene (Darvon). The drugs share a common effect in the brain: they bind to receptors in brain cells to produce drowsiness, pain relief, and euphoria. Dependence on opiates has occurred for centuries, but the effects have been getting more pronounced as new drugs that are increasingly potent are synthesized. Opioid dependence has a deleterious effect on a person's health, relationships, and employment.

For most people who become dependent on oral prescription drugs like codeine, meperidine, or propoxyphene, the appropriate strategy is to achieve and maintain abstinence. This is best accomplished by an intensive program of counseling while stopping your use. This may include an initial two- to four-week inpatient stay at a hospital or detoxification center, especially if there is simultaneous dependence on other drugs, such as alcohol or benzodiazepines. Individual therapy and attendance at Narcotics Anonymous, modeled on Alcoholics Anonymous, are ideal and may be useful for many years until the person develops constructive ways to manage uncomfortable feelings. Medications may be useful to treat an ongoing psychiatric syndrome of anxiety, depression, or mood swings, but no medications have been shown to improve the craving and dependency itself.

Medications for Opiate Dependence

Clonidine (Catapres)
Methadone
Buprenorphine (Buprenex, Suboxone, Subutex)

The physical symptoms that occur when opioids are stopped are very unpleasant, though not generally dangerous, and do not call for any major medical program of detoxification beyond simple tapering. They include increased breathing, increased heart rate, sweating, goose bumps, runny nose, nausea, vomiting, abdominal cramps, tremors, hyperactivity, and irritability over seven to ten days. Clonidine (Catapres), an antihypertensive agent, has been used with some success in inpatient settings to minimize withdrawal symptoms. It has not been as successful when used in outpatient settings because of the side effects of lethargy, dizziness, and oversedation, and the ongoing availability of illicit opioids.

An addiction to intravenous heroin requires a more intense approach. The most common method of detoxification is a one-week to six-month treatment with methadone, which blocks withdrawal effects. Methadone produces mild euphoria, but this effect wanes with regular use. The rapid method is chosen so that counseling can occur in a drug-free state. The longer period of time can be used when a person needs time to address issues in their life relating to the law, employment, and their relationships.

Whether methadone should be prescribed for extended periods is a matter of intense medical, psychiatric, legal, and political controversy. Detractors of methadone maintenance stress the importance of abstinence and a drug-free life. They also note that methadone is often diverted by patients for illicit use. Supporters point to the rather low 15 percent success rate of addicts who attempt abstinence on their own. They also note the decrease in criminal behavior, improved physical health, decreased rate of infection with the HIV virus, and increased employment in addicts who are maintained on methadone. As there is no other treatment that produces these results, many clinicians and addicts feel that while methadone maintenance has its problems, it is worthwhile. Methadone maintenance is available only in federally licensed clinics to people who have been addicted for at least one year.

Buprenorphine is an opioid with a relatively long half-life which has been shown to be as effective as methadone in reducing illicit opioid use. It is available in oral form as Subutex or as Suboxone, in combination with naltrexone.

CHAPTER 12

Eating Disorders

There are a variety of abnormal eating behaviors. The most common is simple overconsumption and the development of obesity. Three disorders have been the focus of psychiatric research and treatment with medication: *bulimia nervosa, anorexia nervosa,* and *binge-eating disorder.*

Bulimia Nervosa

In bulimia nervosa (BN), the individual binges on food many times a week and engages in inappropriate methods to prevent weight gain. The purging type avoids weight gain by purging the body of calories through self-induced vomiting, the excessive use of laxatives, or the repeated use of enemas. The nonpurging type fasts or exercises excessively. In spite of the binge eating and purging, normal body weight is maintained. BN occurs in 1 to 3 percent of the population and is ten times more common in females than males. It usually starts in the teens or early twenties and may last for years. The course of the illness may be chronic, or it may come and go over a period of time. Many people with BN are ashamed of their behavior and may try to conceal it. There is an excessive concern with body shape. Self-esteem and intimate relationships are often impaired. The binges themselves are often accompanied by a feeling of being out of control.

The consequences of vomiting include tooth destruction from stomach acid. Excessive laxative use can damage the bowels so that laxatives are needed just to have a bowel movement. Females may experience menstrual irregularities. Rare but potentially fatal consequences include tears in the esophagus and stomach and heart irregularities.

The etiology and pathogenesis of BN are unknown. There may be an increased rate of BN in parents and siblings of individuals with BN. The marked increase seen around the world in the 1980s, a time when thinness was valued, suggests that there is a strong social component. The abnormal thoughts, feelings, and behaviors suggest a pronounced psychological component.

Treatment Cognitive-behavioral therapy (CBT) has been shown in a variety of studies to significantly improve BN. Treatment lasts about six months. It focuses on normalizing eating behavior and correcting distorted perceptions about body shape and weight.

Antidepressants minimize the purging and binge eating of BN in many people, though not everyone. Both depressed and nondepressed people with BN respond equally well to antidepressants. Many antidepressants have been tested and appear to be about equally effective. The exception is bupropion, which appears to cause a higher rate of seizures in people with BN than would be expected. The dosages of SSRIs may need to be on the high end but are in the same range as those for depression (see chapter 9). Lithium and naltrexone have been studied but have not been shown to be helpful to most people who try them.

Anorexia Nervosa

The syndrome of anorexia nervosa (AN) is characterized by an excessive pursuit of being thin. The individual refuses to maintain a normal body weight, is afraid of gaining weight, and inaccurately believes he or she is obese in spite of objective evidence to the contrary. Low weight is maintained by caloric restriction (the "restricting type"), or self-induced vomiting and the excessive use of laxatives or enemas (the "binge-eating/purging type"). AN occurs in about one-half of one percent of the population and is ten times more common in females. It generally begins in the midteens but can start before puberty. Some people have a time-limited episode and recover fully, while others experience a chronic course with a waxing and waning of symptoms.

Females experience menstrual irregularities and the absence of menstrual cycles. The abnormal dietary intake can result in calcium deficiencies that may lead to brittle bones with fractures and severe osteoporosis. One consequence of vomiting is tooth destruction from stomach acid. Tears in the esophagus and stomach are possible and potentially fatal. Excessive laxative use can damage the bowels so that laxatives are needed to stimulate a bowel movement. Severe dietary restriction can lead to dehydration, heart irregularities, and even death.

The etiology and pathogenesis of AN are unknown, although the first episode is often associated with a stressful life event, such as leaving home. It is more common in industrialized societies in which thinness is perceived to be attractive. There is an increased risk of AN among first-degree relatives of individuals with the disorder.

People with AN have unique thoughts and feelings about themselves and the world that lead to internal distress, conflict with others, and difficulty developing a satisfactory life. The development of healthy self-esteem, sexuality, and relationships with others can be profoundly impaired. There is often an element of despair and depression in daily life.

Treatment   The primary treatment for people with AN is intensive psychodynamic psychotherapy to help them integrate feelings about their bodies, their lives, and the outside world. Individual and group therapy in both outpatient and inpatient settings can be useful, depending on the stage of the illness. Medical hospitalization for nutritional rehabilitation may be necessary during this process if body weight becomes too low. Nutritional support is essential throughout treatment.

Medication plays a minimal role. No medication has a transforming effect on the disorder itself. Cyproheptadine may help hospitalized patients with the restrictive type of AN gain weight more quickly. Antidepressants may help some people eat more but are ineffective for many people. If depression is present, antidepressants should certainly be tried (see chapter 9). SSRIs may provide some benefit if symptoms of obsessive-compulsive disorder are present (see chapter 6). Antipsychotics may be of small value in severe cases. If antipsychotics are used, the newer, atypical antipsychotics probably make the best choice (see chapter 14 for a full discussion of the difference between antipsychotics).

Binge-Eating Disorder

In this disorder, the individual binges on food many times a week but does not engage in inappropriate methods to prevent weight gain, such as self-induced vomiting, excessive use of laxatives, or excessive exercise. Adverse childhood experiences, parental depression, vulnerability to obesity, and repeated exposure to negative comments about shape, weight, and eating predispose a person to developing binge-eating disorder. Research into binge-eating disorder is sparse because it has only recently been recognized. Its relationship to other eating disorders is unclear. Many people with binge-eating disorder are obese.

Treatment　　Cognitive-behavioral therapy has helped some people reduce the frequency of binges. SSRI antidepressants and topiramate have been helpful to some people with binge-eating disorder. Tricyclic antidepressants are helpful for some people with nonpurging bulimia nervosa, a similar disorder, and may also be helpful for binge-eating disorder. (See chapter 9 for details on both classes of drugs.)

CHAPTER 13

Insomnia

Insomnia is common and distressing. It's unpleasant to toss and turn at night, especially if your frustration gets the better of you. You may feel tired during the day. You may find that your thinking is muddled and that it is harder to function effectively. When prolonged for weeks or months, insomnia can worsen your mood and impair your ability to enjoy your life during the day.

From studying people who sleep in a laboratory, we have learned that sleep is a complex activity with a distinct structure. Much of what we have learned derives from the use of the electroencephalograph, a machine that measures the electrical activity of your brain through wires attached to your head. The machine records the electrical activity from your brain by moving a pen back and forth along a moving piece of paper, creating wavelike formations. The recording is called an electroencephalogram (EEG). The number of waves per second are measured in hertz (Hz).

Sleep is divided into non-REM and REM periods. Non-REM sleep consists of four stages characterized by different types of EEG activity. Stage 1 occurs when sleep starts. It is the lightest stage of sleep, in which the EEG shows theta waves of 3.5–7.5 Hz. Stage 2 shows sleep spindles of 12–14 Hz, which are short bursts of waves, and k complexes, which are sudden sharp wave forms. Stage 3 shows 20–50 percent delta waves of less than 3.5 Hz. Stage 4 is the deepest sleep and contains more than 50 percent delta waves. A person goes through these stages in the first ninety minutes of sleep.

After the first cycle into Stage 4, there are periods characterized by rapid eye movements (REM), changes in pulse, blood pressure, and respiration, penile erections, and a general lack of muscle movements with occasional twitching. People awakened during this stage commonly report dreams. REM sleep occurs about every ninety minutes, lasts ten to twenty minutes, and constitutes about 20 percent of sleep time.

Causes of Insomnia

There are many causes of insomnia.

Poor Sleep Habits   Many people have difficulty sleeping, primarily because they have poor sleep habits. Irregular hours, frequent naps, poor nutrition, and a lack of exercise can all contribute to insomnia.

Stress   Sudden bad news or the knowledge that you need to do something difficult in the future may make it difficult to sleep.

Drugs   Caffeine, alcohol, and other recreational drugs can cause insomnia. Even
a cup or two of coffee in the morning can worsen insomnia. Alcohol may make you
drowsy as you begin to sleep, but you will awaken later in the night when the effects
wear off. Recreational drugs like marijuana, cocaine, amphetamines, and narcotics
can also disrupt sleep during the period of intoxication and during the period of
withdrawal.

Primary Sleep Disorders   Primary sleep disorders are disturbances in sleep itself. *Night terrors,* most common in children, are episodes, lasting a few minutes,
of intense fearfulness, sweating, screaming, elevated pulse, and rapid breathing.
They typically occur during the early part of sleeping in non-REM sleep Stages
1–4. In *Sleepwalking* (somnambulism), the individual gets out of bed and engages
in activity while still asleep. These episodes also occur in non-REM sleep. *Sleep
apnea* is a condition in which the individual stops breathing for brief periods during the night. This disrupts sleep and causes fatigue the next day. In *restless legs
syndrome,* sleep is disrupted because of uncomfortable sensations that lead to an
intense urge to move the legs. In *periodic limb movements,* the limbs jerk, preventing the start of sleep or awakening the individual from sleep.

Medical Conditions   Medical conditions that may cause insomnia include hyperthyroidism, heart problems, breathing difficulties, and even colds. If you think
a medical problem may be causing your insomnia, it is essential to seek out a full
medical evaluation, including a physical examination.

Medications   Many medications used for the relief of asthma and colds contain
stimulants like albuterol (Proventyl, Ventolin), metaproterenol (Alupent), terbu-
taline (Brethine), and pseudoephedrine (Sudafed), which can produce insomnia.

Psychiatric Syndromes   Insomnia commonly occurs in the psychiatric syndromes of depression, anxiety, schizophrenia, and bipolar disorder. It is important
to consider psychiatric syndromes in order to ensure that any disorder you have re-
ceives proper attention and treatment. Many people with depression are treated
only with sleeping pills because there has not been an adequate evaluation of their
mood and the possibility of a depressive syndrome. Don't settle for a sleeping pill
without a thorough assessment.

Treatment Options for Insomnia

There are many treatment options to help you sleep better.

Improve Your Sleep Habits   If you experience insomnia for more than a few
days, do everything you can to get the most out of the time you are in bed.

First, establish a regular sleep schedule such that you go to bed and get up at the same time each day. Varied schedules, like the jet lag people get when they travel to other time zones, can interfere with the development of a routine that promotes good sleep. This can occur if you vary your sleep hours because of your work schedule or any other reason.

Avoid caffeine, alcohol, tobacco, and recreational drugs. Avoid nonprescription preparations that contain stimulating adrenaline-like decongestants like pseudoephedrine (Sudafed), phenylephrine, or phenylpropranolamine. If you have asthma, work with your physician to find medications that will not impair your sleep.

Avoid foods high in sugar, like ice cream and cookies, especially in the evening. After the two or three hours your body takes to metabolize the sugar, it increases its adrenaline output. This will worsen insomnia.

Avoid naps during the day. Although you may "catch up" on your sleep, it disrupts the normal rhythms of your brain and makes it harder to fall asleep in the evening. You will probably not feel tired at bedtime if you just awoke from a nap several hours before.

Exercise during the day to enhance sleep. A brisk thirty-minute walk each day can be helpful. However, avoid exercising for three to four hours prior to bedtime, as the adrenaline released during exercise will interfere with sleep.

Minimize Stress   Insomnia can be a signal from your body that you are under too much stress. Perhaps you need to cut down on the amount of work you are doing. You may need to work on resolving conflicts in relationships with people who are close to you.

Obtain an Evaluation   There are three possible parts to a formal evaluation if your insomnia doesn't respond to improving your sleep habits. First, obtain a complete physical examination from your doctor to ensure that there is no medical condition that needs treatment. Second, evaluate the possibility that the insomnia is part of a depressive or anxiety syndrome that needs treatment. You will benefit from educating yourself about any disorder you may think you have and a consultation with a psychiatrist if you have symptoms that suggest an anxiety or depressive disorder. Finally, you may need an evaluation in a sleep laboratory to investigate the possibility that you have a primary sleep disorder. This commonly involves an overnight stay in a sleep laboratory at a hospital.

Medications   A variety of medications have been tried over many centuries to aid sleep. Chloral hydrate was used in the nineteenth century and is still on the market today. Barbiturates like secobarbital (Seconal) and pentobarbital (Nembutal) were introduced in the early twentieth century and are still on the market. Ethinamate (Valmid), ethchlorvynol (Placidyl), glutethimide (Doriden), and others were developed and used widely in the 1950s. These drugs are rarely used these days because they are addictive, lose their effectiveness within a week or two, and can be lethal when used in an overdose. The medications described below are much better alternatives.

Medications for Insomnia

Benzodiazepines
   Alprazolam (Xanax)
   Chlordiazepoxide (Librium)
   Clonazepam (Klonopin)
   Clorazepate (Tranxene)
   Diazepam (Valium)
   Estazolam (ProSom)
   Flurazepam (Dalmane)
   Lorazepam (Ativan)
   Oxazepam (Serax)
   Quazepam (Doral)
   Temazepam (Restoril)
   Triazolam (Halcion)
Antidepressants
   Amitriptyline (Elavil)
   Mirtazapine (Remeron)
   Trazodone (Desyrel)
Antihistamines
   Diphenhydramine (Benadryl)
Antipsychotics
   Chlorpromazine (Thorazine)
   Thioridazine (Mellaril)
   Quetiapine (Seroquel)
Miscellaneous Hypnotics
   Eszopiclone (Lunesta)
   Ramelteon (Rozerem)
   Zaleplon (Sonata)
   Zolpidem (Ambien)

Benzodiazepines   Named for their chemical structure, they are the most frequently used class of medication for insomnia because of their effectiveness and their minimal side effects with short-term use. Common side effects include short-term memory problems and poor coordination, but these are usually minimal. Due to the marketing pitches of drug companies, several have become popular for sleep, but all the drugs in this class can be used.

Some make better choices than others. Both lorazepam and temazepam have a relatively short half-life so there is a minimal morning hangover. Clonazepam has a longer half-life, which can be useful if you tend to wake up too early in the morn-ing. A breakdown product of flurazepam lasts several days, so this is a poor choice.

There are two main problems with benzodiazepines. First, they are habit-forming. With prolonged use you may experience difficulty getting to sleep if you stop taking them. Second, their effectiveness diminishes over time. You may find that they help you get to sleep, but their effectiveness wanes quite quickly, leaving you awake for many hours during the remainder of the night. The best way to avoid these problems is to limit use to less than four weeks.

Antidepressants   Amitriptyline and trazodone cause such pronounced sedation that they are seldom used as antidepressants now that there are other antidepres-sants on the market with fewer side effects (see chapter 9). The pronounced seda-tion they cause makes them effective sleeping aids however. They make good alternatives to benzodiazepines for chronic insomnia because they are not habit-forming and they do not lose their effectiveness. They tend to cause dry mouth, low blood pressure, and may cause weight gain. They are effective for only about 50 percent of people who try them, however. Mirtazapine is also an antidepressant that causes pronounced sedation. Rarely, it can cause agranulocytosis, a poten-tially life-threatening blood disorder, so it should not be used routinely.

Antihistamines   Named for their ability to block the effects of histamine, a chemical released in the body in response to infection or allergies, these medica-tions decrease secretions in your respiratory tract. They also cause sedation. Diphenhydramine is the agent usually used. It is not habit-forming and doesn't lose its effectiveness over time. The effects are generally quite mild, however, and most people do not find antihistamines significantly helpful.

Antipsychotics   Named for their effects on psychotic symptoms, these medica-tions are powerful tranquilizers and often cause pronounced sedation. They can be helpful to induce sleep. However, they have many other possible side effects. These include stiffness, tremor, weight gain, dry mouth, and tardive dyskinesia, an irreversible neurological condition of involuntary, persistent motor movements of the mouth, tongue, hands, trunk, and toes. These potential side effects make them appropriate only for people who are taking them already for psychotic symptoms.

Miscellaneous Hypnotics   An hypnotic induces sleep. Eszopiclone, zaleplon, and zolpidem are structurally different from benzodiazepines, but act in a similar manner in the brain. The chief difference among them is the amount of time they last in your body. Eszopiclone lasts well into the next day, leading to a morning "hangover" as well as impairment of memory and muscle coordination. Zaleplon lasts for only a few hours, so there is no morning hangover or impairment of mem-ory or muscle coordination, but you may wake up in the middle of the night. Zolpi-dem is in the middle. Although these medicines don't appear to lose their effectiveness, most people find that they experience insomnia if they stop them af-ter regular use for more than a few weeks. Ramelteon works differently from ben-zodiazepines and the three described above. It interacts with receptors that respond to melatonin, not GABA. There does not appear to be any rebound insomnia or a withdrawal syndrome if discontinued.

Herbal Remedies   Hops and valerian may be useful for mild insomnia.

Tryptophan   Tryptophan, an amino acid found in many foods, was used in recent years as a "natural" sleeping aid because it causes mild drowsiness. However, some people who took tryptophan developed a potentially fatal disorder called eosinophilia-myalgia syndrome (EMS). Whether EMS is caused by tryptophan, a manufacturing contaminant, or some other factor isn't clear. It is prudent to avoid tryptophan until the issue is resolved.

Treatment of Insomnia in Medical and Psychiatric Conditions

No matter what the cause of your insomnia, it is worth making the changes described in the previous section to improve your sleep, enhance your quality of life, and avoid taking medication with all its attendant difficulties. Further treatment of insomnia depends on its etiology and its duration.

Stress   If a sudden stressful situation is impairing your sleep, medication may be the fastest and best way to get the rest you need. Hypnotics or benzodiazepines are invariably effective. Both can cause short-term memory problems, and benzodiazepines can impair muscle coordination (leading to an increased risk of car accidents and falls). Benzodiazepines are habit-forming and lose their effectiveness with nightly use, so don't take them for more than four weeks.

For prolonged stress that contributes to insomnia, antidepressants may make the most sense. Trazodone has fewer side effects than amitriptyline and is generally well tolerated. Many people don't find it effective, however.

Primary Sleep Disorders   Medical evaluation is indicated if you believe that you have a primary sleep disorder. This evaluation may include overnight evaluation at a sleep laboratory.

Medical Conditions   Medical conditions obviously need appropriate treatment. Hyperthyroidism may take weeks to get under control when first diagnosed. Hypnotics or benzodiazepines may improve sleep and your quality of life while this is occurring. Cardiac and respiratory problems can impair sleep because they may interfere with the amount of oxygen you are getting. Obviously the primary medical problem needs to be treated. Pain may make it hard to sleep, and analgesics may not be enough help. Hypnotics and benzodiazepines may be helpful in the short run. If you experience chronic pain, antidepressants make a more sensible choice.

Medications   If you take stimulant decongestants for asthma or colds, work with your physician to find alternatives.

Psychiatric Syndromes   Insomnia is an unfortunate component of many psychiatric syndromes. Treatment varies depending on what the problem is.

Anxiety   Insomnia often accompanies acute anxiety about an issue in your life. Hypnotics and benzodiazepines are reasonable aids in acute anxiety. Both can cause short-term memory problems, and benzodiazepines can impair muscle coordination (leading to an increased risk of car accidents and falls). Benzodiazepines are habit-forming and lose their effectiveness with nightly use, so don't take them for more than four weeks.

The symptoms of panic disorder, generalized anxiety disorder, posttraumatic stress disorder, and obsessive-compulsive disorder are not short-lived, so zolpidem and benzodiazepines are unlikely to be of long-term benefit. Antidepressants make a much sounder choice.

Depression   Insomnia is common in depression. You may have difficulty falling asleep, you may awake frequently throughout the night only to go back to sleep, or you may wake up after only a few hours and be unable to go back to sleep.

In general, when depression is adequately treated with antidepressants, sleep will improve. In severe depression, however, the lack of sleep can be so troubling that it makes sense to address it directly. Hypnotics and benzodiazepines are invariably effective and well-tolerated. Both can cause short-term memory problems, and benzodiazepines can impair muscle coordination (leading to an increased risk of car accidents and falls). Benzodiazepines are habit-forming and lose their effectiveness with nightly use, so don't take them for more than four weeks.

Some antidepressants are more likely to help you sleep than others. Amitriptyline and trazodone are the two most likely to cause sedation. Unfortunately, they tend to cause pronounced daytime drowsiness at the doses for which they are effective for depression. They can often be used successfully, however, in combination with another antidepressant to improve sleep. Trazodone is perhaps the better choice because it causes less daytime drowsiness and fewer other side effects.

Bipolar Disorder   Insomnia invariably accompanies an episode of mania and may be one of the first signs of an exacerbation of mania. Benzodiazepines can be enormously helpful to induce sleep. Clonazepam is frequently used because its long half-life enhances sleep throughout the night and slows you down during the day, but other benzodiazepines are helpful too. Antipsychotics can be helpful if you have bipolar disorder and you experience psychotic symptoms in addition to insomnia. Antidepressants should be avoided because they may worsen manic symptoms.

Schizophrenia   Insomnia is a common problem for people with schizophrenia, especially during an exacerbation of psychotic symptoms. Most antipsychotics cause some sedation and can be taken in the evening, so the first step is to choose an antipsychotic and dosing schedule that will be the most helpful. If you continue to experience insomnia regularly, the addition of a second antipsychotic with sedative qualities may make some sense. Chlorpromazine, thioridazine, and quetiapine cause the most sedation.

Hypnotics and benzodiazepines can be reasonable choices. Both can cause short-term memory problems, and benzodiazepines can impair muscle coordination (leading to an increased risk of car accidents and falls). Benzodiazepines are habit-forming and tend to lose their effectiveness with nightly use, however. Some people find their psychotic symptoms so intrusive and distressing that they tolerate the side effects for the brief sleep they are able to achieve with chronic use of benzodiazepines.

CHAPTER 14

Psychosis

Psychosis refers to thinking that is not based in reality. Such thinking can take many forms. You may hear voices when no one is there. You may have a belief about yourself or the world which is untrue, such as the belief that aliens from space are sending powerful rays into your body and harming you. Your thoughts may be disorganized so that it is hard to figure out what's going on.

Psychotic thinking can be an overwhelming experience. You may feel terrified by the perceptions and beliefs that appear to threaten your very existence. You may be disoriented, so that you don't know what to believe about your environment, yourself, or the people around you. You may feel alone and unable to trust other people. Your judgment may be so impaired that you find it hard to take care of yourself. When the symptoms are severe, other people may need to intervene to ensure your health and safety.

For centuries, many different societies have confined people to asylums when they became psychotic. One goal was to protect the person from harming himself or anyone else. A less laudable goal was to separate mentally ill people from "normal" society. There were no effective treatments for people with psychotic disorders, so little was done other than preventing people from harming themselves or others. Outlandish treatments like lobotomy and insulin shock therapy were tried earlier in the twentieth century, but they actually caused more harm than good. Physical and mental abuses were rampant in many institutions that cared for those with psychotic disorders.

The number of people confined to mental hospitals rose until the middle of the twentieth century. Two developments altered the practice of long-term confinement of people with psychotic disorders. First, payment for services outside a mental hospital became possible through the creation of Medicare and Medicaid in the 1960s. As a result, nursing homes, short-term psychiatric units at general hospitals, community mental health centers, and outpatient providers sprang up to provide services to people with severe psychiatric problems. These groups endeavored to keep people out of long-term institutions to promote a more satisfying life and avoid the abuses endemic to institutions.

The second change was the improvement in the understanding of psychiatric problems and the development of effective treatments. Instead of lumping all people with psychotic thinking into the "hopeless" category and sticking them in an institution for the rest of their lives, clinicians became increasingly able to distinguish among different psychotic disorders (described below) and choose treatments appropriate for each disorder. New medications, different forms of psychotherapy, and rehabilitation programs focusing on skill development, interpersonal skills, and symptom management all provided significant benefit to many people.

Treatment options for psychotic disorders continue to improve. For the first time in history there is now a wide range of effective treatments. You should feel hopeful about your future or that of a loved one suffering from psychosis. It will take effort on your part, but there is every reason to hope and expect that you can develop a satisfying and meaningful life.

Symptoms

Psychosis is primarily a disorder of thought, but emotions and behavior can also be affected.

Hallucinations   Hallucinations are false perceptions. Auditory hallucinations ("hearing voices") are the most common, but visual, olfactory (smell), tactile (touch), and gustatory (taste) hallucinations occur as well.

Delusions   A delusion is a false belief. Persecutory, religious, somatic (a false belief about your body), and grandiose delusions are most common. Delusions can appear to have some semblance of truth, such as the belief that one is the target of a conspiracy. Other delusions can be bizarre, such as the belief that one's internal organs have been removed and replaced by worms.

Disorganized Thinking   Disorganized thinking occurs when the usual flow of thoughts is disrupted. It is manifested primarily through incoherent speech. When marked, speech becomes incomprehensible and is sometimes called "word salad."

Loose Associations   This form of disorganized thinking occurs when your thoughts follow such a rapid flow of associations that the focus becomes lost.

Thought Broadcasting   The belief that your thoughts can be perceived by others.

Thought Insertion   The belief that other people are putting thoughts into your head.

Ideas of Reference   The belief that events in the environment are specifically directed at you. A common idea of reference is the belief that the radio or television is sending special messages only to you.

Alogia   Alogia, derived from Greek and meaning "without words," is a pronounced decrease in the amount of thoughts and speech.

Avolition   Avolition is the lack of motivation and willingness to pursue goal-directed activities.

Paranoia   Intense fearfulness that is greater than warranted.

Impaired Insight   You may have difficulty accurately perceiving and understanding yourself and the world if your thinking is affected by delusional or disorganized thinking. For example, you may believe that your voices are part of a religious experience and not a symptom of a mental illness.

Impaired Judgment   Your decisions may be so affected by psychotic thinking that you inaccurately assess what is happening in your life and how you should act. For example, if you are paranoid and fear attack from any direction, you may think medication is a poison and refuse it.

Flat Affect   *Affect* refers to the facial expression of emotion. Flat affect is the description given to a face that is largely immobile and unresponsive.

Inappropriate Affect   Inappropriate affect is the facial expression of an emotion that doesn't fit the content of thought. Examples include smiling calmly when talking about painful experiences, giggling continuously no matter what the subject, or crying for hours when there is nothing to be sad about.

Catatonic Behavior   Catatonic behavior occurs if you are so preoccupied with your thoughts that you move in odd ways. You may assume rigid postures and remain still, in spite of efforts by others.

Treatment Options for Psychotic Disorders

The treatment for psychotic disorders has advanced tremendously over the last two decades. Although beneficial medications have been around for more than forty years, many different treatment options can aid your recovery so that you can lead a satisfying and meaningful life.

Diet   You need to maintain a diet that provides adequate caloric intake and contains enough variety to ensure that you are getting the nutrients you need. If you eat so poorly that you lose weight, you may have difficulty motivating yourself and getting things back on track because you are so tired and run-down physically.

Recreational Drugs   Although marijuana, cocaine, heroin, hallucinogenics, and pain relievers can worsen your distress and should be avoided, the drugs that will probably cause you the most harm in the long run are alcohol, caffeine, and tobacco. Alcohol impairs your physical health, fuels despair, and lowers your motivation to pursue your life energetically and enthusiastically. Caffeine makes you more anxious and can worsen psychotic symptoms. The ritual of smoking tobacco may soothe you when you are upset, but smoking contributes to many health problems, including breathing difficulties, respiratory infections, heart disease, and cancer.

Exercise   Regular exercise can improve your energy during the day as well as your sleep at night. The physical feelings of increased energy, elevated heart rate, and powerful exertion help you to feel competent and strong in at least one area of your life, especially when other areas may be in some disarray. Maintaining the discipline to perform regular exercise helps to counteract the paralysis that you may feel with psychotic symptoms because you are getting up and doing something each day.

Psychotherapy   Different kinds of psychotherapy, described in chapter 5, can be very helpful. Work with a therapist can help you learn about yourself, your symptoms, and ways to reduce their influence in your life. Behavior therapy can help you engage in new activities that can become a source of enjoyment and satisfaction. Group therapy with other people can help you learn new strategies for managing the symptoms of your illness. It can also improve your ability to relate positively with other people.

Education   Educate yourself as much as you can about your illness, the problems it causes you, and the benefits from different treatments. Read books, access the Internet, talk to other people with psychotic symptoms, and join the National Alliance for the Mentally Ill.

WRAP   Create a Wellness Recovery Action Plan (WRAP) described in chapter 5. A WRAP organizes all the different steps you can take to promote your mental health, as well as helping you get the care you need when you are having difficulty.

Case Management   A case manager can help you shop for food, seek and maintain housing, keep appointments, obtain psychiatric treatment, and fill out the paperwork necessary to obtain Medicaid, food stamps, Section Eight housing benefits, and Social Security Disability. A case manager can also help you pursue work, new activities, and interests, and perhaps even form relationships with peers.

A Safe Haven   You may find it difficult to live independently. For example, you may find that your symptoms got worse when you tried to leave your parents' home. This is a transition that is hard for many people with psychotic symptoms. While you are coming to terms with your illness and developing a life for yourself, you may find that the most helpful aid is to live in a safe haven.

A haven is an environment where your basic needs for food, clothing, and shelter are met with little expected of you. A haven allows you to focus on integrating your abilities, the symptoms of your illness, and your goals for yourself as you grow and mature.

A haven is most commonly a house with other peers who have psychiatric difficulties and staff. Your parents' home can be a haven, although the natural tensions between parents and adult children sometimes lead to so much conflict that you may not find this a supportive environment.

Day Treatment   You may prefer to live on your own but go to a program during the day that helps you manage your symptoms. Some programs are intensive, short-term, and oriented toward helping you overcome a crisis. Others focus on long-term recovery issues. Both kinds are usually run by professionally trained staff. Many programs are now being developed and run by people who have psychiatric problems themselves. Drop-in centers exist in many areas if you want to socialize with peers and don't want a formal structured program. "Warm lines" in which you speak to other peers over the telephone can be helpful if you want to talk to someone but aren't in crisis.

Crisis Bed   A crisis bed can be helpful if you need a brief respite from your living situation. It can be helpful if your symptoms worsen and you don't feel able to function where you are living. It can also be helpful if there is some disruption at home and you need some space for a few days. Many people prefer to go to a crisis bed with professional staff available, but others prefer to stay with friends or family members.

Hospitalization   If your thinking is so disordered that you are unable to eat appropriately, maintain your hygiene, or maintain housing, hospitalization may be sensible. Hospitalization is most helpful when it allows you to stabilize a medication regime and address the issues in your life that trouble you. Sometimes being in a different environment itself can help to alleviate your distress. Additionally, the care that you get in the hospital can ensure that you eat adequately, exercise regularly, and attend to any medical problems.

An Alternate Decision Maker   If your symptoms are severe enough to interfere with your judgment about medical decisions, it may be useful to designate someone else to make decisions for you. Family and friends can sometimes play this role. It may make sense to obtain a public guardian with full power to make all medical decisions for you. The authority of some guardians is limited to financial decisions.

Job Training   Although work may seem overwhelming when you first experience symptoms, it can provide enormous satisfaction in the long run. Besides the financial benefit, employment can provide a daily structure, interaction with other people, and achievements of which you can be proud.

Vocational rehabilitation programs can assist you in finding employment. Most assess your abilities and prior work experience and offer a range of training options in your areas of interest. This may include classes at a school or training in a specific skill. They may be able to place you at a job and provide coaching when

---

Medications for Psychosis

Antipsychotics

Standard antipsychotics

Phenothiazines

Chlorpromazine (Thorazine)

Fluphenazine (Prolixin)

Mesoridazine (Serentil)

Perphenazine (Trilafon)

Thioridazine (Mellaril)

Trifluoperazine (Stelazine)

Haloperidol (Haldol)

Loxapine (Loxitane)

Molindone (Moban)

Pimozide (Orap)

Thiothixene (Navane)

Atypical antipsychotics

Aripiprazole (Abilify)

Clozapine (Clozaril, Fazaclo)

Olanzapine (Zyprexa, Zyprexa Zydis)

Quetiapine (Seroquel)

Risperidone (Risperdal, Risperdal Consta, and Risperdal M-tabs)

Ziprasidone (Geodon)

Side-effect medications

Antihistamines

Diphenhydramine (Benadryl)

Antiparkinsonian agents

Amantadine (Symmetrel)

Benztropine (Cogentin)

Biperiden (Akineton)

Procyclidine (Kemadrin)

Trihexyphenidyl (Artane)

Medications for Psychosis (continued)

Benzodiazepines
    Alprazolam (Xanax)
    Chlordiazepoxide (Librium)
    Clonazepam (Klonopin)
    Clorazepate (Tranxene)
    Diazepam (Valium)
    Lorazepam (Ativan)
    Oxazepam (Serax)
Beta-blockers
    Nadolol (Corgard)
    Propranolol (Inderal)
Vitamin E

---

you first begin. Vocational counselors often help you anticipate difficulties you may experience and develop strategies to overcome them. Some will speak directly to your employer if there are problems.

You may fear the loss of Medicaid and other benefits if you bring in too much money at your job. This is an unfortunate reality. Most states now allow at least partial temporary employment before reducing your benefits, but you do need to be careful. You may want to work at a volunteer job to avoid the threat to your benefits but still derive satisfaction from work.

Medications   Many medications improve psychotic symptoms. Unfortunately, antipsychotics often cause side effects that require treatment with other drugs. It is useful to educate yourself about the different medications and their side effects in order to make the choice that works best for you.

Antipsychotics   Since the first use of chlorpromazine in the 1950s, many antipsychotic drugs, also called neuroleptics, have been marketed. They are often referred to as "major" tranquilizers to differentiate them from benzodiazepines and other antianxiety agents. They vary in their chemical structure.

Antipsychotics improve many of the symptoms of psychosis. They are quickly effective for inappropriate, agitated, or aggressive behavior. After some days, the inappropriate expression of emotion is generally improved. The disorganized thinking begins to improve within a matter of days, but the full benefit may not be seen for many weeks, or even months. The intensity of delusions and hallucinations usually diminishes within days or weeks, but they rarely go away entirely. Antipsychotics are less helpful for the flat affect and lack of motivation often seen in schizophrenia, the most common psychotic disorder. Antipsychotics are not a cure, but they can improve the symptoms and allow you to take advantage of many other forms of treatment.

Standard antipsychotics, released before 1985, block the neurotransmitter dopamine. Standard antipsychotics need to be taken every day to give you the maximum benefit. A single dose at bedtime is usually sufficient, although you may prefer to split the dose over the course of the day if it minimizes a particular side effect you find troubling. You may prefer to take a dose during the day if the side effect of sedation is helpful. These medications generally begin to work within a matter of days, although you may notice some effects one to two hours after just one dose. You may find it helpful to take an extra dose when stressed.

Standard antipsychotics cause a variety of unpleasant day-to-day side effects: emotional blunting, fatigue, weight gain, sexual dysfunction, and dry mouth. Muscular side effects are often the most unpleasant and include decreased muscle movements, rigidity, tremor, muscle spasms, and restlessness.

Standard antipsychotics can also cause tardive dyskinesia. Tardive dyskinesia is a disorder of abnormal, involuntary, constant, rhythmical muscle movements. The movements usually affect the tongue, mouth, hands, fingers, trunk, and toes. Mouth movements can look a little bit as if you are chewing gum. Trunk movements can appear as a constant rocking. The movements are usually mild but can be severe. The symptoms of tardive dyskinesia can persist even if you stop the medication. There is no cure for tardive dyskinesia if you get it, although vitamin E can sometimes reduce the severity of the symptoms. You have a 10 to 30 percent chance of developing tardive dyskinesia if you take a standard antipsychotic for more than one year. Women, the elderly, and those with brain injury are at higher risk.

Standard antipsychotics are often divided into three groups depending on their potency, or the number of milligrams needed for effectiveness. Haloperidol and fluphenazine, the two "high-potency" drugs, commonly cause muscular side effects. Chlorpromazine and thioridazine, the two "low-potency" drugs, cause the most sedation and low blood pressure. Thioridazine causes the most pronounced QTc prolongation (see chapter 19), so is rarely used anymore. The others are "mid-potency" drugs. They have the potential to cause any of the side effects, but these effects tend to be less severe, especially at low doses.

Six antipsychotic drugs have been marketed in the last decade. These atypical antipsychotics exert effects on other neurotransmitters besides dopamine, which may account for a number of effects that are different from standard antipsychotics. First, they cause fewer muscular side effects. Second, the rate of tardive dyskinesia is much lower, approximately 1 to 5 percent. Finally, some people find them more effective than standard antipsychotics. These medications are also much more expensive than the older drugs.

All atypical antipsychotics can cause substantial weight gain (an increase of 10 to 20% of your current body weight in the first couple of months), diabetes, and elevations of cholesterol or triglycerides (another form of fat in the blood). People with a family history of diabetes are at a higher risk for developing these complications. These serious complications are associated with high blood pressure, heart attacks, strokes, and gallbladder problems. It's not clear if high doses are more likely to cause these problems than low doses. It's not clear if atypical antipsychotics cause these changes in metabolism directly or whether the changes result from weight gain. In either case, it is important to monitor your weight and be tested regularly for the presence of high cholesterol and diabetes. Careful dieting and exercise can minimize weight gain and even permit weight loss in people who have gained weight.

Atypical antipsychotics must also be taken every day to give you the most help. A single nightly dose is usually sufficient, although you may prefer to divide the dose over the course of the day to minimize side effects. Taking an extra dose on days when you feel stressed and your symptoms are worse appears to work only with quetiapine.

Many people with psychotic symptoms do not take their medication every day. Pharmaceutical companies have come up with two different kinds of drug formulations to help with this problem. First, risperidone, fluphenazine, and haloperidol come in formulations in which you receive an injection every one to four weeks. This eliminates the need for daily dosing and ensures that you get the medication you need consistently. Second, clozapine (Fazaclo), olanzapine (Zyprexa Zydis), and risperidone (Risperdal M-tabs) come in tablets that disintegrate in your mouth within seconds upon ingestion. These formulations ensure that you swallow and absorb the medication without being tempted to spit it out after putting it in your mouth.

There are significant differences among the six atypical antipsychotics. Aripiprazole appears to be the least likely to cause weight gain, high cholesterol, and diabetes. However, approximately 25 percent of people who take it experience agitation, insomnia, and a worsening of their psychotic symptoms. Ziprasidone is the most likely of the atypical antipsychotics to cause an abnormal heart condition called QTc prolongation (see chapter 19). This condition is infrequent, even with ziprasidone (less than 1%), but is potentially serious. Ziprasidone must be taken twice a day because the body metabolizes it quickly. This is a problem if you have difficulty taking medication regularly. It should be taken with meals to enhance absorption by the intestines—taken without food causes roughly 50 percent less absorption. Risperidone tends to cause stiffness and restlessness at dosages above 6 mg a day. Although many people improve on doses lower than 6 mg a day, many people need more. Quetiapine causes pronounced sedation. Olanzapine and clozapine appear to cause the most pronounced weight gain and problems with cholesterol and diabetes.

Clozapine is qualitatively different from all other antipsychotics. Many studies have shown that it is more effective than any of the other antipsychotics. It helps people who derive little benefit from any of the others, and increases the improvement of those who get some relief.

Unfortunately, clozapine also causes relatively severe side effects. If you try clozapine, you will probably notice marked sedation, pronounced weight gain, severe constipation, and drooling at night to the point your pillow is wet. Most troubling, however, is that it causes agranulocytosis, a disorder in which your body stops making the white blood cells necessary to fight infection. Without these cells, an infection may overwhelm your body's defenses and you may die. In fact, some people have died from taking clozapine.

Clozapine causes agranulocytosis in about 0.4 to 1 percent of people who take it. It almost always occurs in the first six months of use. To protect you, the Federal Drug Administration (FDA) requires you to get your blood drawn every week for the first six months of use and twice monthly thereafter. Since the FDA made this requirement, many cases of agranulocytosis were caught very early, allowing the person to stop the clozapine and recover. A few people have died in spite of getting their blood drawn regularly, however.

Although the side effects of clozapine sound terrible, most people tolerate them because they find it much more helpful than the other drugs.

Side-Effect Medications   Antipsychotics cause six separate muscular side effects (see chapter 19 for a more detailed discussion of each one). Atypical antipsychotics tend to cause them less frequently. *Akathisia* is an inner restlessness that is intensely uncomfortable. It is relieved somewhat by walking, but the incessant pacing can be distressing as well. *Dystonia* is a muscle spasm, often of the neck, jaw, mouth, and eyes, which usually occurs when antipsychotics are first begun. Sometimes dystonia occurs in the limbs instead. *Pseudoparkinsonism* is a constellation of several symptoms that mimic Parkinson's disease: *akinesia,* a lack of muscle movements, *rigidity,* and *tremor. Tardive dyskinesia* is a form of regular, rhythmical, involuntary muscle movements, usually of the mouth, tongue, hands and toes. It is unsightly, but not painful.

Antihistamines   Antihistamines can rapidly relieve dystonia. They can be helpful for akathisia and pseudoparkinsonian symptoms, although the sedation they cause makes them less advantageous than beta-blockers and antiparkinsonian agents.

Antiparkinsonian Agents   These agents can significantly improve dystonia and pseudoparkinsonian symptoms. They can also improve akathisia, although beta-blockers and benzodiazepines tend to be more effective.

Benzodiazepines   Named for their chemical structure, this class of drugs is generally used for anxiety. Benzodiazepines can provide significant relief of akathisia.

Beta-Blockers   Named for their ability to block the effect of adrenaline on beta-receptors in the heart, lung, and muscles, they are very helpful for akathisia.

Vitamin E   Vitamin E can minimize the symptoms of tardive dyskinesia in some people but can cause heart problems.

Syndromes of Psychosis and Their Treatment

Psychotic symptoms can be a secondary phenomenon originating in another disorder. Thyroid conditions, epilepsy, brain tumors, multiple sclerosis, and syphilis can cause psychotic symptoms. It is important to exclude these causes before treatment. Steroids, stimulants, amphetamines, cocaine, hallucinogens, marijuana, and PCP can also cause psychotic symptoms. It is essential to stop taking any drug that may be causing psychotic symptoms. Psychotic symptoms can also occur in bipolar disorder, depression, dementia, and posttraumatic stress disorder.

There are four disorders in which the primary problem is psychotic thinking.

Acute Psychosis   The syndrome of time-limited psychotic symptoms is called brief reactive psychosis if the symptoms last less than four weeks, and schizophreniform disorder if the symptoms last less than six months, according to DSM-IV, the standard diagnostic manual of the American Psychiatric Association. Whichever term is used, the disorder is distinguished from schizophrenia primarily by the rapid onset and brief duration of the symptoms.

Acute psychotic episodes generally occur in response to stressful situations. They sometimes follow the prolonged use of marijuana, cocaine, PCP, or other hallucinogenic drugs. People generally return to their usual ability to function once the symptoms have resolved.

Ensuring your safety while your symptoms resolve is the main goal of time-limited psychotic symptoms. This can occur at home, but is commonly done in the hospital in order to provide any needed medical treatment.

Antipsychotic medications can be useful until the symptoms resolve. Olanzapine and risperidone are probably the best choices.

Schizophrenia   Schizophrenia is a lifelong illness characterized by a waxing and waning of psychotic symptoms. It occurs equally in men and women in about 1 percent of the population of the world in all societies. It generally starts in the late teens or early twenties in males, and in the late twenties in females. It generally impairs your ability to lead a satisfying life when the symptoms first develop. If symptoms are severe, impairment may be lifelong.

The most common symptoms are auditory hallucinations, disorganized thinking, paranoia, and delusions. Other symptoms include restrictions in the range and intensity of emotional expressions (affective flattening), the flow and production of thought (alogia), and the initiation of goal-directed activity (avolition). These symptoms can cause considerable disruption in your life. When symptoms are at their worst, you may find it hard to maintain hygiene, nutrition, housing, work, and even your own safety. They may impair your insight and judgment, interfering with your ability to develop enduring relationships and work.

There is no accepted etiology or pathogenesis of schizophrenia. Based on the higher rate of schizophrenia among relatives of individuals who have the disease, there appears to be a genetic component. The precise genetic defect has not been identified, however. A mother's infection with the influenza virus during pregnancy may be related to the development of the disorder in the offspring. Many people have proposed that life stresses or bad parenting can cause schizophrenia. Although exacerbations of psychotic thinking are often due to stressful experiences, there is no research to support the belief that stress or bad parenting causes schizophrenia.

Many different kinds of treatment can be helpful if you have schizophrenia. Which treatments will be helpful depends on where you are in the course of your illness.

First, Seek a Full Evaluation   If your symptoms started a short time ago, or if you have only recently realized that your perceptions and thoughts are interfering with your life, the first step is to seek evaluation from a psychiatrist. While many professionals can aid you, psychiatrists are familiar with your illness, know the medical conditions that need to be ruled out, and have the authority to prescribe medication. Don't forget that while the psychiatrist is asking you questions about your symptoms, you are interviewing too! Make sure you feel comfortable with the age, training, and personality of anyone you decide to see again.

It is important to ensure that you don't have one of the medical problems listed above. You should have a physical exam, blood tests of your thyroid, liver, kidneys, electrolytes, calcium, glucose, and a complete blood count (CBC). At some point you should have an EEG to check for seizures and a CT scan or MRI to look for brain abnormalities.

Be Nice to Yourself   It is important to put supports into place. You will likely benefit from support from your family and friends. Maintain your diet to ensure adequate intake and nutrients. Try to get enough sleep. Educate yourself about schizophrenia by reading books, accessing the Internet, and talking with other people who have the illness.

Avoid caffeine, alcohol, marijuana, tobacco, and other recreational drugs. It is maddeningly easy to use these substances to provide some momentary soothing, but they will impair your physical *and* mental health and sabotage any efforts you make to improve your life.

Create a safe haven for yourself so that your day-to-day struggle to manage the illness doesn't turn into a day-to-day struggle to survive in life.

Try to develop a structure for yourself during the day. If work seems too much for you, consider school or a volunteer job. If any sustained activity seems too much, improve the skills you will need to lead your life: maintain your hygiene, shop and prepare food, clean laundry, manage money, and keep appointments. Try to maintain old friendships and develop new ones.

Develop some diversionary activities to reduce the focus on your symptoms. Listening to music, especially on a Walkman, often reduces the awareness of hallucinations. You may enjoy having a pet. Reading, movies, taking a daily walk, hobbies, and meeting regularly with friends can create periods of relative satisfaction even when your symptoms are most troubling.

Consider Medication   Most people find that medication significantly improves the ability to function. Of the medications listed above, I recommend starting with an atypical antipsychotic because they are generally more effective. Each drug has its pluses and minuses. Aripiprazole makes a good first choice because it is the least likely to cause weight gain, diabetes, or elevations in cholesterol or triglycerides. However, about 25 percent of people experience anxiety, insomnia, and a worsening of their psychotic symptoms within days of starting aripiprazole. This choice may be unwise if psychotic symptoms are already quite pronounced or your ability to function and stay safe is significantly compromised. For people without heart problems, ziprasidone may make a good first choice as it appears to be less likely to cause weight gain, diabetes, or elevations in cholesterol. Quetiapine generally makes people tired, and can be a good choice if you have significant agitation or insomnia. Olanzapine and risperidone are generally tolerated fairly well (although they generally cause weight gain). If one atypical antipsychotic is ineffective, it's worthwhile trying the others. It may take two or three tries to find one that feels right to you, but you'll do much better if you genuinely feel that the medication is helpful for you.

If these are ineffective, it is worth trying standard antipsychotics. Fluphenazine, haloperidol, thiothixene, and trifluoperazine are often used because they tend to cause relatively little sedation. If none of these produce significant benefits, consider clozapine. Although the side effects may seem scary and unpleasant, you may find that the improvement in your thinking and functioning is worth the trouble.

You may find it helpful to augment an atypical antipsychotic with a standard antipsychotic. As the drugs have different actions in the brain, combinations are reasonable.

Seek Other Treatments   You will probably benefit from a case manager to help you arrange the details of life. You may find it helpful to meet with a therapist to talk about your symptoms, how they affect your life, and what you can do about them. Group therapy with other people who also have psychotic symptoms can help you feel less alone, help you to develop a support network, and give you ideas about how to handle your symptoms. Consider living with other people who are also coming to terms with schizophrenia, with or without professional staff onsite.

If your symptoms are severe, you may require a crisis bed, day program, residential treatment, or even a hospital to provide the moment-to-moment help you need to keep yourself safe and healthy.

Create a WRAP (described in chapter 5) to help when you begin to feel overwhelmed.

Schizoaffective Disorder   The term *schizoaffective disorder* is often used to describe your illness if you have chronic psychotic symptoms and also experience recurrent manic or depressive episodes (the suffix -*affective* denotes a disturbance of mood or emotion). Schizoaffective disorder is generally more severe than schizophrenia. Not only must you deal with chronic psychotic thinking, but the intermittent disruption of manic symptoms or the feelings of despair from depression can add significantly to your burden.

Treatment generally involves a more complex regimen of medications in order to treat the additional symptoms. If you primarily experience manic symptoms, you may benefit from the treatment for mania described in chapter 8. Mood stabilizers such as valproate, lithium, and carbamazepine may be useful. You should give serious consideration to clozapine, which may be more effective than other antipsychotics for schizoaffective disorder. If you experience periodic or chronic depression, you may benefit from the treatment for depression described in chapter 9. Antidepressants often worsen psychotic symptoms, so use them with extra caution.

Delusional Disorder   Delusional disorder is the label applied if your only psychotic symptom is a delusion. In general, the delusions in this condition are more realistic than those in schizophrenia, although this can be a hard distinction to make. Examples of delusions include the belief that another person is in love with you, that you have a special talent, that your spouse is unfaithful, or that you are being conspired against. You may hold these beliefs based on your interpretation of "evidence" that others find totally insufficient. Your functioning may be minimally or substantially impaired, depending on the degree to which you act on the belief itself.

Treatment is only moderately effective. Medication and psychotherapy are of little benefit in changing the belief itself, although they may help you function more effectively. If your beliefs interfere with work only, you may be able to find relief with a new job.

CHAPTER 15

Alzheimer's Disease

*D*ementia refers to the loss of intellectual functioning. Alzheimer's disease is the most common form of dementia in the elderly. This devastating illness affects more than two and a half million people in the United States. It also exacts a heavy toll on family members' time, emotions, and financial well-being. There is no cure at this time.

Diagnosis

It can be difficult to distinguish the earliest stages of Alzheimer's disease from the mild cognitive decline seen in normal aging. The syndrome starts with a gradual progressive decline in cognitive abilities. There is first an impaired ability to remember new information or recent events, such as the placement of keys or wallet and conversations with others. Other common symptoms include a shortened attention span, trouble with simple math, difficulty in expressing thoughts, and reluctance to try new things or meet new people. The overlap of symptoms of early Alzheimer's with the diminution in abilities often seen with advanced age can delay the realization that dementia is occurring.

As the decline progresses, however, functioning becomes increasingly impaired, and it becomes clear that the problem is not a natural aging phenomenon. Memory loss becomes severe. People may have difficulty dressing, preparing food, or remembering the names of family members. A person may be unable to perform routine household tasks or take care of personal hygiene. There can be mood and personality changes with outbursts of anger or suspiciousness. Judgment and concentration become quite impaired. The cognitive decline progresses to include a severe memory impairment, poor judgment, difficulty speaking, disorientation, and physical decline. Hallucinations and delusions may develop. In its late stages, there are often behavioral abnormalities. These include hyperactivity, agitation, physical and verbal aggressive behaviors, uncooperativeness with caregivers, and wandering. The decline is usually over a matter of many years but can be more rapid.

There is no proven etiology of Alzheimer's. Several abnormal genes have been demonstrated in families whose members develop Alzheimer's at an early age. There appear to be different genetic abnormalities in people with the more common later onset. Age obviously plays a role as well, although it is not clear why this is so.

The pathogenesis is unclear as well. How these abnormal genes, and the abnormal proteins that are formed as a result, cause the destruction of neurons is unclear. The gradual decline in functioning is probably due to progressive impairment of brain cell functioning.

There is no clear diagnostic test that unequivocally establishes the diagnosis of Alzheimer's during a person's life. Cognitive deficits can be documented on sophisticated neuropsychological testing once symptoms have begun. In late stages of the illness, brain atrophy is seen on brain scans. Microscopic examination of the brain at autopsy shows abnormal features called *senile plaques* and *neurofibrillary tangles* in neurons.

It can also be difficult to distinguish Alzheimer's from other causes of dementia. Many people experience cognitive decline that is more than would be expected by age but is different from Alzheimer's. For example, insight and judgment may be quite impaired while memory appears largely preserved. The definitive diagnosis of Alzheimer's cannot be made except by finding the characteristic microscopic abnormalities in brain cells of the brain at the time of death.

If you are concerned that you or someone you love has Alzheimer's, the first step is to seek a full evaluation. This will include a complete physical exam by a physician, as well as blood work and a CT scan or MRI to ensure that other causes of dementia are excluded. Consultation with a neurologist should be sought at some point to rule out rare causes of dementia. Objective testing of cognitive abilities should be performed to establish the degree of impairment and provide a baseline for comparison with measurements in the future.

Treatment

The goal of treatment for anyone with Alzheimer's is to maximize independent, pleasurable functioning as long as possible. To that end there are many aspects to good treatment.

Maintain a good diet. Maintain or begin daily exercise to promote good physical and mental health, after getting clearance from the doctor. Stay as active as possible: get or stay involved in groups with others; maintain any hobbies; take recreational trips to parks, museums, and ball games; and maintain your daily routine to the extent that it is possible. Use memory aids like calendars, lists, written reminders, labels, and safety instructions.

If you are caring for someone with Alzheimer's, you may feel overwhelmed with all that needs to be done. You will probably benefit from the education and support provided by groups organized at the national, state, and local levels for the treatment of Alzheimer's. These groups can often be accessed through a doctor or hospital.

Medications for Alzheimer's

Cognitive enhancers
    Donepezil (Aricept)
    Galantamine (Reminyl)
    Rivastigmine (Exelon)
    Tacrine (Cognex)
    Vitamin E

Antipsychotics
    Standard antipsychotics
        Phenothiazines
            Chlorpromazine (Thorazine)
            Fluphenazine (Prolixin)
            Mesoridazine (Serentil)
            Perphenazine (Trilafon)
            Thioridazine (Mellaril)
            Trifluoperazine (Stelazine)
        Haloperidol (Haldol)
        Loxapine (Loxitane)
        Molindone (Moban)
        Thiothixene (Navane)
    Atypical antipsychotics
        Aripiprazole (Abilify)
        Olanzapine (Zyprexa)
        Quetiapine (Seroquel)
        Risperidone (Risperdal)
        Ziprasidone (Geodon)

Benzodiazepines
    Alprazolam (Xanax)
    Chlordiazepoxide (Librium)
    Clonazepam (Klonopin)
    Clorazepate (Tranxene)
    Diazepam (Valium)
    Lorazepam (Ativan)
    Oxazepam (Serax)

Miscellaneous
    Buspirone (Buspar)

Antidepressants

Medications   Many medications are used in the treatment of Alzheimer's be-cause of the wide variety of symptoms at different stages of the illness.

Cognitive Enhancers   Donepezil, galantamine, and rivastigmine slow the rate of cognitive decline in some people with Alzheimer's disease, but do not change the final outcome for people with Alzheimer's disease. Tacrine is as effective as the other three, but can cause liver problems and is rarely used. Vitamin E can cause heart problems and its benefits are minimal, so it also is rarely used.

Antipsychotics   Antipsychotic medications are used for psychotic thinking and disorganized, agitated, or assaultive behavior.

Psychotic thinking is usually manifested by hallucinations (false perceptions, such as hearing voices or seeing visions) or delusions (false beliefs). The delusions sometimes seen in Alzheimer's tend to be caused in part by poor memory. For ex-ample, a person may believe that someone is stealing their things because they can't find them. There is rarely the elaborate or bizarre delusional thinking seen in schizophrenia.

Acute agitation and disruptive or assaultive behavior may be due to a med-ical illness such as infection, and therefore always require a careful medical evaluation. If no medical cause can be found, it may be due to a change in a per-son's environment. Close personal attention can often provide a calming effect, but sometimes this isn't enough.

Psychotic thinking and behavioral disturbances can be distressing and even dangerous. If no other intervention is effective, antipsychotics may provide some relief. These medications, commonly used in schizophrenia, are often referred to as "major" tranquilizers to differentiate them from benzodiazepines and other an-tianxiety agents. They vary in their chemical structure, but all improve disordered behavior, reduce disorganized thinking, and decrease the intensity of hallucina-tions and delusions.

Following the first use of chlorpromazine in the 1950s, many antipsychotic drugs have been marketed. Standard antipsychotics, released before 1985, block the neurotransmitter dopamine.

Standard antipsychotics need to be taken every day. A single dose at bedtime is usually sufficient, although the dose is sometimes divided over the course of a day to minimize a particular side effect. They generally begin to work within a matter of days, although some effects may be noticeable one to two hours after just one dose.

Standard antipsychotics cause a variety of unpleasant day-to-day side effects. They cause emotional blunting, fatigue, weight gain, sexual dysfunction, and dry mouth. Muscular side effects are often the most unpleasant and include decreased muscle movements, rigidity, tremor, muscle spasms, and restlessness.

Standard antipsychotics can also cause tardive dyskinesia. Tardive dyskinesia is a disorder of abnormal, involuntary, constant, rhythmical muscle movements. The movements usually affect the tongue, mouth, hands, fingers, trunk, and toes.

Mouth movements can look a little bit like chewing gum. Trunk movements can appear as a constant rocking. The movements are usually mild but can be severe. The symptoms of tardive dyskinesia can persist even if the medication is stopped. There is no cure for tardive dyskinesia, although vitamin E can sometimes reduce the severity of the symptoms. There is a 10 to 30 percent chance of developing tardive dyskinesia after using a standard antipsychotic for more than one year. Women, the elderly, and those with brain injury are at higher risk.

Standard antipsychotics are often divided into three groups, depending on their potency (the number of milligrams needed for effectiveness). Though this classification scheme cuts across different chemical classes, its usefulness is that drugs of the same potency tend to have the same side effects. Haloperidol and fluphenazine, the two "high-potency" drugs, commonly cause minimal sedation, but have the most muscular side effects. Chlorpromazine and thioridazine, the two "low-potency" drugs, cause the most sedation and low blood pressure. The others are "mid-potency" drugs. They have the potential to cause any of the side effects, but these effects tend to be less severe, especially at low doses.

A number of antipsychotic drugs have been marketed in the last decade. These "atypical" antipsychotics exert effects on neurotransmitters other than dopamine, which may account for several differences from standard antipsychotics. First, they cause fewer muscular side effects. Second, there is a much lower rate of tardive dyskinesia. Finally, some people find them more effective than standard antipsychotics. Atypical antipsychotics must also be taken every day. A single nightly dose is usually sufficient. They are much more expensive than the older drugs.

All atypical antipsychotics are associated with a higher risk of strokes and sudden death in people over sixty-five with dementia. They also can cause substantial weight gain (an increase of 10 to 20% of your current body weight in the first couple of months), diabetes, and elevations of cholesterol or triglycerides (another form of fat in the blood). People with a family history of diabetes are at a higher risk for developing these complications. These serious complications are associated with high blood pressure, heart attacks, strokes, and gallbladder problems. It's not clear if high doses are more likely to cause these problems than low doses. It's not clear if atypical antipsychotics cause these changes in metabolism directly or whether the changes result from weight gain. In either case, it is important to monitor your weight and be tested regularly for the presence of high cholesterol and diabetes. Careful dieting and exercise can minimize weight gain and even permit weight loss in people who have gained weight.

There are significant differences among atypical antipsychotics. Aripiprazole appears to be the least likely to cause weight gain, high cholesterol, and diabetes. However, approximately 25 percent of people who take it experience agitation, insomnia, and a worsening of their symptoms. Ziprasidone is the most likely of the atypical antipsychotics to cause an abnormal heart condition called QTc prolongation (see chapter 19). This condition is infrequent, even with ziprasidone (less than 1%), but is potentially serious. Ziprasidone must be taken twice a day because the body metabolizes it quickly. This is a problem if you have difficulty taking medication regularly. It should be taken with meals to enhance absorption by the intestines—taken without food causes roughly 50 percent less absorption. Risperidone tends to cause stiffness and restlessness at dosages above 6 mg a day. Although many people improve on doses lower than 6 mg a day, many people need more. Quetiapine causes pronounced sedation. Olanzapine appears to cause the most pronounced weight gain and problems with cholesterol and diabetes.

Benzodiazepines   Named for their chemical structure, benzodiazepines are frequently used for the acute symptoms of anxiety because they are very effective and work within an hour. They can be used intermittently, an attribute that some people find attractive.

Immediate side effects include sedation, poor physical coordination, and impairment of memory and cognition. Daily use for months can dull emotions and contribute to depression. They are also habit-forming. If used daily for more than four weeks, people can experience rebound anxiety when a dose wears off as part of a withdrawal syndrome. This can lead to recurrent symptoms of anxiety.

Because of the memory impairment, cognitive difficulties, and the problems associated with rebound anxiety, benzodiazepines are best used for brief periods (less than four weeks) until other supportive measures can be instituted.

Buspirone   Used for anxiety, buspirone takes two to four weeks to work, so it is not useful in an acute situation. It avoids the problems of the benzodiazepines if something is needed for an extended basis. Only some people with anxiety derive benefit from buspirone.

Antidepressants   It can be hard to differentiate depression and dementia because of the overlap of symptoms. Depression may be experienced early in the illness. It may be due to some awareness over the gravity of the situation, but it may also be due to the illness itself. It is definitely worth treating this with antidepressants (see chapter 9). They may not change the course of the illness but may enhance one's quality of life. Doses should start as low as possible to minimize side effects and any further impairment of cognitive functioning.

PART IV

How to Use Medications

CHAPTER 16

How to Start, Monitor, and Stop Your Medication

Most of us have developed an approach that helps us negotiate the demands of life. This personal philosophy may be centered in religious beliefs or cultural practices. Some people focus their daily lives on moral values or financial concerns. Terrible experiences in life may direct people toward choices that allow them to avoid the feelings that arose in response to those experiences. Some people guide their lives by a wish to maintain their individuality, autonomy, and personal freedom. Some people express all their feelings no matter what the consequences, while others exert tremendous effort to hide the same feelings. Most of us have a variety of beliefs that shape the day-to-day decisions we make in our life. These beliefs may be somewhat contradictory, but we are usually able to resolve the contradictions.

Your Approach to Medication

Your beliefs will play a significant role in your willingness to seek psychiatric treatment and pursue different forms of treatment, particularly medication. Whatever your personality and beliefs, the ingestion of medication will have a particular meaning to you. It is important to identify what that meaning is, so that you approach medications most sensibly.

Use Medication as an Aid   Medications are best used on a strictly pragmatic basis: they can help you to run your life more satisfactorily. While there is no compelling evidence that they cure any biological abnormality, they can be used to substantially alleviate the symptoms of many illnesses and allow you to function better.

Don't Give Medication More Power Than It Warrants   There are several approaches to psychiatric medications that will not serve you well because they attribute power to medication that it simply does not have. Followed blindly, these approaches can cause you harm because you won't get the benefit you are looking for. Instead, you may waste your time and money and neglect forms of treatment that could be beneficial.

Using Medication to Fix an Illness   Don't take medication primarily because it seems like a cure for your "illness." Depression and panic attacks may or may not be helped by medication, but they will not be "cured" even if you take medication. Your symptoms of schizophrenia or bipolar disorder will improve on medication, but they will not go away. You can enhance your life immeasurably if you engage in psychotherapy, social skills training, and vocational training to aid your recovery.

Using Medication to Fill an Inner Incompleteness   Medication will not "fill up" an emptiness or incompleteness you feel inside. Searching for a drug that will compensate a sense of inner incompleteness can be urgent and long-lasting, but is generally self-destructive and futile. I have seen many people insist on taking medication after medication of dubious benefit in an attempt to fix something that medication simply cannot fix. Although this inner feeling of incompleteness can lead people to be anxious or depressed, and medications can help the anxiety and depression, this inner hunger is not resolved through the use of medication.

If you suffer from chronic feelings of incompleteness and emptiness, try to address the inner dissatisfaction in ways that are likely to be successful. Develop relationships with other people in the world instead. Engage in work, religion, and leisure activities to give you satisfaction and meaning.

Avoiding Medication to Avoid Shame   You may avoid medication because you don't want to admit to yourself that you are having a problem. This is putting the cart before the horse, however. Medication doesn't change the reality of whether you have a problem, just what you are going to do about it. It may be reasonable to manage your difficulties with methods other than medication, but it shouldn't change your assessment of what is going on.

Avoiding Medication to Preserve Autonomy   You may not want to "become dependent" on medication. Although some medications are habit-forming and many have withdrawal symptoms if you stop them abruptly after prolonged use, a fear of dependency can be detrimental when carried too far.

For example, many people in their teens and early twenties dislike medication, contact with the medical profession, or any authority that they perceive as controlling. Although this is a common stance among young adults, the refusal to take medication can have devastating consequences for those with schizophrenia. Not only are their psychotic symptoms more intense and terrifying to them, but their ability to function in life, form relationships, work, and develop a satisfying life for themselves becomes significantly impaired.

If you see medication primarily as a threat to your autonomy and your individuality, try to be honest with yourself about whether the medication might help you to further your individuality in constructive and productive ways. Many people with long-standing psychiatric problems such as depression, schizophrenia, and bipolar disorder find that they are more capable of leading an energized and enthusiastic life when they take medication.

Establish a Good Relationship with Your Psychiatrist   No matter what medication you use, it is important that you have a good working relationship with your psychiatrist. Ideally you will feel that your psychiatrist understands you, cares about you, and has your best interests in mind. The fact that there may be some areas of disagreement doesn't mean that you can't work effectively with someone, as long as you can keep those areas of disagreement from sabotaging the relationship.

If you have decided that you want to try medication, it is important that you use the medication sensibly and to your best advantage. Although there are many psychiatric problems and many different medications used to treat them, sensible use is guided by a number of principles that can enable you to get the most out of the medication.

Preliminary Guidelines

Pregnancy and Breastfeeding   You need to be careful about the use of psychiatric medications if you are pregnant or breastfeeding. If you are unsure whether or not you are pregnant it is important to get a pregnancy test prior to beginning any psychiatric medications. Neither pregnancy nor breastfeeding precludes medications, but they must be used with extra caution. This is discussed in more detail in chapter 4.

Driving or Operating Heavy Machinery   Your ability to operate a car or heavy machinery can be impaired by the use of some psychiatric medications. Psychiatric medications can cloud judgment, impair muscular coordination, and make you dizzy by lowering your blood pressure. Make sure you know how you react to any medication before you drive or operate machinery.

Interaction with Other Medications   Discuss *all* medications that you take on even the most casual basis with your doctor, including vitamins, dietary supplements, herbal remedies, and over-the-counter medications. For example, ibuprofen and other anti-inflammatory agents can cause you to become toxic on lithium on even a single dose. Many antihypertensives have the potential to worsen depression. St. John's wort can cause toxic symptoms when combined with some antidepressants. Know what medications you can and cannot take with whatever psychiatric medication you have decided to try (described in part IV).

Caffeine   It may surprise you to learn that caffeine can have a negative impact on many psychiatric problems, but it does! It worsens the symptoms of anxiety, manic thinking and behavior, psychotic thinking, and insomnia. It impairs the sleep of people who are depressed and lowers their energy and mood when the buzz wears off. The effects are mild but can appreciably affect how you feel.

You may experience some withdrawal symptoms when you cut down or stop your caffeine use. Headaches and fatigue are the two most common effects.

You will feel more alert and energetic once you have stopped your caffeine use for some weeks. You will sleep better. You will be calmer and less irritable. If you are considering medication for symptoms that trouble you, you will function better and perhaps need a lower dose if you are able to stop your caffeine use.

Stopping your caffeine use may require a change in your lifestyle. If you use coffee to wake up in the morning, you may need to give yourself a little extra time to get going. If you enjoy having a mug of something to sip all day, you will need to search for other things to enjoy. Many people find herbal teas pleasing.

Alcohol   Besides liver damage, ulcers, heart problems, seizures, and blood problems, alcohol can also exacerbate symptoms of anxiety, depression, and insomnia. Although the euphoria of alcohol can temporarily help you feel better, your distress often returns in a more intense form once the alcohol wears off. This can last some days and is not limited merely to the "morning hangover."

Alcohol causes sedation. When combined with the sedative effects of other drugs, this can lead to marked physical impairment, impaired level of consciousness, and impaired judgment. In combination with benzodiazepines such as Valium, Klonopin, Xanax, or Ativan, it can be especially dangerous. The combination of alcohol and benzodiazepines has caused death in some people and is a not infrequent cause of suicide.

Alcohol can interfere with the effectiveness of some psychiatric drugs by changing the way your body metabolizes them, rendering them ineffective and even potentially dangerous. For example, the regular use of alcohol induces the liver to metabolize alcohol and some other drugs much more rapidly. As a result the usual dose of a psychiatric drug is insufficient. If you compensate by increasing your daily dose of medication but then stop drinking alcohol, you can develop symptoms of drug toxicity from the increased amount of drug in your system.

Regular use of alcohol can overwhelm the benefits derived from psychiatric medications. If you regularly ingest alcohol and find that antidepressants are ineffective for you, it may be that the alcohol itself is impairing the effectiveness of the antidepressants. Many people find that their medication is much more effective when they achieve and maintain sobriety.

Alcohol use prevents an accurate assessment of the effectiveness of whatever medication you are taking. For example, if you take an antidepressant and find that you continue to be depressed, it is difficult to know whether this is due to the alcohol or the ineffectiveness of the antidepressant. Similarly, if you drink alcohol and your anxiety waxes and wanes, it is difficult to know whether the variability in the level of anxiety is due to the ineffectiveness of medication or the brief periods of euphoria from the alcohol alternating with the rebound anxiety when the alcohol wears off.

Most important, alcohol sabotages your willingness and ability to manage your psychological problems in ways that are constructive and effective, and that will lead to long-standing improvement. Alcohol is a most pernicious drug in this regard, because it is so easily available and its effects are so quick. Although it may provide a respite from unpleasant feelings, it is essential that you learn more constructive ways of managing your feelings.

The best way to approach alcohol if you are taking psychiatric medication: *don't use it.*

Recreational Drugs   Recreational drugs can negatively impact your health, any psychiatric problems you experience, and the effectiveness of medication you take. The issues are somewhat different depending on which drugs are involved.

Marijuana   Although the physical effects of marijuana are relatively mild and are generally not dangerous when used with psychiatric medications, the use of marijuana to induce euphoria or relief from psychological distress has the same pernicious effect as alcohol. It sabotages your willingness and ability to engage in other activities that are more constructive for you. Marijuana also prevents an accurate assessment of the effectiveness of any psychiatric drug. It can intensify psychotic thinking in people with psychotic thinking. The only sensible way to use marijuana is the same as alcohol—don't use it at all.

Narcotic Painkillers   Codeine, Darvocet, Darvon, Demerol, Fioricet, Percocet, Talwin, Vicodin, and other opiates are commonly used painkillers. Although occasional use of them is not particularly troublesome, they are habit-forming. Regular use can exacerbate depression and anxiety. Regular use can also impair the effectiveness of psychiatric drugs and impair your ability to assess their effectiveness. If you are taking painkillers for a chronic medical condition, you, your medical doctor, and your psychiatrist need to be in good communication to ensure that your use of pain medication is kept to a minimum in order to avoid exacerbating your psychological symptoms.

Other Drugs   Heroin, cocaine, crack, hallucinogenic drugs such as LSD, mescaline and PCP, and amphetamines such as methedrine (speed) have significant harmful effects on your body. They are dangerous when used by themselves and especially in combination with psychiatric medications. The effects of these powerful drugs virtually overwhelm any noticeable effect from most psychiatric medications and make it impossible to assess the effectiveness of any psychiatric medication.

How to Start Medication

Choose a Medication   After you have decided that you want to try medication, review with your psychiatrist the alternatives for the psychiatric syndrome that best fits your symptoms and choose a medication. Your choice will be affected by the assessment process described in chapter 3, the symptoms themselves, the psychiatric syndrome of which they are a part, and the specific qualities of whatever medication you believe will help you best.

New Medications   Drug companies have realized in the last decade that there is an enormous demand for psychiatric drugs. As a result, they are actively working on many drugs for a wide variety of problems. When they bring out a new drug, they advertise aggressively. However, premarketing trials, performed to satisfy the Food and Drug Administration's requirements to market a new medication, test at most a few thousand people in a highly structured situation. As a result, there are two issues to keep in mind when considering taking a drug that has just been introduced onto the market.

First, the claim for effectiveness is just that—a claim. The effectiveness of any medication cannot be reliably assessed when the only source of information is the company marketing the drug. The company designs the study to make their drug look as good as possible, and there may be subtleties in the design of the study that make the drug look better than it really is. Research by independent investigators is necessary to establish a drug's true value.

Second, the side effects you experience may be different from those advertised by the drug company. Drug company studies estimate the frequency of side effects based upon the self-report of patients in their studies, not by a systematic survey of possible side effects. If patients are unaware of, or too embarrassed to describe, a specific side effect, it will not be noted.

Brand-Name versus Generic Medications   There are no inherent differences between generic and brand-name preparations. Because of differences in the inactive ingredients necessary to place the medication into pill form, there may be slight differences in the total amount that gets absorbed. It is important to maintain the same preparation, however, in order to avoid changes in the amount of medication absorbed.

The exception to this general rule is methylphenidate. Many, though not all, people notice that Ritalin, the brand-name preparation, is more effective than a generic preparation.

Learn about the Medication   There are a number of factors that influence how a medication is handled by the body, including *absorption* in the intestines, *distribution* and storage in the body, *time of onset of action, metabolism, half-life,* and *excretion.* While you don't need to become a psychopharmacologist to benefit from medication, knowing the facts about your medication can help you use it most sensibly.

First, how should you take it so that *absorption* will be most effective? Some drugs need to be taken on an empty stomach. This is not true of most psychiatric medications. Because many psychiatric medications cause mild stomach upset, ingesting these medications with food helps you tolerate the medication more easily.

Second, how long does the medication take to work? The *time to onset of action* varies tremendously. Methylphenidate and lorazepam can begin to work within thirty to sixty minutes, lithium may take one to two weeks, and fluoxetine, paroxetine, and imipramine may take many weeks. Knowing when to expect the onset of action can help you to be realistic about when you can expect to feel better, allowing you to coordinate other treatments sensibly.

Third, how long does the medication treat your symptoms? The *duration of action* also varies widely. Antiparkinsonian agents, antihistamines, benzodiazepines, and beta-blockers treat symptoms directly. You will feel the effectiveness wane as the dose wears off, though different drugs last different amounts of times. For example, alprazolam may help your anxiety for only a couple of hours, but an injection of haloperidol decanoate can be effective for psychotic symptoms for many weeks. Methylphenidate may last for only two to four hours, while the same amount of the sustained-release preparation lasts twice as long. Mood stabilizers and antidepressants work only if taken consistently, and you will not notice when a single dose wears off.

The duration of action is affected by the rate of absorption, the time to onset of action, the half-life, where the drug is stored in your body, and its specific chemical effects. Drugs that are highly fat-soluble are widely distributed in your fat tissue and may take a long time to be metabolized. As a result, the duration of action may be most pronounced in the first few hours, but some effects may linger for days and weeks.

Fourth, how long does the drug last in your body? Drugs are *metabolized,* broken down into smaller parts, so that they can be excreted by the body. Because of the complex process involved in metabolizing any drug, the time a drug lasts in your body is measured by its *half-life.* The half-life is the amount of time required for your body to break down 50 percent of the drug in your body. The half-life remains constant no matter how much of the medication is in your body. Thus, if the half-life of a drug is twenty-four hours, 50 percent of the drug will be left after one day if no more doses are taken, 25 percent after two days, 12.5 percent after three days, and so on. After six half-lives more than 98 percent will be gone.

The level of a drug in your body will obviously increase if you take a dose before the previous dose has been metabolized. A "steady state" level in your body, such that the amount ingested equals the amount excreted, is generally reached after six half-lives with steady dosing.

Some drugs, like methylphenidate and lorazepam, have a short half-life. As a result, their effects are relatively transitory, and effective treatment may require several daily doses. Other drugs, like sertraline and risperidone, have much longer half-lives, and once-daily dosing is sufficient.

Some psychiatric drugs are metabolized into chemicals that also have potent psychological effects. For example, amitriptylene is broken down into nortriptyline. Nortriptyline also has antidepressant effects and is marketed on its own as Pamelor. These breakdown products are also metabolized by the body into further breakdown products and have their own half-lives. For example, flurazepam has a half-life of only two to three hours, but its breakdown product, N-desalkylflurazepam, has a half-life of more than fifty hours. This is why many people notice a hangover after several days of flurazepam use.

Surprisingly, nicotine from smoking affects the metabolism of many drugs. Drug levels can be higher or lower, depending on which drug it is. If you start or stop smoking while taking a psychiatric drug, you may notice reduced effectiveness or more pronounced side effects.

Some medications are metabolized more quickly by your body if you stay on them for an extended time. For example, the half-life of carbamazepine, a mood stabilizer used for bipolar disorder, is 25–65 hours initially, but with steady use it decreases to 12–17 hours. Obtaining a blood level once you've been on it can ensure that the dose you are on is therapeutic.

The effect of medication may last long after the disappearance of the medication from the body. For example, lithium is generally gone from the body after a few days, but a return of symptoms may not occur for one to two weeks. This is probably because it takes this long for the brain to return to the state it was in without lithium.

Identify Target Symptoms   It is important not to confuse the effects of medication on a psychiatric syndrome with the effects on the *target symptoms*. Most psychiatric syndromes are a constellation of thoughts, emotions, physical sensations, and behaviors that wax and wane over time in a complex fashion. No medication cures a psychiatric syndrome, but it can minimize some of the distressing symptoms of some of the disorder. For example, many people with depression have insomnia, tearfulness, poor energy, and feelings of hopelessness. Medication may help you sleep better, stop crying, and give you the energy to get out of bed, but only you can make your life improve to the point where you feel good about it.

Identify which target symptoms you are attempting to treat. The target symptom does not have to be a single symptom. Often one looks at a number of symptoms that are part of the psychiatric syndrome that one hopes will improve on medication. For example, mood stabilizers for the manic phase of the bipolar disorder commonly improve and slow down a person's thoughts, decrease the amount and rapidity of speech, normalize a person's euphoric or irritable mood, and decrease their hyperactivity. All of these would be considered part of the target symptom complex.

Develop a Sensible Dosing Regimen   The dosing regimen that you arrive at should take into consideration how quickly the drug takes effect and how quickly it is metabolized by the body. It is best to try to simplify your drug regimen in order to make it easier for you to take it regularly. Although many psychiatric drugs are prescribed numerous times a day in the hospital, because the drugs are more easily tolerated in smaller doses when they first are begun and because the nursing staff is available to administer them at the correct times, complicated dosing regimens are often impractical outside the hospital.

Avoid Polypharmacy   Polypharmacy is the simultaneous use of two or more psychiatric medications. Although it can be reasonable to take different psychiatric medications simultaneously, it is important to be sensible about their use. For example, different antipsychotic medications used to treat delusions and hallucinations have very different pharmacological and physical effects, and many people with schizophrenia take more than one in order to gain more benefit than they would get from either one alone. On the other hand, benzodiazepines all have about the same effects, so using two different ones makes little sense.

With so many drugs on the market, and more drugs that work in different ways due to come out over the next few years, different combinations may be sensible in the future. Balancing safety, reason, and a desire for help should lead you to be creative, but reasonable.

Coordinate Medications with Other Treatments   It is important to coordinate the use of medication with other treatments such as psychotherapy, behavior plans, or hospitalization. For example, it makes little sense to talk about anxiety-provoking issues if you are overwhelmed with anxiety. You will probably find it more helpful to first get the symptoms of anxiety under control with medication. Many children and adults with attention deficit disorder find behavioral interventions quite effective for some of their difficulties. It may be useful to first try either behavioral treatments or the medication, but not both simultaneously. By starting with one and then adding the second, you can be clear about the effectiveness of each treatment.

How to Monitor Your Progress

The use of psychiatric medications requires careful evaluation to ensure their effectiveness and safety. Always arrange a follow-up appointment with your doctor to go over your response to the medication. There are many issues to consider.

Evaluate Effectiveness   Obviously the most important issue is whether the medication improves the target symptoms. Although it is certainly valid to believe that a medication makes you "feel better," it can be enlightening to know exactly how. You may find it only improves one or two symptoms, or you may find them all better. For example, you may feel that lorazepam helps you feel less anxious and that you no longer have panic attacks. However, since the effect of lorazepam wears off after a few hours, you will soon feel anxious and need another pill. If you think you are "better," you are probably only focusing on one aspect of your experience, the time when the medication is working, and neglecting the periods of rising anxiety that lead you to take another pill.

Observe Physical and Psychological Changes   It is important to notice all the various effects the medication has on you. If you notice any difficulties when you are taking medication in regards to your thoughts, feelings, behaviors or physical condition, it is important to bring this up with your doctor so that it can be addressed as effectively as possible. For example, antidepressants such as fluoxetine, paroxetine, and sertraline often cause significant sexual dysfunction. Even if your physician doesn't ask about it, bring it up so that you can discuss how you might handle it.

Changes in your condition will affect your relationship with your family, friends and, most especially, your partner. Ideally, these will be positive changes that will enhance your relationships. Sometimes however, these changes can require unforeseen adjustments. For example, if sildenafil (Viagra) improves your sexual functioning, the change may be disconcerting to someone who has grown accustomed to your previous level of sexual interest. If fluoxetine has improved your anxiety and depression to the point that you want to start working, your partner's role as provider or caregiver may no longer be the same. This may lead to distress if your partner felt satisfaction with your previous level of functioning. Make sure you communicate with your partner and family about the changes you notice and how those changes may affect your relationship with them.

Complete a Full Trial   You need to give any drug a full trial before deciding whether it is going to be effective for you. This means that you need to take it at an adequate dose for an adequate period of time to produce a therapeutic response. The dosage size and time period for each drug is different, so there is not a uniform standard as to what constitutes an adequate trial. If you stop before you've finished a complete trial, you gain little information about your response to that drug. I have seen countless people switch drugs prematurely, only to go back to the first drug when subsequent ones were ineffective, resulting in needless distress from symptoms because of the time delay.

Use Blood Levels as Servants, Not Masters   Lithium, valproate, and many antidepressants and antipsychotics can be measured in the blood. Although therapeutic ranges for effective doses have been proposed, many people respond to levels that are above or below the supposedly "therapeutic" range. It is important to use blood levels as a guide to treatment, but not to believe them so blindly that you ignore the most important aspect of any drug treatment: how *you* are doing.

There are times when a blood level is important. First, it can ensure that your dosage is not so high as to be dangerous. For example, imipramine and amitriptyline can cause cardiac arrhythmias when the blood level gets too high in the absence of any physical symptoms that might alert you to any problems. Second, a blood level can provide useful information if a drug appears to be ineffective at the maximum recommended dose. If it turns out that the level is too low, it may make sense to proceed beyond the usual upper limit of dosing size to ensure that you get an adequate trial. Third, blood levels can be essential when you are adding or removing another psychiatric or medical drug that interacts with your psychiatric medication. For example, fluoxetine, paroxetine, and fluvoxamine can raise the level of other antidepressants and antipsychotics in the blood to dangerous levels. A blood level check can guide you to the appropriate dose of the other medication after you add one of these medications.

Monitor Side Effects   *All* medications have side effects. Aspirin can cause ulcers. It can even cause severe brain damage in infants when ingested during the course of a viral illness. Acetaminophen can cause liver damage. Amoxicillin, the most common antibiotic given to ward off ear infections, can cause allergic reactions that are potentially fatal. There is no way to introduce a chemical into the body that induces only the alteration that helps you. They all cause other changes that may result in side effects.

You should be aware of the common side effects. It is important to know how the more dangerous ones might manifest themselves so that you can alert your doctor right away. For example, some medications can impair your bone marrow's ability to make blood cells. This can result in an infection, anemia, or problems with clotting, problems that are potentially life-threatening. If you take a medication such as this, you should be on the lookout for easy bruisability or sores on the mouth, so that you and your doctor can be alert to the possibility that you are experiencing an unusual but potentially dangerous side effect as soon as possible. (Side effects are listed in part IV.)

Second, you should know what you can do about any side effects that do occur. Some side effects occur only when you first start a drug, while others are long-lasting. Know which is which. You need to alert your prescribing practitioner if you are experiencing any dangerous side effect. Many of the more common side effects, however, can be anticipated so that you can manage them when they arise. (Methods to minimize different side effects are discussed in part IV.)

How to Stop Medication

Issues to Consider in Stopping Medication   You will want to stop taking the medication if it has not been effective for you. Even if it has been effective for you, however, the question still arises: how long do you need to stay on it? There are three issues you need to consider in making the decision about whether or not to stop medication.

The Nature of the Disorder   Different psychiatric disorders require treatment for different periods of time. Crises such as distress over the loss of a loved one may require short-term use of medication, whereas an ongoing illness such as schizophrenia or bipolar disorder may require medication indefinitely. Some people with depression may stop medication without difficulty once the life circumstances that led to the depression have resolved. Others find that they get more depressed when they go off their medication and elect to stay on them for many years.

The Positive and Negative Effects of the Medication   You must weigh the effectiveness of the medication against the side effects you experience. Weight gain from imipramine and the need to diet may be unpleasant, but the diminished anxiety and depression may be worth the price. The potential for a life-threatening blood disorder may seem terrible, but that may be better than being stuck in a hospital overwhelmed by hallucinations and delusions. On the other hand, the sexual dysfunction caused by fluoxetine may be enough to dissuade you from its use even though you feel somewhat better on it. Methylphenidate may help your son's disruptiveness in school, but his headaches, stomach cramps, and the potential for stunted growth may override any benefits you see.

The Effectiveness of Other Treatments   You need to judge the effectiveness of alternative treatments. Are there other treatments that would allow you to get off the medication at some point? For example, panic attacks often resolve with a combination of brief psychotherapy, relaxation exercises, and lifestyle changes. While taking medication during the first few weeks after they've started may provide enormous relief, taking them for many years without even trying these treatments makes little sense.

Drug Holidays   There are times when it makes sense to stop the medications on a regular basis for brief periods. For example, some children with ADHD take methylphenidate only on school days, not on weekends or during vacation. This minimizes the retarding effect methylphenidate can have on growth. Some people find that omitting one or two doses of their antidepressant improves the impairment the drug causes to their sexual functioning. A drug holiday needs to take the above issues into account, however, and should never be undertaken without consulting with your doctor.

Steps to Stop Your Medication   There are four things to do if you decide to stop your medication.

Consult with Your Doctor   It is vital to consult your doctor. You will cause yourself needless distress if you don't learn about the effects you may experience when you stop the medication. Use the benefit of your doctor's training and experience with other people who have stopped their medication to help you go through the process.

Educate Yourself about What to Expect   First, you may experience transitory physical and psychological changes that are primarily due to the withdrawal of the drug. As long as you are aware of these, they should not cause you to doubt the wisdom of your decision to stop, though they may be unpleasant. You may also experience a reemergence of the symptoms that led you to go on the medication in the first place. If this occurs, you will need to reconsider your decision to stop, reevaluating the nature of your disorder, the positive and negative effects of medication, and the usefulness of other treatments.

Taper Gradually   You need to take into account the physical effects of withdrawal and the psychological changes you will experience. For example, benzodiazepines and antidepressants cause a variety of physical and emotional changes. These changes are far more easily tolerated when there has been a small decrease in the total amount you are taking rather than a complete cessation. Make sure your body has adapted to one change before you undertake another. In the case of some antidepressants, this may take months.

Monitor All Changes   You should expect physical and psychological changes as you taper your medications. Ideally these will be transitory, but you will feel confident that this is the case only if you've educated yourself about what you may experience and if you monitor yourself during the process.

Call your doctor if you notice a change for which you are unprepared. It is much better to address any problems when they first arise, rather than waiting until they've gotten significantly worse. Err on the side of a phone call that may turn out to be unnecessary rather than waiting until a problem arises that overwhelms you.

CHAPTER 17

The Medications

All drugs used as treatments for a disorder are described here. The focus is on information that will be useful as you consider or use a drug. The information is derived from the manufacturer's prescribing information (listed in the *Physician's Desk Reference* and enclosed with all prescriptions), psychopharmacology textbooks, journal articles, consultation with colleagues, and my own clinical experience. The drugs are listed in alphabetical order by their generic names.

General information lists the brand-name preparation. The **class** of a medication refers to the shorthand label applied to other drugs that are similar in chemical structure, pharmacological action, or the uses to which they are put. Conditions **used in** includes psychiatric conditions, not other medical problems. The primary uses of the drug are listed first. These are the conditions for which the drug is commonly employed and exerts a substantial clinical effect. The secondary conditions for which a drug is used are listed in parentheses. These are conditions in which the drug is used infrequently because it is minimally effective, either because others of its class are more effective, or because the severity of side effects makes it a less than desirable first choice. The **mechanism of action** is a description of the known effect in the brain. The therapeutic benefit of a drug is assumed to be due to this action, but how this action causes cognitive and emotional changes is unclear for all psychiatric drugs.

Precautions are issues you should be aware of *before* you start any drug. Liver disease can impair the metabolism of any drug, and kidney disease can impair its excretion. Use extra caution with dosing if you have any impairment of your liver or kidney to avoid pronounced or prolonged effect. There are no studies establishing the safety of *any drug* during *pregnancy* or *breastfeeding*. Specific birth defects associated with a particular drug will be noted, but the absence of any specific defect doesn't mean that the drug is safe—merely that nothing harmful has been linked to the drug. Almost all drugs are passed in the breast milk, so you should refrain from breastfeeding if you take any drug until you discuss it with your pediatrician and psychiatrist. Always notify your physician if you are pregnant, are considering pregnancy, or are breastfeeding. Use extra caution if you are over sixty-five, as you may be more sensitive than younger people to the effects of medication.

Drug interactions can occur in different ways that affect you adversely. Some occur because the effects of the two drugs are additive and potentially dangerous, such as pronounced sedation from the combination of benzodiazepines and sedating antidepressants. These interactions will be noted. Another occurs when a second drug is added to one you are already taking. Either drug may affect the rate of metabolic breakdown of the other, leading you to experience more side effects or decreased effectiveness of either drug. This second type of interaction is complex and beyond the scope of this book. You should *always* inform your physician of any prescription drug you take, to ensure that interactions won't harm you.

Dosing is given in milligrams (mg), or milligrams per kilogram of body weight (mg/kg). The safety and effectiveness for most psychiatric drugs have not been established for children (those under 18). Nevertheless, there is increasing use of drugs in children. The dosages listed for children are either approved by the FDA or commonly employed by child psychiatrists. Specific dosages for the elderly (those over 65) are not noted unless there is a recommendation by the manufacturer for this age group. In general, lower doses should be used (see chapter 4). Almost all psychiatric drugs can cause some mild stomach upset. It is generally relieved by taking the pills with food. This may slow the rate of absorption, which may make stimulants less effective, but rarely alters the effectiveness of other drugs.

Monitoring your use describes a number of useful facts about the medication. **Half-lives** vary from one individual to another because of differences in how drugs are metabolized in the liver. Some drugs are broken down into *active metabolites* that are also effective in treating symptoms.

Side effects are listed by their frequency of occurrence. Those listed are most common or are known to be associated with a particular drug. Many side effects listed by a drug's manufacturer in the package insert or in the *Physician's Desk Reference* are not listed here because they are uncommon or the connection between the side effect and the drug has not been established. Consult your physician if you experience anything which concerns you, whether or not it is listed here. It is wise to remember that *any drug can cause any side effect.*

What to expect when you stop a medication needs to be considered before you stop your use. Abrupt cessation may cause a rapid return of symptoms and can sometimes lead to serious medical complications. These complications are noted here. Never stop medication without consulting your psychiatrist to ensure that your decision to stop and the tapering schedule you choose won't cause you harm.

Generic Name/Brand Name

The generic name of a drug is derived from its chemical structure. Pharmaceutical companies who produce a drug often give it a unique brand name in order to generate recognition and loyalty to their product.

The use of two names for the same drug can generate confusion. For reference, all the drugs described in this book are listed alphabetically by generic *and* brand name. Next to each name is the corresponding brand name or generic name. Generic names are in lowercase and brand names are capitalized and set in italics. A full description of each drug appears in this chapter under the generic name.

Abilify	aripiprazole
acamprosate	*Campral*
Adderall	combination of amphetamine and dextroamphetamine
Akineton	biperiden
alprazolam	*Xanax*
amantadine	*Symmetrel*
Ambien	zolpidem
amitriptyline	*Elavil*
amoxapine	*Asendin*
Anafranil	clomipramine
Antabuse	disulfiram
Aricept	donepezil
aripiprazole	*Abilify*
Artane	trihexyphenidyl
Asendin	amoxapine
Atarax	hydroxyzine
Ativan	lorazepam
atomoxetine	*Strattera*
Aventyl	nortriptyline
Benadryl	diphenhydramine
benztropine	*Cogentin*
biperiden	*Akineton*
Buprenex	buprenorphine
buprenorphine	*Buprenex, Suboxone, Subutex*
bupropion	*Wellbutrin, Zyban*
Buspar	buspirone
buspirone	*Buspar*
Campral	acamprosate
carbamazepine	*Tegretol*
Catapres	clonidine
Celexa	citalopram
chlordiazepoxide	*Librium*
chlorpromazine	*Thorazine*
Cialis	tadalafil
citalopram	*Celexa*
clomipramine	*Anafranil*
clonazepam	*Klonopin*
clonidine	*Catapres*

clorazepate	*Tranxene*
clozapine	*Clozaril, Fazaclo*
Clozaril	clozapine
Cogentin	benztropine
Cognex	tacrine
Concerta	methylphenidate
Corgard	nadolol
Cylert	pemoline
Cymbalta	duloxetine
cyproheptadine	*Periactin*
Dalmane	flurazepam
Depade	naltrexone
Depakene	valproate
Depakote	valproate
desipramine	*Norpramin*
Desoxyn Gradumet	methamphetamine
Desyrel	trazodone
Dexedrine	dextroamphetamine
dextroamphetamine	*Dexedrine*
diazepam	*Valium*
diphenhydramine	*Benadryl*
disulfiram	*Antabuse*
Dolophine	methadone
donepezil	*Aricept*
Doral	quazepam
doxepin	*Sinequan*
duloxetine	*Cymbalta*
Effexor	venlafaxine
Elavil	amitriptyline
Eldepryl	selegiline
escitalopram	*Lexapro*
Eskalith	lithium
estazolam	*Prosom*
eszopiclone	*Lunesta*
Exelon	rivastigmine
Fazaclo	clozapine
fluoxetine	*Prozac, Sarafem, Symbyax*
fluphenazine	*Prolixin*
flurazepam	*Dalmane*
fluvoxamine	*Luvox*
Focalin	methylphenidate
gabapentin	*Neurontin*
galantamine	*Reminyl*

Geodon	ziprasidone
guanfacine	*Tenex*
Halcion	triazolam
Haldol	haloperidol
haloperidol	*Haldol*
hydroxyzine	*Atarax, Vistaril*
imipramine	*Tofranil*
Inderal	propranolol
isocarboxazid	*Marplan*
Kemadrin	procyclidine
Klonopin	clonazepam
Lamictal	lamotrigine
lamotrigine	*Lamictal*
Lexapro	escitalopram
Levitra	vardenafil
Librium	chlordiazepoxide
lithium	*Eskalith, Lithobid, Lithonate*
Lithobid	lithium
Lithonate	lithium
lorazepam	*Ativan*
loxapine	*Loxitane*
Loxitane	loxapine
Ludiomil	maprotiline
Lunesta	eszopiclone
Luvox	fluvoxamine
maprotiline	*Ludiomil*
Marplan	isocarboxazid
Mellaril	thioridazine
mesoridazine	*Serentil*
Metadate	methylphenidate
methadone	*Dolophine*
methamphetamine	*Desoxyn Gradumet*
methylphenidate	*Concerta, Focalin, Metadate, Ritalin*
mirtazapine	*Remeron*
Moban	molindone
molindone	*Moban*
nadolol	*Corgard*
naltrexone	*Depade, Revia, Trexan*
Nardil	phenelzine
Navane	thiothixene
nefazodone	*Serzone*
Neurontin	gabapentin
Norpramin	desipramine

nortriptyline	*Aventyl, Pamelor*
olanzapine	*Symbyax, Zyprexa, Zyprexa Zydis*
Orap	pimozide
oxazepam	*Serax*
oxcarbazepine	*Trileptal*
Pamelor	nortriptyline
Parnate	tranylcypromine
paroxetine	*Paxil*
Paxil	paroxetine
pemoline	*Cylert*
Periactin	cyproheptadine
perphenazine	*Trilafon*
phenelzine	*Nardil*
pimozide	*Orap*
procyclidine	*Kemadrin*
Prolixin	fluphenazine
propranolol	*Inderal*
Prosom	estazolam
protriptyline	*Vivactil*
Prozac	fluoxetine
quazepam	*Doral*
quetiapine	*Seroquel*
ramelteon	*Rozerem*
Remeron	mirtazapine
Reminyl	galantamine
Restoril	temazepam
ReVia	naltrexone
Risperdal (Consta and M-tabs)	risperidone
risperidone	*Risperdal (Consta and M-tabs)*
Ritalin	methylphenidate
rivastigmine	*Exelon*
Rozerem	ramelteon
selegiline	*Eldepryl*
Serax	oxazepam
Serentil	mesoridazine
Seroquel	quetiapine
sertraline	*Zoloft*
Serzone	nefazodone
sildenafil	*Viagra*
Sinequan	doxepin
Sonata	zaleplon
Stelazine	trifluoperazine
Strattera	atomoxetine

Suboxone	buprenorphine and naloxone
Subutex	buprenorphine
Surmontil	trimipramine
Symbyax	fluoxetine and olanzapine
Symmetrel	amantadine
tacrine	*Cognex*
tadalafil	*Cialis*
Tegretol	carbamazepine
temazepam	*Restoril*
Tenex	guanfacine
thioridazine	*Mellaril*
thiothixene	*Navane*
Thorazine	chlorpromazine
Tofranil	imipramine
Topamax	topiramate
topiramate	*Topamax*
Tranxene	clorazepate
tranylcypromine	*Parnate*
trazodone	*Desyrel*
Trexan	naltrexone
triazolam	*Halcion*
trifluoperazine	*Stelazine*
trihexyphenidyl	*Artane*
Trilafon	perphenazine
Trileptal	oxcarbazepine
trimipramine	*Surmontil*
Valium	diazepam
valproate	*Depakene, Depakote*
vardenafil	*Levitra*
venlafaxine	*Effexor*
Viagra	sildenafil
Vistaril	hydroxyzine
Vivactil	protriptyline
Wellbutrin	bupropion
Xanax	alprazolam
Yocon	yohimbine
yohimbine	*Yocon*
zaleplon	*Sonata*
ziprasidone	*Geodon*
Zoloft	sertraline
zolpidem	*Ambien*
Zyban	bupropion
Zyprexa (Zydis)	olanzapine

Acamprosate

GENERAL   **Preparations:** Brand name Campral only in pills. **Class:** Alcohol deterrent. **Used in:** Alcohol dependence. **Mechanism of action:** Interacts with glutamate and GABA receptors.

PRECAUTIONS   **Warning:** Some people taking acamprosate have experienced suicidal thoughts and behavior; the reason for this is unclear, and may be related to prior alcohol use and/or depression. **Use extra caution if you have:** *Kidney* problems, as lower acamprosate dosages may be needed. **Tests before starting:** None. **Alcohol:** Should be avoided, but the simultaneous use of both is not medically dangerous.

DRUG INTERACTIONS   No specific precautions are needed with other medications.

DOSING   **Adults:** The starting dose is 666 mg three times daily. **Children:** Not FDA-approved for under 18.

MONITORING YOUR USE   **Time to effectiveness:** 3–8 hours. **A full trial is:** Determined by its effectiveness in maintaining abstinence. **Half-life of drug and active metabolites:** 20–33 hours with no active metabolites. **How to monitor dosage:** The optimal dose is determined by its effectiveness in maintaining abstinence. **How to monitor safety:** No specific tests are needed. **If you miss a dose:** Take a missed dose if it's within an hour or two. Do not try to make up for a missed dose by doubling your next dose; just continue with your regular dosing schedule.

SIDE EFFECTS   **Less common (1–10%):** Diarrhea. **Those requiring attention by your physician:** Any other physical or emotional changes not described here.

WHAT TO EXPECT IF YOU STOP   You may notice an increase in your desire to drink alcohol. **If stopped abruptly:** There is no acute withdrawal syndrome.

Alprazolam

GENERAL   **Preparations:** Generic, brand name Xanax, and long-acting Xanax XR. **Class:** Benzodiazepine. **Used in:** Anxiety disorders, bipolar disorder (Alzheimer's disease, alcohol withdrawal, antipsychotic-induced akathisia [restlessness], insomnia). **Mechanism of action:** Intensifies the effects of gamma-aminobutyric acid (GABA).

PRECAUTIONS   Warnings: *It is habit-forming.* Alprazolam, like all benzo-diazepines, is physically and psychologically habit-forming. People who have experienced traumatic events in their lives and have chronic anxiety are especially prone to developing dependence. Prolonged use is associated with a range of problems. Use for more than four weeks is *not* recommended. If you stop alprazolam after more than four weeks of daily use, you will probably experience withdrawal symptoms (see below). *Seizures can occur if it is stopped abruptly,* so consultation with your physician is essential if you wish to stop. **Tests needed before starting:** None. **Alcohol:** Alcohol must be avoided entirely. The simultaneous use of alprazolam and alcohol is extremely dangerous because it can cause you to stop breathing. The combination can cause death. **Use in pregnancy:** There is a higher rate of babies born with a cleft palate to mothers who took benzodiazepines during pregnancy. **The elderly** are especially sensitive to the effects of benzodiazepines and may experience pronounced side effects at low doses (see chapter 4).

DRUG INTERACTIONS   Use with extra caution and notify your physician if you take: *Anticonvulsants, antidepressants, antihistamines, antipsychotics, barbiturates,* or any drug that causes sedation or central nervous system depression, because the combination can cause pronounced sedation. **Use extra caution if you take:** *Erythromycin, fluoxetine (Prozac), fluvoxamine (Luvox), itraconazole, ketoconazole, or nefazodone (Serzone)*, as they increase alprazolam blood levels; *carbamazepine,* as it may decrease alprazolam blood levels.

DOSING   Adults: The usual starting dose is 0.25–1.0 mg three times a day, depending on the severity of the symptoms. Increases of 0.5 mg/day can occur every few days, up to a maximum dose of 4 mg/day. **Dosing of Xanax XR:** Once-daily dosing of 3 to 6 mg in the morning, although some individuals may require 10 mg a day to achieve a successful response. **Children:** Not FDA-approved for under 18.

MONITORING YOUR USE   Time to effectiveness: 15–30 minutes. **A full trial is:** A few doses, which are generally enough to establish whether it will be helpful. **Half-life of drug and active metabolites:** 6–26 hours with active metabolites. **How to monitor dosage:** The optimal dose is determined by its effectiveness in alleviating the target symptoms. **If you miss a dose:** Do *not* try to make up for a missed dose, just continue with your regular dosing schedule. **How to monitor safety:** No specific medical tests are needed to monitor safety.

SIDE EFFECTS   Common (10–50%): Sedation, memory impairment, poor muscle coordination (causing a higher rate of falls in the elderly and a higher risk of motor vehicle accidents in all adults). **Infrequent (less than 1%):** Paradoxical agitation and insomnia. **Those requiring attention from your physician:** Any physical or emotional changes not described here. **Side effects associated with use longer than four weeks:** Use of alprazolam for longer than four weeks may cause physical and psychological dependence, and you may notice the desire for another dose as each one wears off. Ongoing anxiety, reduced effectiveness of each dose, depression, emotional blunting, and impairment of memory and cognition may occur with use longer than one year.

WHAT TO EXPECT WHEN YOU STOP   You may notice a return of your symptoms if alprazolam is tapered gradually. Other withdrawal symptoms include anxiety, insomnia, irritability, headaches, tremors, nausea, diarrhea, sweating, and confusion. The rate at which you should taper it is affected by the duration of your use and the size of your dose, but it may take months if you have been on it for an extended period of time. **If stopped abruptly:** *Seizures* can occur if alprazolam is stopped abruptly. They are potentially life-threatening. You should never stop alprazolam abruptly, and you should always work with your physician to taper it gradually.

Amantadine

GENERAL   **Preparations:** Generic and brand name Symmetrel in pills and liquid. **Class:** Antiparkinsonian agent. **Used in:** The treatment of side effects induced by antipsychotics: akathisia, dystonia, and pseudoparkinsonism (tremor, rigidity, akinesia). **Mechanism of action:** Causes the release of dopamine and norepinephrine from presynaptic neurons. At high doses it also causes the release of serotonin.

PRECAUTIONS   **Use extra caution if you have:** *Congestive heart failure, edema, epilepsy, glaucoma, low blood pressure, prostatic hypertrophy,* or *urinary retention,* as amantadine may worsen the symptoms of the disorder; a *psychotic disorder* that is not being treated with antipsychotic medication, as amantadine may make psychotic symptoms worse. **Tests needed before starting:** None. **Alcohol:** Should be avoided, as the simultaneous use of amantadine and alcohol can lower blood pressure significantly and cause confusion. Also, alcohol worsens anxiety and depression and impairs insight and judgment. **Use in pregnancy:** Infants born to mothers taking amantadine may have an increased risk of heart abnormalities.

DRUG INTERACTIONS   **Do not use if you take:** *Antihypertensives,* as they may combine to lower blood pressure excessively; *antihistamines, phenothiazines,* or *tricyclic antidepressants,* as they may combine to produce pronounced dry mouth, blurry vision, constipation, low blood pressure, rapid heart rate, and even mental confusion.

DOSING   **Adults:** The usual starting dose is 100 mg twice daily with an increase of 100 mg/day up to a maximum of 300 mg/day. **Children:** The dosage for children for the treatment of antipsychotic-induced muscular side effects has not been established.

MONITORING YOUR USE **Time to effectiveness:** 1–2 hours. **A full trial is:** A few days. **Half-life of drug and active metabolites:** 17 hours with no active metabolites. **How to monitor dosage:** The optimal dose is determined by its effectiveness in alleviating the target symptoms. **How to monitor safety:** No special medical tests are needed. **If you miss a dose:** Take a missed dose if it's within an hour or two. Do not try to make up for a missed dose by doubling your next dose; just continue with your regular dosing schedule.

SIDE EFFECTS **Usual (50–100%):** Blurry vision, constipation, dry mouth. **Less common (1–10%):** Anxiety, depression, dizziness, headache, insomnia, low blood pressure, mental status changes, nausea, sedation. **Infrequent:** Urinary difficulty. **Those requiring attention from your physician:** Hallucinations, physical or emotional changes not listed.

WHAT TO EXPECT WHEN YOU STOP You may notice a return of your symptoms if amantadine is stopped. Neuroleptic malignant syndrome, a potentially severe reaction with symptoms of fever, muscular rigidity, and mental status changes has been reported upon cessation of amantadine (see chapter 19).

Amitriptyline

GENERAL **Preparations:** Generic and brand name Elavil. **Class:** Tricyclic antidepressant. **Used in:** Depression, insomnia (anxiety disorders, bulimia). **Mechanism of action:** Blocks the reuptake of norepinephrine and serotonin into presynaptic neurons.

PRECAUTIONS **Don't use if you have:** *Heart block* (an abnormal heart rhythm) or if you recently had a *heart attack,* as amitriptyline may worsen heart block and dangerously affect heart function. **Use extra caution if you have:** *Bipolar disorder,* as amitriptyline may cause a manic episode; *epilepsy,* as amitriptyline may increase the frequency of seizures; *glaucoma;* as amitriptyline can worsen the symptoms of untreated angle closure glaucoma, *low blood pressure,* as amitriptyline may lower blood pressure further; a *psychotic disorder,* as amitriptyline may make psychotic symptoms worse; *hyperthyroidism,* as amitriptyline may cause irregular heart rhythms; *prostatic hypertrophy* or *urinary retention,* as amitriptyline may worsen urinary retention. **Tests needed before starting:** An electrocardiogram (EKG) if you are over 35, to ensure that you do not have any form of heart block. **Alcohol:** Should be avoided, as the simultaneous use of amitriptyline and alcohol can lower blood pressure significantly and cause confusion. Also, alcohol worsens anxiety and depression and impairs insight and judgment. **Use in pregnancy:** There is a higher rate of miscarriages born to women who take tricyclics, but no specific defect is associated with their use.

DRUG INTERACTIONS   **Do not use if you take:** *MAOI antidepressants,* as their use with amitriptyline can cause pronounced hypertension and the potential for strokes. **Use with extra caution if you take:** *Phenothiazines,* as the combination may cause irregular heart rhythms that are potentially fatal; *antihypertensives:* as they may combine to lower blood pressure excessively; *antihistamines, phenothiazines,* and *antiparkinsonian agents* as they may combine to produce pronounced dry mouth, blurry vision, constipation, low blood pressure, rapid heart rate, and even mental confusion; *guanethadine* to lower blood pressure, as amitriptyline may block its effects.

DOSING   **Adults:** For depression, the usual starting dose is 25 mg at bedtime with increases every other day up to 150 mg/day. The maximum recommended dose is 300 mg/day. For insomnia, the usual starting dose is 25 mg at bedtime with increases every other day up to a maximum of 100 mg/day. **Children:** Not FDA-approved for under 12. Some child psychiatrists use a starting dose of 25 mg at bedtime with increases of 25 mg/day every few days up to a maximum dose of 100 mg/day for those over 12. **The elderly:** For depression, the usual starting dose is 10 mg at bedtime with increases every few days up to 50–100 mg/day. For insomnia, the usual starting dose is 10 mg at bedtime with increases every other day up to a maximum of 50 mg/day.

MONITORING YOUR USE   **Time to effectiveness:** Sedative effects are generally noticeable within a few doses, but the antidepressant effect may take 2–4 weeks. **A full trial is:** Four weeks at the maximum tolerated dosage. **Half-life of drug and active metabolites:** 20–46 hours. It is metabolized into nortriptyline, a metabolite with antidepressant activity, whose half-life is 16–90 hours. **How to monitor dosage:** The optimal dose is determined by its effectiveness in alleviating the target symptoms. The therapeutic effect of amitriptyline is more likely when the concentration in the blood is between 150 and 300 micrograms. A blood level check may be useful to assist in determining the best dosage if you do not respond or if your side effects are more pronounced than expected. **How to monitor safety:** A blood level should be obtained if doses go over 150 mg/day. An EKG may be useful to ensure that heart function is not impaired. **If you miss a dose:** Take a missed dose if it's within an hour or two. Do not try to make up for a missed dose by doubling your next dose; just continue with your regular dosing schedule.

SIDE EFFECTS   **Usual (50–100%):** Blurry vision, constipation, dry mouth, fatigue, increased heart rate, low blood pressure. **Common (10–50%):** Sweating, weight gain. **Less common (1–10%):** Sexual dysfunction, urinary difficulty. **Those requiring attention from your physician:** Physical or emotional changes not listed, such as suicidal thoughts or behavior.

WHAT TO EXPECT WHEN YOU STOP   You may notice a return of your symptoms if amitriptyline is stopped. **If stopped abruptly:** You may experience agitation, headaches, insomnia, and nausea, as well as depression. Amitriptyline should be slowly tapered if you decide to stop it. The rate of discontinuation is different for each person and is determined by the clinical situation necessitating the change, your age, severity of symptoms, dosage size, and your duration of use.

Amoxapine

GENERAL **Preparations:** Generic and brand name Asendin. **Class:** Tricyclic antidepressant. **Used in:** Bulimia, depression. **Mechanism of action:** Blocks the reuptake of norepinephrine and serotonin into presynaptic neurons. It also blocks the response of dopamine receptors to dopamine on postsynaptic neurons.

PRECAUTIONS **Warnings:** Although amoxapine is used as an antidepressant, its action of blocking dopamine gives it antipsychotic-like activity, and the potential to cause side effects common to other antipsychotics. All antipsychotics can cause *neuroleptic malignant syndrome,* a rare but severe and potentially fatal reaction consisting of fever, muscle rigidity, mental status changes, and alterations in pulse and blood pressure. They can also cause *tardive dyskinesia,* a potentially irreversible disorder of rhythmical, involuntary muscle movements (see chapter 19 for details of both conditions). **Don't use if you have:** *Heart block* (an abnormal heart rhythm) or if you recently had a *heart attack,* as amoxapine may worsen heart block and dangerously affect heart function. **Use extra caution if you have:** *Breast cancer,* as amoxapine can elevate prolactin, a hormone released by the pituitary that may cause breast cancer to grow faster; *bipolar disorder,* as amoxapine may cause a manic episode; *epilepsy,* as amoxapine may increase the frequency of seizures; *glaucoma,* as amoxapine can worsen the symptoms of untreated angle closure glaucoma; *low blood pressure,* as amoxapine may lower blood pressure further; a *psychotic disorder,* as amoxapine may make psychotic symptoms worse (although it may improve them); *hyperthyroidism,* as amoxapine may cause irregular heart rhythms; *prostatic hypertrophy* or *urinary retention,* as amoxapine may worsen urinary retention. **Tests needed before starting:** An electrocardiogram (EKG) if you are over 35, to ensure you do not have any form of heart block. **Alcohol:** Should be avoided, as the simultaneous use of amoxapine and alcohol can lower blood pressure significantly and cause confusion. Also, alcohol worsens anxiety and depression, and impairs insight and judgment. **Use in pregnancy:** There is a higher rate of miscarriages born to women who take tricyclics, but no specific defect is associated with their use.

DRUG INTERACTIONS **Do not use if you take:** *MAOI antidepressants,* as their use with amoxapine can cause pronounced hypertension and the potential for strokes. **Use with extra caution if you take:** *Phenothiazines,* as the combination may cause irregular heart rhythms that are potentially fatal; *antihypertensives,* as they may combine to lower blood pressure excessively; *antihistamines, phenothiazines,* and *antiparkinsonian agents,* as they may combine to produce pronounced dry mouth, blurry vision, constipation, low blood pressure, rapid heart rate, and even mental confusion; *guanethadine* to lower blood pressure, as amoxapine may block its effects.

DOSING   **Adults:** The usual starting dose is 25 mg at bedtime, with increases every other day up to150 mg. The maximum recommended dose is 300 mg/day. **Children:** Not FDA-approved for under 16. **The elderly:** For depression, the usual starting dose is 10 mg at bedtime with increases every few days up to a maximum of 50–100 mg/day.

MONITORING YOUR USE   **Time to effectiveness:** Side effects are generally noticeable within a few doses, but the therapeutic effect may take 2–4 weeks. **A full trial is:** Four weeks at the maximum tolerated dosage. **Half-life of drug and active metabolites:** 8–18 hours with two active metabolites with half-lives of 6 and 30 hours. **How to monitor dosage:** The optimal dose is determined by its effectiveness in alleviating the target symptoms. The therapeutic effect of amoxapine is more likely when the concentration in the blood is between 150 and 300 micrograms. A blood level may be useful to assist in determining the best dosage if you do not respond or if your side effects are more pronounced than expected. **How to monitor safety:** A blood level should be obtained if doses go over 150 mg/day. An EKG may be useful to ensure that heart function is not impaired. **If you miss a dose:** Take a missed dose if it's within an hour or two. Do not try to make up for a missed dose by doubling your next dose; just continue with your regular dosing schedule.

SIDE EFFECTS   **Usual (50–100%):** Blurry vision, constipation, dry mouth, fatigue, increased heart rate, low blood pressure. **Common (10–50%):** Sweating, weight gain. **Less common (1–10%):** Insomnia, mental status changes, nausea, palpitations, rash, sexual dysfunction, tremor. **Infrequent (less than 1%):** Tardive dyskinesia, urinary difficulty. **Those requiring attention from your physician:** Symptoms of fever, muscular rigidity, and mental status changes, as you may have neuroleptic malignant syndrome, a potentially severe reaction; any abnormal involuntary movements that suggest tardive dyskinesia, any physical or emotional changes not listed, such as suicidal thoughts or behavior.

WHAT TO EXPECT WHEN YOU STOP   You may notice a return of your symptoms if amoxapine is stopped. **If stopped abruptly:** You may experience agitation, headaches, insomnia, and nausea, as well as depression. Amoxapine should be slowly tapered if you decide to stop it. The rate of discontinuation is different for each person and is determined by the clinical situation necessitating the change, your age, severity of symptoms, dosage size, and your duration of use.

Aripiprazole

GENERAL   **Preparations:** Brand name Abilify only in pills. **Class:** Atypical antipsychotic. **Used in:** Bipolar disorder, psychotic disorders (Alzheimer's disease, severe anxiety, developmental disorders). **Mechanism of action:** Blocks a subset of dopamine and serotonin receptors.

PRECAUTIONS   **Warnings:** All antipsychotics can cause *neuroleptic malignant syndrome*, a rare but severe and potentially fatal reaction consisting of fever, muscle rigidity, mental status changes, and alterations in pulse and blood pressure. They can also cause *tardive dyskinesia,* a potentially irreversible disorder of rhythmical, involuntary muscle movements. Aripiprazole and other atypical antipsychotics are associated with the development of *weight gain, high cholesterol, and diabetes mellitus.* Aripiprazole and other atypical antipsychotics are also associated with a higher incidence of *strokes* and *sudden death* in elderly people with dementia. **Use extra caution if you have:** *Breast cancer,* as aripiprazole may elevate prolactin, a hormone released by the pituitary that may cause breast cancer to grow faster; *epilepsy,* as aripiprazole may increase the frequency of seizures; *heart problems,* as aripiprazole can worsen heart function further. **Tests before starting:** Weight measurement. **Alcohol:** Should be avoided, as the simultaneous use of aripiprazole and alcohol can cause confusion. Also, alcohol worsens anxiety and depression, and impairs insight and judgment.

DRUG INTERACTIONS   **Use with extra caution if you take:** *Anticonvulsants, antidepressants, antihistamines, antipsychotics, barbiturates, benzodiazepines,* or any drug that causes sedation or central nervous system depression, because the combination can cause pronounced sedation; *antihypertensives,* as aripiprazole may combine to lower blood pressure excessively; *antihistamines* or *antiparkinsonian agents,* as they may combine to produce pronounced dry mouth, blurry vision, constipation, low blood pressure, rapid heart rate, or mental confusion.

DOSING   **Adults:** The starting dose is 5–15 mg a day, with increases every week of 5–10 mg up to a maximum of 30 mg a day. **Children:** Not FDA-approved for under 18.

MONITORING YOUR USE   **Time to effectiveness:** The first effects may be noticed within some days, but it may be one to three weeks to notice a pronounced change. It may take several months to derive full benefit. **A full trial is:** Four weeks at no less than 30 mg a day. **Half-life of drug and active metabolites:** 75–94 hours with one active metabolite. **How to monitor dosage:** The optimal dose is determined by its effectiveness in alleviating the target symptoms. **How to monitor safety:** Pretreatment and periodic weight measurements should be performed to assess weight gain; blood glucose, cholesterol, and lipid profiles should be obtained within three months and yearly thereafter to check for diabetes and elevations in cholesterol or triglycerides; a physical examination for the presence of tardive dyskinesia should be done twice yearly. **If you miss a dose:** Take a missed dose if it's within an hour or two. Do not try to make up for a missed dose the next day by doubling your dose; just continue with your regular dosing schedule.

SIDE EFFECTS   **Common (10–50%):** Agitation, low blood pressure (light-headedness, dizziness), headaches. **Less common (1–10%):** Akathisia (restlessness), constipation, fatigue, menstrual irregularities, nausea, sedation, sexual dysfunction, pseudoparkinsonism (muscular tremor, rigidity, akinesia), tardive dyskinesia, weight gain. **Those requiring attention by your physician:** Symptoms of fever, muscular rigidity, and mental status changes, as you may have neuroleptic malignant syndrome, a potentially severe reaction; any abnormal involuntary movements that suggest tardive dyskinesia; any other physical or emotional changes not described here.

WHAT TO EXPECT IF YOU STOP: You may notice a return of your symptoms if aripiprazole is tapered gradually. **If stopped abruptly:** There is no acute withdrawal syndrome, but symptoms may return quickly.

Atomoxetine

GENERAL   **Preparations:** Brand name Strattera only in pills. **Class:** Norepinepherine reuptake inhibitor **Used in:** ADD. **Mechanism of action:** Blocks norepinepherine reuptake.

PRECAUTIONS   **Warning:** Rarely, atomoxetine can cause liver failure. Also rarely, some people experience suicidal thoughts on atomoxetine. **Use extra caution if you have:** *Bipolar disorder,* as atomoxetine can exacerbate mood swings; *cardiovascular disease, hypertension,* or *tachycardia,* as atomoxetine can raise your heart rate and blood pressure; *glaucoma,* as atomoxetine can exacerbate the symptoms; *liver problems,* as atomoxetine can build up in your system to excessive levels; *low blood pressure,* as atomoxetine can cause dizziness or fainting; *prostatic hypertrophy or urinary retention,* as atomoxetine may worsen urinary retention; *schizophrenia or other psychotic disorders,* as atomoxetine can worsen psychotic symptoms. **Tests before starting:** None. **Alcohol:** The simultaneous use of atomoxetine and alcohol causes no specific adverse consequences, but alcohol should be avoided because it can impair attention and concentration, decreasing the effectiveness of atomoxetine.

DRUG INTERACTIONS   **Use with extra caution if you take:** *Albuterol (Combivent, Ventolin)* for asthma or other breathing problems, as atomoxetine can increase the effect of albuterol on the cardiovascular system, raising heart rate and blood pressure; *MAOI antidepressants,* as their use with atomoxetine can cause a serious, sometimes fatal, reaction of agitation, fever, cardiovascular changes, and mental status changes.

DOSING **Adults:** The starting dose is 25 mg a day with increases every week of 20 mg up to a maximum of 100 mg a day. **Children:** The starting dose is 0.5 mg/kg, increased after three days to 1.2 mg/kg. The total daily dose should not exceed 1.4 mg/kg/day or 100 mg/day, whichever is less.

MONITORING YOUR USE **Time to effectiveness:** The first effects may be noticed within some days, but it may be one to three weeks at the full dose to notice a pronounced change. It may take several months to derive full benefit. **A full trial is:** Four weeks at no less than 80 mg/day for adults, and 1.2 mg/kg of body weight for children. **Half-life of drug and active metabolites:** 5 hours with no active metabolites. **How to monitor dosage:** The optimal dose is determined by its effectiveness in alleviating the target symptoms. **How to monitor safety:** Pretreatment and periodic weight and height measurements should be performed to assess weight gain and growth. **If you miss a dose:** Take a missed dose if it's within an hour or two. Do not try to make up for a missed dose the next day by doubling your dose; just continue with your regular dosing schedule.

SIDE EFFECTS **Common (10–50%):** Abdominal pain, constipation, decreased appetite, dry mouth, headaches, nausea, vomiting. **Less common (1–10%):** Fatigue, insomnia, sexual dysfunction (erectile difficulties), menstrual cramps, urinary hesitancy. **Those requiring attention by your physician:** Any physical or emotional changes not described here.

WHAT TO EXPECT IF YOU STOP: You may notice a return of your symptoms if atomoxetine is stopped, but there is no acute withdrawal syndrome.

Benztropine

GENERAL **Preparations:** Generic and brand name Cogentin. **Class:** Antiparkinsonian agent. **Used in:** The treatment of side effects induced by antipsychotics: akathisia, dystonia, and pseudoparkinsonism (tremor, rigidity, akinesia, nighttime drooling caused by clozapine). **Mechanism of action:** Blocks postsynaptic acetyl choline receptors.

PRECAUTIONS **Use extra caution if you have:** *Congestive heart failure, edema, epilepsy, glaucoma, low blood pressure, prostatic hypertrophy,* or *urinary retention,* as benztropine may worsen the symptoms of the disorder. **Tests needed before starting:** None. **Alcohol:** Should be avoided as the simultaneous use of benztropine and alcohol can lower blood pressure significantly and cause confusion. Also, alcohol worsens anxiety and depression and impairs insight and judgment.

DRUG INTERACTIONS   **Do not use if you take:** *Antihypertensives,* as they may combine to lower blood pressure excessively; *antihistamines, phenothiazines,* or *tricyclic antidepressants,* as they may combine to produce pronounced dry mouth, blurry vision, constipation, low blood pressure, rapid heart rate, and even mental confusion.

DOSING   **Adults:** The usual starting dose is 1–2 mg twice daily with a weekly increase of 2 mg/day up to 8 mg/day. Some people may need higher dosages. **Children:** 1–2 mg once or twice a day.

MONITORING YOUR USE   **Time to effectiveness:** 1–2 hours, but the full effect may take 2–3 days. **A full trial is:** A few days at the maximum recommended dose. **Half-life of drug and active metabolites:** The half-life and metabolism of benztropine are unknown, but the effects generally last for a day or two upon cessation. **How to monitor dosage:** The optimal dose is determined by its effectiveness in alleviating the target symptoms. **How to monitor safety:** No special medical tests are needed. **If you miss a dose:** Take a missed dose if it's within an hour or two. Do not try to make up for a missed dose by doubling your next dose; just continue with your regular dosing schedule.

SIDE EFFECTS   **Usual (50–100%):** Blurry vision, constipation, dry mouth. **Less common (1–10%):** Heart rate elevation, low blood pressure, nausea, vomiting. **Infrequent (less than 1%):** Rash, urinary difficulty. **Those requiring attention from your physician:** Any physical or emotional changes not listed.

WHAT TO EXPECT WHEN YOU STOP   You may notice a return of your symptoms if benztropine is stopped. **If stopped abruptly:** There are no acute withdrawal effects.

Biperiden

GENERAL   **Preparations:** Brand name Akineton only. **Class:** Antiparkinsonian agent. **Used in:** The treatment of muscular side effects induced by antipsychotics: akathisia, dystonia, and pseudoparkinsonism (tremor, rigidity, akinesia). **Mechanism of action:** Blocks postsynaptic acetylcholine receptors.

PRECAUTIONS   **Use extra caution if you have:** *Congestive heart failure, edema, epilepsy, glaucoma, low blood pressure, prostatic hypertrophy* or *urinary retention,* as biperiden may worsen the symptoms of these disorders. **Tests needed before starting:** None. **Alcohol:** Should be avoided as the simultaneous use of biperiden and alcohol can lower blood pressure significantly and cause confusion. Also, alcohol worsens anxiety and depression and impairs insight and judgment.

DRUG INTERACTIONS **Do not use if you take:** *Antihypertensives,* as they may combine to lower blood pressure excessively; *antihistamines, phenothiazines,* or *tricyclic antidepressants,* as they may combine to produce pronounced dry mouth, blurry vision, constipation, low blood pressure, rapid heart rate, and even mental confusion.

DOSING **Adults:** The usual starting dose is 2 mg twice daily with an increase every few days of 4 mg/day up to 16 mg/day. **Children:** Dosages, safety, and effectiveness in children have not been established.

MONITORING YOUR USE **Time to effectiveness:** 1–2 hours, but the full effect may take 2–3 days. **A full trial is:** A few days at the maximum recommended dose. **Half-life of drug and active metabolites:** The half-life and metabolism of biperiden are unknown, but the effects generally last for a day or two upon cessation. **How to monitor dosage:** The optimal dose is determined by its effectiveness in alleviating the target symptoms. **How to monitor safety:** No special medical tests are needed. **If you miss a dose:** Take a missed dose if it's within an hour or two. Do not try to make up for a missed dose by doubling your next dose, just continue with your regular dosing schedule.

SIDE EFFECTS **Usual (50–100%):** Blurry vision, constipation, dry mouth. **Less common (1–10%):** Heart rate elevation, low blood pressure, nausea, vomiting. **Infrequent (less than 1%):** Rash, urinary difficulty. **Those requiring attention from your physician:** Any physical or emotional changes not listed.

WHAT TO EXPECT WHEN YOU STOP You may notice a return of your symptoms if biperiden is stopped. **If stopped abruptly:** There are no acute withdrawal effects.

Buprenorphine

GENERAL **Preparations:** Brand name Buprenex for injection and brand name Subutex sublingual tablets. Brand name Suboxone is a combination of buprenorphine and naloxone. **Class:** Narcotic. **Used in:** Narcotic withdrawal. **Mechanism of action:** Stimulates postsynaptic opiate receptors.

PRECAUTIONS **Warning:** Buprenorphine is addictive in its own right. It produces euphoria when first begun, although much less than heroin. **Use extra caution if you have:** *Asthma* or *other breathing problems,* as buprenorphine may impair breathing further; *low blood pressure,* as buprenorphine may lower blood pressure further; *urinary retention* or *prostatic hypertrophy,* as buprenorphine may worsen urinary retention. **Tests needed before starting:** None. **Alcohol:**

Alcohol should be avoided as the combination may lower blood pressure and may impair breathing, as well as worsen anxiety and depression and cause confusion. **Use in pregnancy:** Babies born to mothers on buprenorphine go through a withdrawal syndrome.

DRUG INTERACTIONS   **Do not use if you take:** *MAOI antidepressants,* as the combination of narcotics and MAOIs can impair breathing, lower blood pressure, and impair your level of consciousness. On occasion, the combination has been fatal. **Use with extra caution if you take:** *Pentazocine, phenytoin,* or *rifampin,* as the combination may cause withdrawal symptoms; *anticonvulsants, antidepressants, antihistamines, antipsychotics, barbiturates, benzodiazepines,* or any drug that causes sedation or central nervous system depression, because the combination with buprenorphine can cause pronounced sedation, breathing problems, and death; *erythromycin, indinavir, itraconazole, ketoconazole, ritonavir,* or *saquinavir,* as these drugs may increase blood levels of buprenorphine.

DOSING   **Adults:** The analgesic dose is 0.3 mg per intramuscular injection at 6-hour intervals. Some adults may need 0.6 mg per injection, 12–16 mg a day Subutex, or Suboxone taken orally.

MONITORING YOUR USE   **Time to effectiveness:** 30–60 minutes. **A full trial is:** Determined by adherence to the treatment program and abstinence from other substance use. **Half-life of drug:** 1–7 hours. **How to monitor dosage:** Dosage size is determined by the ability to suppress withdrawal symptoms. **How to monitor safety:** No specific medical tests are needed. **If you miss a dose:** Don't double up on the next dose; continue with the regular dosing schedule.

SIDE EFFECTS   **Usual (50–100%):** Constipation, decreased appetite, dry mouth, euphoria, sedation, sexual dysfunction, urinary difficulty. **Less common (1–10%):** Agitation, fainting, headache, insomnia, nausea and vomiting, low heart rate, rash. **Those requiring attention from your physician:** Any emotional, cognitive, and physical changes not listed here.

WHAT TO EXPECT WHEN YOU STOP   You will experience narcotic withdrawal symptoms: runny nose, sneezing, sweating, goose bumps, fever, chills, restlessness, irritability, weakness, anxiety, depression, dilated pupils, rapid heart beat, abdominal cramps, body aches, twitching, decreased appetite, nausea, vomiting, diarrhea, and weight loss. The severity of these symptoms depends on the length of time you have taken buprenorphine, how much you took each day, whether you also take other drugs, and the rate of tapering. There may be psychological dependence and a craving for narcotics long after the last dose is taken. **If stopped abruptly:** The withdrawal symptoms will be pronounced.

Bupropion

GENERAL **Preparations:** Generic, and brand names Wellbutrin, Wellbutrin SR (sustained release), Wellbutrin XL (extended release), and Zyban. **Class:** Antidepressant. **Used in:** Depression, nicotine dependence (ADHD). **Mechanism of action:** Inhibits reuptake of norepinephrine and dopamine by presynaptic neurons.

PRECAUTIONS **Don't use if you have:** *Epilepsy,* as bupropion may increase the frequency of seizures. **Use extra caution if you have:** *Anorexia* or *bulimia,* as there is a higher incidence of seizures if you take bupropion; *bipolar disorder,* as bupropion can cause a manic episode; *Parkinson's,* as bupropion may worsen agitation and lead to confusion; a *psychotic disorder,* as bupropion can worsen psychotic symptoms. **Tests needed before starting:** None. **Alcohol:** Should be avoided because its use with bupropion puts you at higher risk for seizures. Also, alcohol worsens anxiety and depression.

DRUG INTERACTIONS **Do not use if you take:** *MAOI antidepressants* because of the high potential for seizures. **Use with extra caution if you take:** *Antidepressants, antipsychotics, theophylline,* and *steroids,* because of the higher risk of seizures.

DOSING **Adults:** *For depression:* The usual starting dose is 75–100 mg twice daily with weekly increases of 100 mg/day up to a maximum of 450 mg/day. No dose should be more than 150 mg, as the incidence of seizures is much higher over this dose. Thus the highest dose is 150 mg three times a day with at least 4 hours between doses. The maximum dose of the sustained release preparation is 200 mg twice daily; the dose of the XL formulation is 450 mg once daily. *For smoking cessation:* 150 mg twice daily of the *sustained-release* preparation. **Children:** Not FDA-approved for under 18.

MONITORING YOUR USE **Time to effectiveness:** You may notice some side effects within one to two days, but any improvement in depression generally takes two to four weeks. **A full trial is:** Four weeks at the maximum dose. **Half-life of drug and active metabolites:** 8–24 hours with several active metabolites, two of which have half-lives longer than bupropion. **How to monitor dosage:** The optimal dose is determined by its effectiveness in alleviating the target symptoms. **How to monitor safety:** No specific tests are needed to monitor your health while on bupropion. **If you miss a dose:** Take a missed dose if it's within an hour or two, but always maintain 4 hours between doses to minimize the risk of seizures. Do not try to make up for a missed dose by doubling your next dose; just continue with your regular dosing schedule.

SIDE EFFECTS **Common (10–50%):** Agitation, anxiety, dizziness, decreased appetite, insomnia, and weight loss. **Less common (1–10%):** Constipation, dry mouth, headaches, rash, sweating, and tremor. **Those requiring attention from your physician:** Seizures; any physical or emotional changes not listed, such as suicidal thoughts or behavior.

WHAT TO EXPECT WHEN YOU STOP You may notice a return of your symptoms if bupropion is tapered gradually. **If stopped abruptly:** You may experience pronounced depression. A withdrawal syndrome has not been reported, but physical symptoms may occur.

Buspirone

GENERAL **Preparations:** Brand name Buspar only. **Class:** Antianxiety agent. **Used in:** Anxiety disorders (Alzheimer's disease, developmental disorders, tardive dyskinesia). **Mechanism of action:** Blocks a subset of presynaptic and post-synaptic serotonin and dopamine receptors.

PRECAUTIONS **Tests needed before starting:** None. **Alcohol:** The simultaneous use of buspirone and alcohol causes no specific adverse consequences, but alcohol should be avoided because it worsens anxiety and depression.

DRUG INTERACTIONS **Do not use if you take:** *MAOI antidepressants,* as their use with buspirone can cause an elevation of blood pressure, which could potentially lead to a stroke.

DOSING **Adults:** The usual starting dose is 5 mg three times daily with increases of 5 mg/day every few days up to a maximum of 30 mg/day. Dosages up to 40 mg three times daily can be helpful for tardive dyskinesia. **Children:** Not FDA-approved for under 18. Some child psychiatrists recommend a starting dose of 2.5–5 mg once daily, with increases every 3–4 days of 2.5–5 mg up to a maximum of 20 mg/day in children under 12.

MONITORING YOUR USE **Time to effectiveness:** You may notice some side effects within one to two days, but any improvement in symptoms generally takes two to four weeks. **A full trial is:** Four weeks at the maximum dose. **Half-life of drug and active metabolites:** Two to three hours, with no active metabolites present in sufficient concentration to affect your response. **How to monitor dosage:** The optimal dose is determined by its effectiveness in alleviating the target symptoms. **How to monitor safety:** No specific tests are needed to monitor your health while on buspirone. **If you miss a dose:** Take a missed dose if it's within an hour or two. Do not try to make up for a missed dose by doubling your next dose; just continue with your regular dosing schedule.

SIDE EFFECTS   Common (10–50%): Dizziness, and drowsiness. **Less common (1–10%):** Headaches, nausea. **Those requiring attention from your physician:** Any physical or emotional changes not listed.

WHAT TO EXPECT WHEN YOU STOP   You may notice a return of your symptoms if buspirone is tapered gradually.

Carbamazepine

GENERAL   Preparations: Generic and brand names Tegretol and Tegretol XR (extended release) in pills and liquid form. **Class:** Mood stabilizer. **Used in:** Bipolar disorder. **Mechanism of action:** Carbamazepine has many actions in the brain on receptors, neurotransmitter concentrations, ion channels, and second messenger systems, but it is unknown which effect stabilizes mood.

PRECAUTIONS   Warnings: Carbamazepine can cause *aplastic anemia* and *agranulocytosis,* two blood disorders that are potentially fatal (see chapter 19). Although the likelihood of these disorders is quite low, close monitoring is necessary during treatment. **Use extra caution if you have:** *Glaucoma,* as carbamazepine can worsen the symptoms. **Tests needed before starting:** Complete blood count (CBC). **Alcohol:** Should be avoided as it may impair the effectiveness of carbamazepine. Alcohol should also be avoided because it can worsen depression and cause confusion in bipolar disorder. **Use in pregnancy:** It may cause spina bifida, a defect in the spinal cord. There may be seizures, vomiting, and diarrhea in babies born to mothers who took carbamazepine during pregnancy. These symptoms may be due to a withdrawal syndrome.

DRUG INTERACTIONS   Do not use if you take: *Clozapine,* as they can both cause agranulocytosis; *MAOI antidepressants,* as their use with carbamazepine can cause a dangerous elevation of blood pressure and a stroke. **Use with extra caution if you take:** *Anticonvulsants, antidepressants, antihistamines, antipsychotics, barbiturates, benzodiazepines,* or any drug that causes sedation or central nervous system depression, because the combination can cause pronounced sedation. *Oral or subdermal implant contraceptives,* as breakthrough bleeding may occur and their reliability may be affected.

DOSING   Adults: The usual starting dose is 100–200 mg twice daily with weekly increases of 100–200 mg/day up to a maximum of 1200 mg/day. 1600 mg/day has been used in rare instances. **Children:** Over 12: the same as adults. Ages 6–12: the usual starting dose is 100 mg twice daily or 50 mg four times daily, with weekly increases of 100 mg/day up to a maximum of 1000 mg/day. Under 6: 10 mg/kg/day in divided doses.

MONITORING YOUR USE   Time to effectiveness: You may notice some side effects within one to two days, but any improvement in symptoms generally takes one to two weeks if you are manic. **A full trial is:** Three weeks at the maximum therapeutic level if you are manic. There is no set period of time with which to determine effectiveness if you start carbamazepine when your mood is stable, as manic symptoms are often absent for extended periods of time. Essentially, you stay on the drug and watch for any symptoms of mania. If none appear, or if they are milder than usual, then carbamazepine is at least partially effective. **Half-life of drug and active metabolites:** 25–65 hours initially, but with steady use it decreases to 12–17 hours. There are active metabolites, but what role they may play in the treatment of bipolar disorder is unclear. **How to monitor dosage:** The optimal dose is determined by a blood level of 4–12 micrograms/ml of blood. Improved effectiveness can sometimes be achieved by maintaining the level at the higher end of the therapeutic range. **How to monitor safety:** Periodic CBCs when you first begin are essential to screen for agranulocytosis and aplastic anemia. **If you miss a dose:** Take a missed dose if it's within a few hours. Do not try to make up for a missed dose by doubling your next dose; just continue with your regular dosing schedule.

SIDE EFFECTS   Common (10–50%): Mild sedation, impaired muscular coordination, an unsteady gait, and nausea are common when you first start, but tend to go away within the first week. **Those requiring attention from your physician:** You should consult your physician immediately if you notice unusual bleeding or bruising, sores in the mouth, fever, or sore throat, which may suggest agranulocytosis or aplastic anemia; physical or emotional changes not listed.

WHAT TO EXPECT WHEN YOU STOP   You may notice a return of your symptoms if carbamazepine is tapered gradually. **If stopped abruptly:** You may develop withdrawal seizures. Carbamazepine should not be stopped abruptly but needs to be gradually tapered in consultation with your physician.

Chlordiazepoxide

GENERAL   Preparations: Generic and brand name Librium. **Class:** Benzodiazepine. **Used in:** Alcohol withdrawal, anxiety disorders, bipolar disorder (Alzheimer's disease, antipsychotic-induced akathisia [restlessness], insomnia). **Mechanism of action:** Intensifies the effects of gamma-aminobutyric acid (GABA).

PRECAUTIONS   Warnings: *It is habit-forming.* Chlordiazepoxide, like all benzodiazepines, is physically and psychologically habit-forming. People who have experienced traumatic events in their lives and have chronic anxiety are especially prone to developing dependence. Prolonged use is associated with a range of problems. Use for more than four weeks is *not* recommended. If you stop chlordiazepoxide after more than four weeks of daily use, you will probably experience withdrawal symptoms (see below). *Seizures can occur if it is stopped abruptly,* so consultation with your physician is essential if you wish to stop. **Tests needed before starting:** None. **Alcohol:** Alcohol must be avoided entirely. The simultaneous use of chlordiazepoxide and alcohol is extremely dangerous because it can cause you to stop breathing. The combination can cause death. **Use in pregnancy:** There is a higher rate of babies born with a cleft palate to mothers who took benzodiazepines during pregnancy. **The elderly** are especially sensitive to the effects of benzodiazepines and may experience pronounced side effects at low doses (see chapter 4).

DRUG INTERACTIONS   **Use with extra caution if you take:** *Anticonvulsants, antidepressants, antihistamines, antipsychotics, barbiturates, benzodiazepines,* or any drug that causes sedation or central nervous system depression, because the combination can cause pronounced sedation.

DOSING   **Adults:** The usual starting dose is 5–25 mg three to four times a day depending on the severity of the symptoms, up to a maximum dose of 100 mg/day. **Children:** Not FDA-approved for under 6. Some child psychiatrists recommend a starting dose of 5 mg two to four times a day with an increase up to a maximum of 30 mg/day in children over 6. **The elderly:** The starting dose is 5 mg two to four times daily, with increases as needed.

MONITORING YOUR USE   **Time to effectiveness:** 30–60 minutes. **A full trial is:** A few doses, which are generally enough to establish whether it will be helpful. **Half-life of drug and active metabolites:** 24–48 hours with several active metabolites. **How to monitor dosage:** The optimal dose is determined by its effectiveness in alleviating the target symptoms. **If you miss a dose:** Do *not* try to make up for a missed dose; just continue with your regular dosing schedule. **How to monitor safety:** No specific medical tests are needed to monitor safety.

SIDE EFFECTS   **Common (10–50%):** Sedation, memory impairment, poor muscle coordination (causing a higher rate of falls in the elderly and a higher risk of motor vehicle accidents). **Infrequent (less than 1%):** Paradoxical agitation and insomnia. **Those requiring attention from your physician:** Any physical or emotional changes not described here. **Side effects associated with use longer than four weeks:** Use of chlordiazepoxide longer than four weeks may cause physical and psychological dependence, and you may notice the desire for another dose as each one wears off. Ongoing anxiety, reduced effectiveness of each dose, depression, emotional blunting, and impairment of memory and cognition may occur with use longer than one year.

WHAT TO EXPECT WHEN YOU STOP   You may notice a return of your symptoms if chlordiazepoxide is tapered gradually. Other withdrawal symptoms include anxiety, insomnia, irritability, headaches, tremors, nausea, diarrhea, sweating, and confusion. The rate at which you should taper is affected by the duration of your use and the size of your dose, but may take months if you have been on it for an extended period of time. **If stopped abruptly:** *Seizures* can occur if chlordiazepoxide is stopped abruptly. They are potentially life-threatening. You should never stop chlordiazepoxide abruptly, and you should always work with your physician to taper it gradually.

Chlorpromazine

GENERAL　　**Preparations:** Generic and brand name Thorazine in pill and liquid form. **Class:** Standard antipsychotic of the phenothiazine group. **Used in:** Psychotic disorders, bipolar disorder (Alzheimer's disease, severe anxiety, severe ADHD, developmental disorders, insomnia). **Mechanism of action:** Blocks postsynaptic dopamine receptors.

PRECAUTIONS　　**Warnings:** All antipsychotics can cause *neuroleptic malignant syndrome,* a rare, but severe and potentially fatal reaction consisting of fever, muscle rigidity, mental status changes, and alterations in pulse and blood pressure. They can also cause *tardive dyskinesia,* a potentially irreversible disorder of rhythmical, involuntary muscle movements (see chapter 19 for details of both conditions). **Use extra caution if you have:** *Breast cancer,* as chlorpromazine can elevate prolactin, a hormone released by the pituitary which may cause breast cancer to grow faster; *epilepsy,* as chlorpromazine may increase the frequency of seizures; *glaucoma, low blood pressure, prostatic hypertrophy,* or *urinary retention,* as the symptoms may worsen. **Tests before starting:** None. **Alcohol:** Should be avoided as the simultaneous use of chlorpromazine and alcohol can lower blood pressure significantly and cause confusion. Also, alcohol worsens anxiety and depression and impairs insight and judgment. **Use in pregnancy:** Phenothiazines have been linked with the "floppy infant syndrome," in which the baby has poor muscle tone. The fetus may experience pseudoparkinsonism and dystonia, muscular side effects that may cause fetal distress before, during, and shortly after birth. **Sunlight:** Severe sunburns can occur if you take chlorpromazine. Avoid sunbathing entirely and avoid casual exposure to the sun for more than thirty minutes. Use a sunblock of a sun protection factor (SPF) of 15 or more if exposure to the sun cannot be avoided.

DRUG INTERACTIONS　　**Use with extra caution if you take:** *Tricyclic antidepressants,* as the combination may cause irregular heart rhythms that are potentially fatal; *anticonvulsants, antidepressants, antihistamines, antipsychotics, barbiturates, benzodiazepines,* or any drug that causes sedation or central nervous system depression, because the combination can cause pronounced sedation; *antihypertensive medication,* as chlorpromazine may combine to lower blood pressure excessively; *antihistamines,* or *antiparkinsonian agents,* as they may combine to produce pronounced dry mouth, blurry vision, constipation, low blood pressure, rapid heart rate, and mental confusion.

DOSING **Adults:** The starting dose is 25–50 mg three times a day for outpatients, with increases of 25–50 mg/day up to a maximum of 400 mg/day. Some people may require doses up to 1000–2000 mg/day. **Children:** 0.25 mg/kg every four to six hours as needed. In severe cases doses up to 200 mg/day may be needed.

MONITORING YOUR USE **Time to effectiveness:** Calming effects are often noticed within one to three hours of a dose, but several days may be needed to notice any effect on psychotic symptoms. A pronounced effect may take one to two weeks. Many months may be needed to derive full benefit. **A full trial is:** Four weeks at no less than 300 mg/day. **Half-life of drug and active metabolites:** 23–37 hours with many active metabolites. **How to monitor dosage:** The optimal dose is determined by its effectiveness in alleviating the target symptoms. **How to monitor safety:** Examination for the presence of tardive dyskinesia (see below) should be performed twice yearly. **If you miss a dose:** Take a missed dose if it's within an hour or two. Do not try to make up for a missed dose by doubling your next dose; just continue with your regular dosing schedule.

SIDE EFFECTS **Usual (50–100%):** Sedation, dry mouth, constipation, blurry vision. **Common (10–50%):** Low blood pressure (light-headedness, dizziness), fatigue, ataraxia (zombielike feeling), weight gain, menstrual irregularities, akathisia (restlessness), sexual dysfunction, pseudoparkinsonism (muscular tremor, rigidity, akinesia), and tardive dyskinesia. **Less common (1–10%):** Dystonia (muscle spasms, usually of the head and neck, face, and jaw), galactorrhea (milk leaking from breasts), sexual dysfunction, cataracts. **Infrequent (less than 1%):** Jaundice (yellow eyes and skin, from liver impairment), urinary difficulty. **Those requiring attention from your physician:** Symptoms of fever, muscular rigidity, and mental status changes, as you may have neuroleptic malignant syndrome, a potentially severe reaction; any abnormal involuntary movements which suggest tardive dyskinesia; any other physical or emotional changes not described here.

WHAT TO EXPECT WHEN YOU STOP You may notice a return of your symptoms if chlorpromazine is tapered gradually. **If stopped abruptly:** You may experience nausea, vomiting, stomach upset, dizziness, and tremor. These effects are unpleasant but not dangerous.

Citalopram

GENERAL **Preparations:** Generic and brand name Celexa. **Class:** SSRI (selective serotonin reuptake inhibitor). **Used in:** Bulimia, depression, panic disorder, and other anxiety disorders (obsessive-compulsive disorder, developmental disorders). **Mechanism of action:** Blocks the reuptake of serotonin by presynaptic neurons.

PRECAUTIONS **Warnings:** When taken with other serotonin reuptake inhibitors, citalopram can cause the *serotonin syndrome,* which consists of potentially dangerous alterations in pulse, blood pressure, hyperactivity, and mental status changes (see chapter 19). Rarely, citalopram can cause hyponatremia, or low sodium in your blood. **Use extra caution if you have:** *Bipolar disorder,* as citalopram can cause a manic episode; *epilepsy,* as citalopram may increase the frequency of seizures; a *psychotic disorder,* as citalopram can worsen psychotic symptoms. **Tests needed before starting:** None. **Alcohol:** The simultaneous use of citalopram and alcohol causes no specific adverse consequences, but alcohol should be avoided because it worsens anxiety and depression. **Use in pregnancy:** There is a higher rate of miscarriages, heart defects, and intestinal defects in the babies of women who take citalopram during pregnancy.

DRUG INTERACTIONS **Do not use if you take:** *Other SSRIs, St. John's wort,* or *tryptophan,* as their use with citalopram can cause the *serotonin syndrome; MAOI antidepressants,* as their use with citalopram can cause a serious, sometimes fatal, reaction of agitation, fever, cardiovascular changes and mental status changes.

DOSING **Adults:** The usual starting dose is 20 mg once daily with weekly increases of 20 mg/day up to a maximum of 60 mg/day. **Children:** Not FDA-approved for under 18. **The elderly:** The starting dose is 10–20 mg/day with an increase of 20 mg after one week up to a maximum of 40 mg/day.

MONITORING YOUR USE **Time to effectiveness:** You may notice some side effects within one to two days, but any improvement in symptoms generally takes two to four weeks. **A full trial is:** Four weeks at the maximum dose. **Half-life of drug and active metabolites:** 33 hours. Metabolites are essentially inactive. **How to monitor dosage:** The optimal dose is determined by its effectiveness in alleviating the target symptoms. **How to monitor safety:** No specific tests are needed to monitor your health while on citalopram. **If you miss a dose:** Take a missed dose if it's the same day. Do not try to make up for a missed dose the next day by doubling your next dose; just continue with your regular dosing schedule.

SIDE EFFECTS **Common (10–50%):** Dry mouth, fatigue, insomnia, nausea, weakness, sweating, and sexual dysfunction. **Less common (1–10%):** Anxiety, diarrhea, headaches, low blood pressure, menstrual irregularities, rash, tremor. **Those requiring attention from your physician:** Hyperactivity, mental status changes, or alterations in your pulse or blood pressure, which suggest the serotonin syndrome. Any physical or emotional changes not listed, such as suicidal thoughts or behavior.

WHAT TO EXPECT WHEN YOU STOP You may notice a return of your symptoms if citalopram is tapered gradually. **If stopped abruptly:** You may notice a flulike syndrome of nausea, vomiting, diarrhea, dizziness, as well as anxiety and depression. Citalopram should not be stopped abruptly but needs to be gradually tapered in consultation with your physician.

Clomipramine

GENERAL   **Preparations:** Generic and brand name Anafranil. **Class:** Tricyclic antidepressant. **Used in:** Bulimia, depression, obsessive-compulsive disorder (other anxiety disorders). **Mechanism of action:** Blocks the reuptake of serotonin by presynaptic neurons.

PRECAUTIONS   **Do not use if you have:** *Heart block* (an abnormal heart rhythm) or if you recently had a *heart attack,* as clomipramine may worsen heart block and dangerously affect heart function. **Use extra caution if you have:** *Bipolar disorder,* as clomipramine may cause a manic episode; *epilepsy,* as clomipramine may increase the frequency of seizures; *glaucoma,* as clomipramine can worsen the symptoms of untreated angle closure glaucoma; *low blood pressure,* as clomipramine may lower blood pressure further; a *psychotic disorder,* as clomipramine may make psychotic symptoms worse; *hyperthyroidism,* as clomipramine may cause irregular heart rhythms; *prostatic hypertrophy* or *urinary retention,* as clomipramine may worsen urinary retention. **Tests needed before starting:** An electrocardiogram (EKG) if you are over 35, to ensure that you do not have any form of heart block. **Alcohol:** Should be avoided, as the simultaneous use of clomipramine and alcohol can lower blood pressure significantly and cause confusion. Also, alcohol worsens anxiety and depression, and impairs insight and judgment. **Use in pregnancy:** There is a higher rate of miscarriages born to women who take tricyclics, but no specific defect is associated with their use. Jitteriness, tremors, and seizures have been reported in babies born to mothers who took clomipramine until birth.

DRUG INTERACTIONS   **Do not use if you take:** *MAOI antidepressants,* as their use with clomipramine can cause pronounced hypertension and the potential for strokes. **Use with extra caution if you take:** *Phenothiazines,* as the combination may cause irregular heart rhythms that are potentially fatal; *antihypertensives,* as they may combine to lower blood pressure excessively; *antihistamines, phenothiazines,* and *antiparkinsonian agents,* as they may combine to produce pronounced dry mouth, blurry vision, constipation, low blood pressure, rapid heart rate, and even mental confusion; *guanethadine* to lower blood pressure, as clomipramine may block its effects.

DOSING   **Adults:** The usual starting dose is 25 mg at bedtime with increases every few days up to 100 mg in two weeks. The maximum recommended dose is 250 mg/day. **Children:** Not FDA-approved for under 10. Some child psychiatrists use a starting dose of 25 mg at bedtime with increases of 25 mg/day every few days up to a maximum dose of 200 mg/day or 3 mg/kg/day for those over 10. **The elderly:** The usual starting dose is 10 mg at bedtime with increases every few days up to 50–100 mg/day.

MONITORING YOUR USE   Time to effectiveness: Side effects are generally noticeable within a few doses, but the therapeutic effect may take two to four weeks. **A full trial is:** Four weeks at the maximum tolerated dosage. **Half-life of drug and active metabolites:** 20–39 hours with active metabolites with half-lives of 54–77 hours. **How to monitor dosage:** The optimal dose is determined by its effectiveness in alleviating the target symptoms. The therapeutic effect of clomipramine is more likely when the concentration in the blood is between 150 and 300 micrograms. A blood level may be useful to assist in determining the best dosage if you do not respond or if your side effects are more pronounced than expected. **How to monitor safety:** A blood level should be obtained if doses go over 150 mg/day. An EKG may be useful to ensure that heart function is not impaired. **If you miss a dose:** Take a missed dose if it's within an hour or two. Do not try to make up for a missed dose by doubling your next dose; just continue with your regular dosing schedule.

SIDE EFFECTS   Usual (50–100%): Blurry vision, constipation, dizziness, dry mouth, fatigue, headache, increased heart rate, low blood pressure, sedation, tremor. **Common (10–50%):** Anxiety, decreased appetite, insomnia, muscle aches, muscle twitching, nausea, sexual dysfunction, sweating, weight gain. **Less common (1–10%):** Cognition impairment, ear ringing, flushing, memory impairment, urinary difficulty. **Those requiring attention from your physician:** Any physical or emotional changes not listed, such as suicidal thoughts or behavior.

WHAT TO EXPECT WHEN YOU STOP   You may notice a return of your symptoms if clomipramine is stopped. **If stopped abruptly:** You may experience agitation, dizziness, headaches, insomnia, and nausea, as well as depression. Clomipramine should be slowly tapered if you decide to stop it. The rate of discontinuation is different for each person and is determined by the clinical situation necessitating the change, your age, severity of symptoms, dosage size, and your duration of use.

Clonazepam

GENERAL   Preparations: Generic and brand name Klonopin. **Class:** Benzodiazepine. **Used in:** Anxiety disorders, bipolar disorder, insomnia (alcohol withdrawal, Alzheimer's disease, and antipsychotic-induced akathisia [restlessness]). **Mechanism of action:** Intensifies the effects of gamma-aminobutyric acid (GABA).

PRECAUTIONS   Warnings: *It is habit-forming.* Clonazepam, like all benzodiazepines, is physically and psychologically habit-forming. People who have experienced traumatic events in their lives and have chronic anxiety are especially prone to developing dependence. Prolonged use is associated with a range of problems. Use for more than four weeks is *not* recommended. If you stop clonazepam after more than four weeks of daily use, you will probably experience withdrawal symptoms (see below). *Seizures can occur if it is stopped abruptly,* so consultation with your physician is essential if you wish to stop. **Tests needed before starting:** None. **Alcohol:** Alcohol must be avoided entirely. The simultaneous use of clonazepam and alcohol is extremely dangerous because it can cause you to stop breathing. The combination can cause death. **Use in pregnancy:** There is a higher rate of babies born with a cleft palate to mothers who took benzodiazepines during pregnancy. **The elderly** are especially sensitive to the effects of benzodiazepines and may experience pronounced side effects at low doses (see chapter 4).

DRUG INTERACTIONS   **Use with extra caution if you take:** *Anticonvulsants, antidepressants, antihistamines, antipsychotics, barbiturates, benzodiazepines,* or any drug that causes sedation or central nervous system depression, because the combination with clonazepam can cause pronounced sedation.

DOSING   **Adults:** The usual starting dose is 0.25–1.0 mg two times a day depending on the severity of the symptoms. Increases of 0.5 mg/day can occur every few days up to a maximum dose of 4 mg/day. **Children:** Not FDA-approved for under 18.

MONITORING YOUR USE   **Time to effectiveness:** 30–60 minutes. **A full trial is:** A few doses, which are generally enough to establish whether it will be helpful. **Half-life of drug and active metabolites:** 18–50 hours with no active metabolites. **How to monitor dosage:** The optimal dose is determined by its effectiveness in alleviating the target symptoms. **If you miss a dose:** Do *not* try to make up for a missed dose; just continue with your regular dosing schedule. **How to monitor safety:** No specific medical tests are needed to monitor safety.

SIDE EFFECTS   **Common (10–50%):** Sedation, memory impairment, poor muscle coordination (causing a higher rate of falls in the elderly and a higher risk of motor vehicle accidents in all adults). **Infrequent (less than 1%):** Paradoxical agitation and insomnia. **Those requiring attention from your physician:** Any physical or emotional changes not described here. **Side effects associated with use longer than four weeks:** Use of clonazepam longer than four weeks may cause physical and psychological dependence, and you may notice the desire for another dose as each one wears off. Ongoing anxiety, reduced effectiveness of each dose, depression, emotional blunting, and impairment of memory and cognition may occur with use longer than one year.

WHAT TO EXPECT WHEN YOU STOP   You may notice a return of your symptoms if clonazepam is tapered gradually. Other withdrawal symptoms include anxiety, insomnia, irritability, headaches, tremors, nausea, diarrhea, sweating, and confusion. The rate at which you should taper is affected by the duration of your use and the size of your dose but may take months if you have been on it for an extended period of time. **If stopped abruptly:** *Seizures* can occur if clonazepam is stopped abruptly. They are potentially life-threatening. You should never stop clonazepam abruptly, and you should always work with your physician to taper it gradually.

Clonidine

GENERAL   **Preparations:** Generic and brand name Catapres. **Class:** A centrally acting alpha-agonist. **Used in:** ADHD, heroin dependence (developmental disorders). **Mechanism of action:** It stimulates postsynaptic alpha adrenergic receptors in the brain, causing lower blood pressure and heart rate.

PRECAUTIONS   **Tests needed before starting:** Measure pulse and blood pressure. **Alcohol:** The simultaneous use of clonidine and alcohol should be avoided because clonidine can cause excessive sedation.

DRUG INTERACTIONS   **Use with extra caution if you take:** *Tricyclic antidepressants* as the combination may lower blood pressure excessively; *diltiazem, digitalis, verapamil,* and *beta-blockers,* as the combination with clonidine may slow the heart rate excessively.

DOSING   Clonidine comes in tablets and three different strengths of a seven-day skin patch. **Adults:** The usual starting dose is 0.1 mg twice a day, with daily increases of 0.1 mg/day. The usual maintenance dose is 0.2–0.6 mg/day, but doses up to 2.4 mg/day have been employed. **Children:** Not FDA-approved for under 12. Some child psychiatrists recommend a starting dose of 0.05–0.1 mg/day, with increases of 0.05 mg/day every few days up to a maximum of 0.4 mg/day in those under 12. **Skin patch:** Use the smallest size, and increase until therapeutic benefit has been established.

MONITORING YOUR USE   **Time to effectiveness:** The effects on pulse and blood pressure are immediate, but the calming effect sought in ADHD and developmental disorders may take a few days until the dose has built up. **A full trial:** In ADHD and developmental disorders is four weeks at the maximum dose. **Half-life of drug and active metabolites:** 12–16 hours with no active metabolites. **How to monitor dosage:** Pulse and blood pressure should be monitored regularly. The optimal dose is determined by its effectiveness in alleviating the target symptoms. **If you miss a dose:** Do *not* try to make up for a missed dose; just continue with the regular dosing schedule.

SIDE EFFECTS   **Usual (50–100%):** Dizziness, dry mouth, sedation. **Common (10–50%):** Constipation, rash (40% with the patch), weakness. **Less common (1–10%):** Anxiety, depression, headaches, nausea, sexual dysfunction, vomiting. **Those requiring attention from your physician:** Any physical or emotional changes not described here.

WHAT TO EXPECT WHEN YOU STOP   You may notice a return of your symptoms if clonidine is tapered gradually. **If stopped abruptly:** You can develop agitation, anxiety, headaches, and tremor. Most important, your pulse and blood pressure can rise rapidly, putting you at risk for a stroke. Clonidine should always be tapered gradually in consultation with your doctor.

Clorazepate

GENERAL   **Preparations:** Generic and brand name Tranxene. **Class:** Benzodiazepine. **Used in:** Anxiety disorders, bipolar disorder (alcohol withdrawal, Alzheimer's disease, antipsychotic-induced akathisia [restlessness], insomnia). **Mechanism of action:** Intensifies the effects of gamma-aminobutyric acid (GABA).

PRECAUTIONS   **Warnings:** *It is habit-forming.* Clorazepate, like all benzodiazepines, is physically and psychologically habit-forming. People who have experienced traumatic events in their lives and have chronic anxiety are especially prone to developing dependence. Prolonged use is associated with a range of problems. Use for more than four weeks is *not* recommended. If you stop clorazepate after more than four weeks of daily use you will probably experience withdrawal symptoms (see below). *Seizures can occur if it is stopped abruptly,* so consultation with your physician is essential if you wish to stop. **Tests needed before starting:** None. **Alcohol:** Alcohol must be avoided entirely. The simultaneous use of clorazepate and alcohol is extremely dangerous because it can cause you to stop breathing. The combination can cause death. **Use in pregnancy:** There is a higher rate of babies born with a cleft palate to mothers who took benzodiazepines during pregnancy. **The elderly** are especially sensitive to the effects of benzodiazepines and may experience pronounced side effects at low doses (see chapter 4).

DRUG INTERACTIONS   **Use with extra caution if you take:** *Anticonvulsants, antidepressants, antihistamines, antipsychotics, barbiturates, benzodiazepines,* or any drug that causes sedation or central nervous system depression, because the combination with clorazepate can cause pronounced sedation.

DOSING   **Adults:** The usual starting dose is 7.5–15 mg twice a day with weekly increases of 7.5 mg up to a maximum of 60 mg/day. **Children:** Not FDA-approved for under 9. Some child psychiatrists recommend the same dosages as adults. **The elderly:** The usual starting dose is 7.5 mg daily with increases of 7.5 mg every few days. The maximum dose for the elderly has not been determined.

MONITORING YOUR USE   **Time to effectiveness:** 30–60 minutes. **A full trial is:** A few doses, which are generally enough to establish whether it will be helpful. **Half-life of drug and active metabolites:** Less than 6 hours, with one metabolite with a half-life of 40–50 hours. **How to monitor dosage:** The optimal dose is determined by its effectiveness in alleviating the target symptoms. **If you miss a dose:** Do *not* try to make up for a missed dose, just continue with your regular dosing schedule. **How to monitor safety:** No specific medical tests are needed to monitor safety.

SIDE EFFECTS   Common (10–50%): Sedation, memory impairment, poor muscle coordination (causing a higher rate of falls in the elderly and a higher risk of motor vehicle accidents in all adults). **Infrequent (less than 1%):** Paradoxical agitation and insomnia. **Those requiring attention from your physician:** Any physical or emotional changes not described here. **Side effects associated with use longer than four weeks:** Use of clorazepate longer than four weeks may cause physical and psychological dependence, and you may notice the desire for another dose as each one wears off. Ongoing anxiety, reduced effectiveness of each dose, depression, emotional blunting, and impairment of memory and cognition may occur with use longer than one year.

WHAT TO EXPECT WHEN YOU STOP   You may notice a return of your symptoms if clorazepate is tapered gradually. Other withdrawal symptoms include anxiety, insomnia, irritability, headaches, tremors, nausea, diarrhea, sweating, and confusion. The rate at which you should taper is affected by the duration of your use and the size of your dose, but may take months if you have been on it for an extended period of time. **If stopped abruptly:** *Seizures* can occur if clorazepate is stopped abruptly. They are potentially life-threatening. You should never stop clorazepate abruptly, and you should always work with your physician to taper it gradually.

Clozapine

GENERAL   **Preparations:** Generic and brand name Clozaril and orally disintegrating Fazaclo. **Class:** Atypical antipsychotic. **Mechanism of action:** Blocks a subset of dopamine and serotonin receptors. **Used in:** Psychotic disorders (bipolar disorder).

PRECAUTIONS   Warnings: Clozapine can cause *agranulocytosis,* a serious and potentially fatal blood disorder, in about 1 percent of people who try it (see chapter 19). About 1 in 3,000 experience severe *low blood pressure,* cardiac arrest, and they stop breathing, a reaction that may be more likely if used in combination with benzodiazepines. Clozapine causes *myocarditis,* a potentially fatal inflammation of the heart in approximately 1 in 3,000 patients. Most cases occur within the first month of therapy. Because of these side effects, clozapine should be used only in people who have not responded to full trials of at least two other antipsychotic medications. All antipsychotics can cause *neuroleptic malignant syndrome,* a rare but severe and potentially fatal reaction consisting of fever, muscle rigidity, mental status changes, and alterations in pulse and blood pressure. They can also cause *tardive dyskinesia,* a potentially irreversible disorder of rhythmical, involuntary muscle movements (see chapter 19 for details of both conditions). Clozapine and other atypical antipsychotics are associated with the development of *weight gain, high cholesterol, and diabetes.* Clozapine and other atypical antipsychotics are also associated with a higher incidence of *strokes* and *sudden death* in elderly people with dementia. **Use extra caution if you have:** *Any bone marrow disorder,* as clozapine can worsen bone marrow function; *breast cancer,* as clozapine can elevate prolactin, a hormone released by the pituitary that may cause breast cancer to grow faster; *epilepsy,* as clozapine may increase the frequency of seizures; *glaucoma,* as clozapine can worsen glaucoma; *liver disease,* as clozapine may worsen impairment of liver functioning; *low blood pressure,* as clozapine can lower blood pressure even further; *heart problems,* as clozapine often causes an elevated heart rate, which can exacerbate heart problems. **Tests before starting:** A complete physical examination, CBC, liver tests, kidney tests, electrolytes, EKG, EEG (optional). **Alcohol:** Should be avoided, as the simultaneous use of clozapine and alcohol can lower blood pressure significantly and cause confusion. Also, alcohol worsens anxiety and depression and impairs insight and judgment.

DRUG INTERACTIONS **Use with extra caution if you take:** *Benzodiazepines,* as the combination may cause you to stop breathing when you first start clozapine. Once stabilized on clozapine, benzodiazepines may be cautiously introduced; *carbamazepine,* as use with clozapine may put you at higher risk of agranulocytosis; *anticonvulsants, antidepressants, antihistamines, antipsychotics, barbiturates,* or any drug that causes sedation or central nervous system depression, because the combination can cause pronounced sedation; *antihypertensives,* as clozapine may lower blood pressure excessively; *antihistamines,* or *antiparkinsonian agents* as they may combine to produce pronounced dry mouth, blurry vision, constipation, low blood pressure, rapid heart rate, and mental confusion.

DOSING Because of the potentially serious side effects that may occur when clozapine is initiated, and the time to onset of effectiveness, many patients and physicians believe clozapine is begun most safely in the hospital. If stopped for more than two days, dosage should be restarted at 12.5 mg/day and increased within a week back to the previous dose. **Adults:** The starting dose is 12.5 mg/day once daily with increases every few days of 25–50 mg/day to achieve a target dose of 300–450 mg/day after two weeks up to a maximum of 900 mg/day. Doses are usually given at night because of sedation, but some people prefer to divide the dose over the course of the day because they find the sedative effect helpful. The incidence of seizures increases with doses over 600 mg/day. Dosages over this amount are sometimes given in combination with an anticonvulsant such as valproate. **Children:** Not FDA-approved for under 18. **The elderly:** The usual starting dose is 12.5 mg/day once a day with increases of

12.5–25 mg every few days. The maximum dose for the elderly has not been determined.

MONITORING YOUR USE **Time to effectiveness:** The first effects may be noticed within some days, but it may take one to three weeks to notice a pronounced change. It may take several months to derive full benefit. **A full trial is:** Eight weeks at no less than 300–500 mg/day. **Half-life of drug and active metabolites:** 8–12 hours. Metabolites are essentially inactive. **How to monitor dosage:** The optimal dose is determined by its effectiveness in alleviating the target symptoms. Blood levels of clozapine may be obtained. A therapeutic range has been suggested, but many people respond best to doses both above and below this range. **How to monitor safety:** (1) A weekly WBC (white blood cell count) every week for six months, then biweekly for six months, then monthly thereafter to monitor for the development of agranulocytosis. If the WBC falls below 3000/microliter or drops more than 3000 over a three-week period, then clozapine should be stopped. Immediate consultation with a hematologist is necessary to manage agranulocytosis and to determine the necessity for treatment with drugs that stimulate the bone marrow to produce more white blood cells. (2) Pretreatment and periodic weight measurements should be performed to assess weight gain; blood glucose, cholesterol, and lipid profiles should be obtained after three months and yearly thereafter to check for diabetes and elevations in cholesterol or triglycerides. (3) A physical examination for the presence of tardive dyskinesia (see below) should be done twice yearly. **If you miss a dose:** Take a missed dose if it's the same day. Do not try to make up for a missed dose the next day by doubling your next dose; just continue with your regular dosing schedule.

SIDE EFFECTS **Usual (50–100%):** Low blood pressure (light-headedness, dizziness), constipation, drooling during sleep, fatigue. **Common (10–50%):** Cholesterol elevations, diabetes, heart rate increase, sexual dysfunction, weight gain. **Less common (1–10%):** Akathisia, bedwetting, dry mouth, headache, menstrual irregularities, nausea, pseudoparkinsonism, sweating, tardive dyskinesia, tremor. **Infrequent (less than 1%):** Pulmonary embolism (a blood clot in your lung, which can impair breathing suddenly—see chapter 19 for details). **Those requiring attention from your physician:** Any sign of infection, such as lethargy, fever, or sore throat, which may be due to agranulocytosis. Symptoms of fever, muscular rigidity, and mental status changes, as you may have neuroleptic malignant syndrome, a potentially severe reaction; any abnormal involuntary movements that suggest tardive dyskinesia; any other physical or emotional changes not described here.

WHAT TO EXPECT IF YOU STOP You may notice a return of your symptoms if clozapine is tapered gradually. **If stopped abruptly:** There is no acute withdrawal syndrome, but symptoms may return quickly.

Cyproheptadine

GENERAL **Preparations:** Generic and brand name Periactin in pills and liquid form. **Class:** Antihistamine. **Used in:** Cyproheptadine improves the ability to achieve orgasm in some people who experience sexual dysfunction induced by SSRIs. It can increase the rate of weight gain in hospitalized patients with anorexia. **Mechanism of action:** Blocks postsynaptic histamine and serotonin receptors.

PRECAUTIONS **Use extra caution if you have:** *Asthma, congestive heart failure, edema, epilepsy, glaucoma, heart disease, hyperthyroidism, low blood pressure, prostatic hypertrophy* or *urinary retention,* as cyproheptadine may worsen the symptoms of these disorders. **Tests needed before starting:** None. **Alcohol:** Should be avoided as the simultaneous use of cyproheptadine and alcohol can lower blood pressure significantly and cause confusion. Also, alcohol worsens anxiety and depression and impairs insight and judgment. **Use in pregnancy:** Infants born to mothers dependent on cyproheptadine may have an increased risk of heart abnormalities.

DRUG INTERACTIONS **Use with extra caution if you take:** *Antihypertensives,* as cyproheptadine may lower blood pressure excessively; *antihistamines, phenothiazines,* or *tricyclic antidepressants,* as they may combine to produce pronounced dry mouth, blurry vision, constipation, low blood pressure, rapid heart rate, and even mental confusion; *MAOI antidepressants,* as they can intensify the side effects of cyproheptadine; *anticonvulsants, antidepressants, antihistamines, antipsychotics, barbiturates, benzodiazepines,* or any drug that causes sedation or central nervous system depression, because the combination can cause pronounced sedation.

DOSING **Adults:** For sexual dysfunction, the usual dose is 4–12 mg one to two hours prior to initiating sexual activity. To increase weight gain in anorexia, amounts up to 32 mg/day in divided doses are used.

MONITORING YOUR USE **Time to effectiveness:** Effects may be noticeable within one to four hours. **A full trial is:** A few tries. **Half-life of drug and active metabolites:** One to four hours with many metabolites of unknown activity. **How to monitor dosage:** The optimal dose is determined by its effectiveness in alleviating the target symptoms. **How to monitor safety:** No special medical tests are needed. **If you miss a dose:** Take a missed dose if it's within an hour or two. Do not try to make up for a missed dose by doubling your next dose; just continue with your regular dosing schedule.

SIDE EFFECTS **Usual (50–100%):** Blurry vision, dizziness, dry mouth, sedation. **Less common (1–10%):** Constipation, headache, low blood pressure, nausea. **Infrequent:** Agitation, urinary retention, visual changes. **Those**

requiring attention from your physician: Any physical or emotional changes not listed.

WHAT TO EXPECT WHEN YOU STOP   You may notice a return of your symptoms if cyproheptadine is stopped.

Desipramine

GENERAL   **Preparations:** Generic and brand name Norpramin. **Class:** Tricyclic antidepressant. **Used in:** ADHD, bulimia, depression, panic disorder, and other anxiety disorders. **Mechanism of action:** Blocks the reuptake of norepinephrine and serotonin into presynaptic neurons.

PRECAUTIONS   **Don't use if you have:** *Heart block* (an abnormal heart rhythm) or if you recently had a *heart attack,* as desipramine may worsen heart block and dangerously affect heart function. **Use extra caution if you have:** *Bipolar disorder,* as desipramine may cause a manic episode; *epilepsy,* as desipramine may increase the frequency of seizures; *glaucoma,* as desipramine can worsen the symptoms of untreated angle closure glaucoma; *low blood pressure;* as desipramine may lower blood pressure further; a *psychotic disorder,* as desipramine may make psychotic symptoms worse; *hyperthyroidism,* as desipramine may cause irregular heart rhythms; *prostatic hypertrophy* or *urinary retention,* as desipramine may worsen urinary retention. **Tests needed before starting:** An electrocardiogram (EKG) if you are over 35, to ensure that you do not have any form of heart block. **Alcohol:** Should be avoided, as the simultaneous use of desipramine and alcohol can lower blood pressure significantly and cause confusion. Also, alcohol worsens anxiety and depression and impairs insight and judgment. **Use in pregnancy:** There is a higher rate of miscarriages born to women who take tricyclics, but no specific defect is associated with their use.

DRUG INTERACTIONS   **Do not use if you take:** *MAOI antidepressants,* as their use with desipramine can cause pronounced hypertension and the potential for strokes. **Use with extra caution if you take:** *Phenothiazines,* as the combination may cause irregular heart rhythms which are potentially fatal; *antihypertensives,* as they may combine to lower blood pressure excessively; *antihistamines, phenothiazines,* and *antiparkinsonian agents,* as they may combine to produce pronounced dry mouth, blurry vision, constipation, low blood pressure, rapid heart rate, and even mental confusion; *guanethadine* to lower blood pressure, as desipramine may block its effects.

DOSING   **Adults:** The usual starting dose is 25 mg at bedtime with increases every other day up to 150 mg. The maximum recommended dose is 300 mg/day. **Children:** It is not recommended for those under 18, as several deaths have been associated with its use. **The elderly:** The usual starting dose is 10 mg at bedtime with increases every few days up to 50–100 mg/day.

MONITORING YOUR USE   **Time to effectiveness:** Side effects are generally noticeable within a few doses, but the therapeutic effect may take two to four weeks. **A full trial is:** Four weeks at the maximum tolerated dosage. **Half-life of drug and active metabolites:** 10–31 hours with no active metabolites. **How to monitor dosage:** The optimal dose is determined by its effectiveness in alleviating the target symptoms. The therapeutic effect of desipramine is more likely when the concentration in the blood is between 150 and 300 micrograms. A blood level may be useful to assist in determining the best dosage if you do not respond or if your side effects are more pronounced than expected. **How to monitor safety:** A blood level should be obtained if doses go over 150 mg/day. An EKG may be useful to ensure that heart function is not impaired. **If you miss a dose:** Take a missed dose if it's within an hour or two. Do not try to make up for a missed dose by doubling your next dose; just continue with your regular dosing schedule.

SIDE EFFECTS   **Usual (50–100%):** Blurry vision, constipation, dry mouth, fatigue, increased heart rate, low blood pressure. **Common (10–50%):** Agitation, sweating, weight gain. **Less common (1–10%):** Insomnia, sexual dysfunction, urinary difficulty. **Those requiring attention from your physician:** Physical or emotional changes not listed, such as suicidal thoughts or behavior.

WHAT TO EXPECT WHEN YOU STOP   You may notice a return of your symptoms if desipramine is stopped. **If stopped abruptly:** You may experience agitation, headaches, insomnia, and nausea, as well as depression. Desipramine should be slowly tapered if you decide to stop it. The rate of discontinuation is different for each person and is determined by the clinical situation necessitating the change, your age, severity of symptoms, dosage size, and your duration of use.

Dextroamphetamine

GENERAL   **Preparations:** Generic and brand name in regular tablets and sustained-release spansules. The brand name Dexedrine contains dextroamphetamine. The brand name Adderall and Adderall XR (extended release) contain dextroamphetamine and amphetamine, which are mirror images of each other. Dextroamphetamine is more potent, but there is some evidence that some people benefit from a combination of both. They will be discussed together as amphetamines, as their properties are virtually equivalent. **Class:** Stimulant. **Used in:** ADD (developmental disorders). **Mechanism of action:** Releases dopamine and norepinephrine from presynaptic neurons. At high doses it also causes the release of serotonin.

PRECAUTIONS   Warnings: *Abuse potential.* Amphetamines have been extensively abused for their stimulant effects of euphoria and increased energy. Extreme psychological dependence has occurred in some individuals, who may exhibit insomnia, irritability, hyperactivity, and personality changes. **Don't use if you have:** *Heart disease,* as amphetamines can cause an elevated heart rate; *hypertension,* as amphetamines can elevate blood pressure; *hyperthyroidism,* as amphetamines can cause a further elevation of heart rate; *glaucoma,* as amphetamines can worsen the symptoms; *Tourette's disorder* or *tics,* as amphetamines can worsen tics. **Use extra caution if you have:** *Bipolar disorder,* as amphetamines can cause a manic episode; *epilepsy,* as amphetamines may increase the frequency of seizures; a *psychotic disorder,* as amphetamines can worsen psychotic symptoms. **Tests needed before starting:** None. **Alcohol:** The simultaneous use of amphetamines and alcohol causes no specific adverse consequences, but alcohol should be avoided because it worsens anxiety and depression and impairs judgment and thinking. **Use in pregnancy:** Infants born to mothers dependent on amphetamines have an increased risk of premature delivery and low birth weight.

DRUG INTERACTIONS   Do not use if you take: *MAOI antidepressants,* as their use with amphetamines can cause pronounced hypertension and the potential for strokes.

DOSING   Adults: The usual starting dose is 5 mg twice daily with weekly increases of 10 mg up to a maximum of 1 mg/kilogram of body weight. **Children:** The usual starting dose for children over age five is 5 mg once or twice daily, with increases of 5 mg/week up to a maximum of 40 mg/day. Children over three are started on 2.5 mg/day, with weekly increases of 2.5 mg/day.

MONITORING YOUR USE   Time to effectiveness: Some effects are noticeable within a few doses. **A full trial is:** Four weeks at the maximum dose. **Half-life of drug and active metabolites:** 6–8 hours in children; 8–10 in adults. There are no active metabolites. **How to monitor dosage:** The optimal dose is determined by its effectiveness in alleviating the target symptoms. **How to monitor safety:** Weight and height should be monitored regularly, as amphetamines may slow growth. Examination for tics should occur regularly. **If you miss a dose:** Take a missed dose if it's within an hour or two. Do not try to make up for a missed dose by doubling your next dose; just continue with your regular dosing schedule.

SIDE EFFECTS   Common (10–50%): Abdominal pain, insomnia, tremor, headaches, dry mouth, decreased appetite with weight loss, palpitations, blood pressure increase. **Less common (1–10%):** Tics, growth suppression, psychosis with prolonged excessive use. **Those requiring attention from your physician:** Physical or emotional changes not listed.

WHAT TO EXPECT WHEN YOU STOP   You may notice a return of your symptoms if amphetamines are stopped. **If stopped abruptly:** After prolonged use at a high dose, abrupt cessation can cause fatigue and depression.

Diazepam

GENERAL   **Preparations:** Generic and brand name Valium. **Class:** Benzodiazepine. **Used in:** Anxiety disorders, bipolar disorder (alcohol withdrawal, Alzheimer's disease, antipsychotic-induced akathisia [restlessness], insomnia). **Mechanism of action:** Intensifies the effects of gamma-aminobutyric acid (GABA).

PRECAUTIONS   **Warnings:** *It is habit-forming.* Diazepam, like all benzodiazepines, is physically and psychologically habit-forming. People who have experienced traumatic events in their lives and have chronic anxiety are especially prone to developing dependence. Prolonged use is associated with a range of problems. Use for more than four weeks is *not* recommended. If you stop diazepam after more than four weeks of daily use you will probably experience withdrawal symptoms (see below). *Seizures can occur if it is stopped abruptly,* so consultation with your physician is essential if you wish to stop. **Tests needed before starting:** None. **Alcohol:** Alcohol must be avoided entirely. The simultaneous use of diazepam and alcohol is extremely dangerous because it can cause you to stop breathing. The combination can cause death. **Use in pregnancy:** There is a higher rate of babies born with a cleft palate to mothers who took benzodiazepines during pregnancy. **The elderly** are especially sensitive to the effects of benzodiazepines and may experience pronounced side effects at low doses (see chapter 4).

DRUG INTERACTIONS   **Use with extra caution if you take:** *Anticonvulsants, antidepressants, antihistamines, antipsychotics, barbiturates, benzodiazepines,* or any drug that causes sedation or central nervous system depression, because the combination with diazepam can cause pronounced sedation.

DOSING   **Adults:** The usual starting dose is 2–10 mg two to four times a day depending on the severity of the symptoms. The maximum dose is 40 mg/day. **Children:** The usual starting dose is 1–2.5 mg three to four times a day only for seizures. The FDA has not approved it for anxiety in children.

MONITORING YOUR USE   **Time to effectiveness:** 30–60 minutes. **A full trial is:** A few doses are generally enough to establish whether it will be helpful. **Half-life of drug and active metabolites:** 30–60 hours with several active metabolites. **How to monitor dosage:** The optimal dose is determined by its effectiveness in alleviating the target symptoms. **If you miss a dose:** Do *not* try to make up for a missed dose; just continue with your regular dosing schedule. **How to monitor safety:** No specific medical tests are needed to monitor safety.

SIDE EFFECTS   Common (10–50%): Sedation, memory impairment, poor muscle coordination (causing a higher rate of falls in the elderly and a higher risk of motor vehicle accidents in all adults). **Infrequent (less than 1%):** Paradoxical agitation and insomnia. **Those requiring attention from your physician:** Any physical or emotional changes not described here. **Side effects associated with use longer than four weeks:** Use of diazepam longer than four weeks may cause physical and psychological dependence, and you may notice the desire for another dose as each one wears off. Ongoing anxiety, reduced effectiveness of each dose, depression, emotional blunting, and impairment of memory and cognition may occur with use longer than one year.

WHAT TO EXPECT WHEN YOU STOP   You may notice a return of your symptoms if diazepam is tapered gradually. Other withdrawal symptoms include anxiety, insomnia, irritability, headaches, tremors, nausea, diarrhea, sweating, and confusion. The rate at which you should taper is affected by the duration of your use and the size of your dose, but may take months if you have been on it for an extended period of time. **If stopped abruptly:** *Seizures* can occur if diazepam is stopped abruptly. They are potentially life-threatening. You should never stop diazepam abruptly and you should always work with your physician to taper it gradually.

Diphenhydramine

GENERAL   **Preparations:** Generic and brand name Benadryl in pills and liquid form. **Class:** Antihistamine. **Used in:** Insomnia, antipsychotic-induced dystonia (pseudoparkinsonism). **Mechanism of action:** Blocks postsynaptic histamine receptors.

PRECAUTIONS   **Use extra caution if you have:** *Asthma, congestive heart failure, edema, epilepsy, glaucoma, heart disease, hyperthyroidism, low blood pressure, peptic ulcer disease, enlarged prostate* or *urinary retention,* as diphenhydramine can worsen the symptoms of these disorders. **Tests needed before starting:** None. **Alcohol:** Should be avoided as the simultaneous use of diphenhydramine and alcohol can lower blood pressure significantly and cause confusion. Also, alcohol worsens anxiety and depression and impairs insight and judgment.

DRUG INTERACTIONS   **Use with extra caution if you take:** *Antihypertensives,* as diphenhydramine may lower blood pressure excessively; *antihistamines, phenothiazines,* or *tricyclic antidepressants,* as they may combine to produce pronounced dry mouth, blurry vision, constipation, low blood pressure, rapid heart rate, and even mental confusion; *MAOI antidepressants,* as they can intensify the side effects of diphenhydramine; *anticonvulsants, antidepressants, antihistamines, antipsychotics, barbiturates, benzodiazepines,* or any drug that causes sedation or central nervous system depression, because the combination can cause pronounced sedation.

DOSING **Adults:** The usual dose for dystonia is 25–50 mg administered by injection either intramuscularly or intravenously, with repeated dosing up to 100 mg if required. The maximum daily dose is 400 mg/day. The usual dose for pseudoparkinsonism is 25–50 mg one to four times a day. The usual dose for insomnia is 25–50 mg 30 minutes before bedtime. **Children:** 5 mg/kg day.

MONITORING YOUR USE **Time to effectiveness:** Effects are noticeable within one hour. **A full trial is:** A few days at the maximum dose. **Half-life of drug and active metabolites:** 2–8 hours with no active metabolites. **How to monitor dosage:** The optimal dose is determined by its effectiveness in alleviating the target symptoms. **How to monitor safety:** No special medical tests are needed. **If you miss a dose:** Take a missed dose if it's within an hour or two. Do not try to make up for a missed dose by doubling your next dose; just continue with your regular dosing schedule.

SIDE EFFECTS **Usual (50–100%):** Dry mouth, sedation. **Less common (1–10%):** Blurry vision, constipation, dizziness, headache, low blood pressure, nausea. **Infrequent:** Agitation, urinary retention, visual changes. **Those requiring attention from your physician:** Any physical or emotional changes not listed.

WHAT TO EXPECT WHEN YOU STOP You may notice a return of your symptoms if it is stopped.

Disulfiram

GENERAL **Preparations:** Generic and brand name Antabuse. **Class:** Alcohol deterrent. **Used in:** Alcohol dependence. **Mechanism of action:** Disulfiram inactivates aldehyde dehydrogenase, thereby changing the way your body metabolizes alcohol.

PRECAUTIONS **Warnings:** If you drink alcohol after taking it, acetaldehyde will build up, leading you to experience flushing, a headache, shortness of breath, nausea, vomiting, sweating, thirst, chest pain, rapid heart rate, agitation, and confusion. When severe, you may experience impairment of breathing and heart function, convulsions, and even death. The severity of the reaction is influenced by the amount of disulfiram and alcohol in your system. **Don't use if you have:** *Heart problems,* as the disulfiram-alcohol reaction can place an extra strain on the heart. **Use with extra caution if you have:** *Diabetes, epilepsy, hypothyroidism, kidney* or *liver problems,* as an accidental disulfiram-alcohol reaction may impair your health further. **Tests needed before starting:** None.

DRUG INTERACTIONS **Don't use if you take:** *Any alcohol-containing medication; isoniazid,* as your gait may be impaired.

DOSING   **Adults:** 250–500 mg daily is the starting and maintenance dose.

MONITORING YOUR USE   **Time to effectiveness:** Immediate. **A full trial:** Lasts until a reaction occurs, in which case disulfiram can be deemed insufficient and too dangerous to try again. It can also be stopped if abstinence can be maintained through other means. **Half-life of drug and active metabolites:** Sensitization to the effects of disulfiram can last as long as two weeks. **How to monitor dosage:** No specific tests are used to adjust dosage. **How to monitor safety:** No tests are needed to monitor safety. If any symptoms of a reaction occur, immediate medical attention is required. **If you miss a dose:** Take a missed dose if it's in the same day. Do not try to make up for a missed dose by doubling your next dose; just continue with your regular dosing schedule.

SIDE EFFECTS   **Less common (1–10%):** Acne, headaches, rash, sedation. **Those requiring attention from your physician:** Symptoms suggesting hepatitis: yellow eyes, yellow skin, abdominal pain. Any other physical or emotional changes not noted.

WHAT TO EXPECT WHEN YOU STOP   There is generally no reaction to stopping disulfiram.

Donepezil

GENERAL   **Preparations:** Brand name Aricept only. **Class:** Cognitive enhancer. **Used in:** Alzheimer's disease. **Mechanism of action:** Inhibits the enzyme cholinesterase, which breaks down acetylcholine.

PRECAUTIONS   **Use extra caution if you have:** *Asthma or other lung disease, epilepsy, heart block,* or *ulcers,* as donepezil may worsen the medical problem; *liver problems,* as it may lead to higher levels of donepezil. **Tests needed before starting:** The diagnosis of Alzheimer's needs to be established through a neurological and physical exam, neuropsychological testing, or a brain imaging study. A complete physical examination should be done to ensure that there are no active medical problems that would preclude the use of donepezil. **Alcohol:** Although there are no specific adverse consequences when alcohol and donepezil are combined, the use of alcohol should be avoided since it impairs thinking and judgment.

DRUG INTERACTIONS   **Use with extra caution if you take:** *Nonsteroidal anti-inflammatory drugs like aspirin, ibuprofen (Motrin),* or *naproxen (Aleve),* as the combination may cause stomach bleeding.

DOSING   **Adults:** The starting and maintenance dose is 5–10 mg once daily. 10 mg/day may or may not be more effective, and it may result in more side effects.

MONITORING YOUR USE   Time to effectiveness: As there is no immediate obvious effect, there is no objective way to assess whether or not it is having a
positive effect. It is reasonable to begin it as soon as the diagnosis is clear and as
long as any memory function remains. **A full trial:** Lasts until there is minimal
memory function remaining. **Half-life of drug and active metabolites:** 70 hours,
with at least two active metabolites. **How to monitor dosage:** The optimal dose is
determined by the absence of side effects. **If you miss a dose:** Do *not* try to make
up for a missed dose; just continue with your regular dosing schedule. **How to
monitor safety:** Monitor weight.

SIDE EFFECTS   Common (10–50%): Diarrhea, headaches, nausea. **Less
common (1–10%):** Decreased appetite, dizziness, insomnia, muscle cramps.
Those requiring attention from your physician: Any physical, cognitive, or
emotional change not noted here.

WHAT TO EXPECT WHEN YOU STOP   There may be a further impairment in memory. **If stopped abruptly:** There is no specific withdrawal syndrome
beyond the loss of effectiveness.

Doxepin

GENERAL   Preparations Generic and brand name Sinequan in pills and liquid
form. **Class:** Tricyclic antidepressant. **Used in:** Bulimia, depression, panic disorder, and other anxiety disorders. **Mechanism of action:** Blocks the reuptake of
norepinephrine and serotonin into presynaptic neurons.

PRECAUTIONS   Don't use if you have: *Heart block* (an abnormal heart
rhythm) or if you recently had a *heart attack,* as doxepin may worsen heart block
and dangerously affect heart function. **Use extra caution if you have:** *Bipolar disorder,* as doxepin may cause a manic episode; *epilepsy,* as doxepin may increase
the frequency of seizures; *glaucoma,* as doxepin can worsen the symptoms of untreated angle closure glaucoma; *low blood pressure,* as doxepin may lower blood
pressure further; a *psychotic disorder,* as doxepin may make psychotic symptoms
worse; *hyperthyroidism,* as doxepin may cause irregular heart rhythms; *prostatic
hypertrophy* or *urinary retention,* as doxepin may worsen urinary retention. **Tests
needed before starting:** An electrocardiogram (EKG) if you are over 35, to ensure that you do not have any form of heart block. **Alcohol:** Should be avoided, as
the simultaneous use of doxepin and alcohol can lower blood pressure significantly and cause confusion. Also, alcohol worsens anxiety and depression, and
impairs insight and judgment. **Use in pregnancy:** There is a higher rate of miscarriages born to women who take tricyclics, but no specific defect is associated with
their use.

DRUG INTERACTIONS   Do not use if you take: *MAOI antidepressants,* as their use with doxepin can cause pronounced hypertension and the potential for strokes. **Use with extra caution if you take:** *Phenothiazines,* as the combination may cause irregular heart rhythms that are potentially fatal; *antihypertensives,* as they may combine to lower blood pressure excessively; *antihistamines, phenothiazines,* and *antiparkinsonian agents,* as they may combine to produce pronounced dry mouth, blurry vision, constipation, low blood pressure, rapid heart rate, and even mental confusion; *guanethadine* to lower blood pressure, as doxepin may block its effects.

DOSING   Adults: The usual starting dose is 25 mg at bedtime with increases every other day up to 150 mg. The maximum recommended dose is 300 mg/day. **Children:** Not FDA-approved for under 12. **The elderly:** The usual starting dose is 10 mg at bedtime with increases every few days up to 50–100 mg/day.

MONITORING YOUR USE   Time to effectiveness: Side effects are generally noticeable within a few doses, but the therapeutic effect may take two to four weeks. **A full trial is:** Four weeks at the maximum tolerated dosage. **Half-life of drug and active metabolites:** 8–47 hours, with several active metabolites. **How to monitor dosage:** The optimal dose is determined by its effectiveness in alleviating the target symptoms. The therapeutic effect of doxepin is more likely when the concentration in the blood is between 150 and 300 micrograms. A blood level may be useful to assist in determining the best dosage if you do not respond or if your side effects are more pronounced than expected. **How to monitor safety:** A blood level should be obtained if doses go over 150 mg/day. An EKG may be useful to ensure that heart function is not impaired. **If you miss a dose:** Take a missed dose if it's within an hour or two. Do not try to make up for a missed dose by doubling your next dose; just continue with your regular dosing schedule.

SIDE EFFECTS   Usual (50–100%): Blurry vision, constipation, dry mouth, fatigue, increased heart rate, low blood pressure. **Common (10–50%):** Agitation, sweating, weight gain. **Less common (1–10%):** Insomnia, sexual dysfunction, urinary retention. **Those requiring attention from your physician:** Physical or emotional changes not listed, such as suicidal thoughts or behavior.

WHAT TO EXPECT WHEN YOU STOP   You may notice a return of your symptoms if doxepin is stopped. **If stopped abruptly:** You may experience agitation, headaches, insomnia, and nausea, as well as depression. Doxepin should be slowly tapered if you decide to stop it. The rate of discontinuation is different for each person and is determined by the clinical situation necessitating the change, your age, severity of symptoms, dosage size, and your duration of use.

Duloxetine

GENERAL **Preparations:** Brand name Cymbalta only in sustained release. **Class:** Antidepressant. **Used in:** Depression. **Mechanism of action:** Blocks the reuptake of norepinephrine and serotonin into presynaptic neurons.

PRECAUTIONS **Use extra caution if you have:** *Bipolar disorder*, as duloxetine can cause a manic episode; e*pilepsy,* as duloxetine may increase the frequency of seizures; *glaucoma,* as duloxetine can worsen the symptoms; *high blood pressure,* as duloxetine can increase blood pressure; *kidney or liver disease,* as levels of duloxetine can build up too high in your system and can cause further liver damage; *a psychotic disorder,* as duloxetine can worsen psychotic symptoms. **Tests needed before starting:** None. **Alcohol:** Duloxetine can cause liver damage in people who drink substantial amounts of alcohol. On its own, alcohol can worsen anxiety and depression. Alcohol should be avoided entirely. **Use in pregnancy:** Some babies exposed during pregnancy to medications similar to duloxetine (such as SSRIs) have developed significant problems upon birth that could be due to the medication or its discontinuance. Reactions can include breathing problems, temperature instability, metabolic abnormalities, seizures, irritability, and constant crying.

DRUG INTERACTIONS **Don't use if you take:** *Other SSRIs, St. John's wort,* or *tryptophan* or other serotonin reuptake inhibitors, as duloxetine can cause the *serotonin syndrome,* which consists of potentially dangerous alterations in pulse, blood pressure, hyperactivity, and mental status changes (see chapter 19); *MAOI antidepressants,* as their use with duloxetine can cause a serious, sometimes fatal, reaction of agitation, fever, cardiovascular changes, and mental status changes.

DOSING **Adults:** The usual starting dose is 20 mg two times daily, with weekly increases of 20 mg/day up to a maximum of 120 mg daily. **Children:** Not FDA-approved for under 18.

MONITORING YOUR USE **Time to effectiveness:** You may notice some side effects within one to two days, but any improvement in symptoms generally takes two to four weeks. **A full trial is:** Four weeks at the maximum dose. **Half-life of drug and active metabolites:** 12 hours. **How to monitor dosage:** The optimal dose is determined by its effectiveness in alleviating the target symptoms. **How to monitor safety:** Pulse and blood pressure should be monitored regularly until the dose is stabilized. **If you miss a dose:** Take a missed dose if it's within an hour or two. Do not try to make up for a missed dose the next day by doubling your dose; just continue with your regular dosing schedule.

SIDE EFFECTS **Common (10–50%):** Decreased appetite, anxiety, constipation, dizziness, dry mouth, fatigue, headache, insomnia, nausea, sweating, sexual dysfunction, urinary hesitancy, and weight loss. **Less common (1–10%):** Blurry vision, tremor. **Rare:** Suicidal thoughts. **Those requiring attention by your physician:** Hyperactivity, mental status changes, or alterations in your pulse or blood pressure, which suggest the serotonin syndrome; any physical or emotional changes not listed, such as suicidal thoughts or behavior.

WHAT TO EXPECT WHEN YOU STOP   You may notice a return of your symptoms if duloxetine is tapered gradually. **If stopped abruptly:** You may notice a flulike syndrome of nausea, vomiting, diarrhea, and dizziness, as well as anxiety and depression. Duloxetine should not be stopped abruptly, but needs to be gradually tapered in consultation with your physician.

Escitalopram

GENERAL   **Preparations:** Brand name Lexapro only. **Class:** SSRI (selective serotonin reuptake inhibitor). **Used in:** Bulimia, depression, panic disorder, and other anxiety disorders (obsessive-compulsive disorder, developmental disorders). **Mechanism of action:** Blocks the reuptake of serotonin by presynaptic neurons.

PRECAUTIONS   **Warnings:** When taken with other serotonin reuptake inhibitors, escitalopram can cause the *serotonin syndrome,* which consists of potentially dangerous alterations in pulse, blood pressure, hyperactivity, and mental status changes (see chapter 19). Rarely, escitalopram can cause *hyponatremia,* or low sodium in your blood. **Use extra caution if you have:** *Bipolar disorder,* as escitalopram can cause a manic episode; *epilepsy,* as escitalopram may increase the frequency of seizures; *a psychotic disorder,* as escitalopram can worsen psychotic symptoms. **Tests needed before starting:** None. **Alcohol:** The simultaneous use of escitalopram and alcohol causes no specific adverse consequences, but alcohol should be avoided because it worsens anxiety and depression. **Use in pregnancy:** There is a higher rate of miscarriages, heart defects, and intestinal defects in the babies of women who take escitalopram during pregnancy.

DRUG INTERACTIONS   **Don't use if you take:** *Other SSRIs, St. John's wort,* or *tryptophan,* as their use with escitalopram can cause the *serotonin syndrome; MAOI antidepressants,* as their use with escitalopram can cause a serious, sometimes fatal, reaction of agitation, fever, cardiovascular changes, and mental status changes.

DOSING   **Adults:** The usual starting dose is 10 mg once daily, with weekly increases of 10 mg/day up to a maximum of 30 mg/day. **Children:** Not FDA-approved for under 18. **The elderly:** The starting dose is 5–10 mg/day, with an increase of 5 mg weekly up to a maximum of 20 mg/day.

MONITORING YOUR USE   Time to effectiveness: You may notice some side effects within one to two days, but any improvement in symptoms generally takes two to four weeks. **A full trial is:** Four weeks at the maximum dose. **Half-life of drug and active metabolites:** 33 hours. Metabolites are essentially inactive. **How to monitor dosage:** The optimal dose is determined by its effectiveness in alleviating the target symptoms. **How to monitor safety:** No specific tests are needed to monitor your health while on escitalopram. **If you miss a dose:** Take a missed dose if it's the same day. Do not try to make up for a missed dose the next day by doubling your next dose; just continue with your regular dosing schedule.

SIDE EFFECTS   Common (10–50%): Dry mouth, fatigue, insomnia, nausea, weakness, sweating, and sexual dysfunction. **Less common (1–10%):** Anxiety, diarrhea, headaches, low blood pressure, menstrual irregularities, rash, tremor. **Those requiring attention by your physician:** Hyperactivity, mental status changes, or alterations in your pulse or blood pressure, which suggest the serotonin syndrome; physical or emotional changes not listed, such as suicidal thoughts or behavior.

WHAT TO EXPECT WHEN YOU STOP   You may notice a return of your symptoms if escitalopram is tapered gradually. **If stopped abruptly:** You may notice a flulike syndrome of nausea, vomiting, diarrhea, and dizziness, as well as anxiety and depression. Escitalopram should not be stopped abruptly, but needs to be gradually tapered in consultation with your physician.

Estazolam

GENERAL   Preparations: Generic and brand name ProSom. **Class:** Benzodiazepine. **Used in:** Insomnia. **Mechanism of action:** Intensifies the effects of gamma-aminobutyric acid (GABA).

PRECAUTIONS   Warnings: *It is habit-forming.* Estazolam, like all benzodiazepines, is physically and psychologically habit-forming. People who have experienced traumatic events in their lives and have chronic anxiety are especially prone to developing dependence. Prolonged use is associated with a range of problems. Use for more than four weeks is *not* recommended. If you stop estazolam after more than four weeks of daily use you will probably experience withdrawal symptoms (see below). **Tests needed before starting:** None. **Alcohol:** Alcohol must be avoided entirely. The simultaneous use of estazolam and alcohol is extremely dangerous because it can cause you to stop breathing. The combination can cause death. **Use in pregnancy:** There is a higher rate of babies born with a cleft palate to mothers who took benzodiazepines during pregnancy. **The elderly** are especially sensitive to the effects of benzodiazepines and may experience pronounced side effects at low doses (see chapter 4).

DRUG INTERACTIONS   Use with extra caution if you take: *Anticonvulsants, antidepressants, antihistamines, antipsychotics, barbiturates, benzodiazepines,* or any drug that causes sedation or central nervous system depression, because the combination with estazolam can cause pronounced sedation.

DOSING   Adults: 1–2 mg at bedtime. **Children:** Not FDA-approved for under 18. **The elderly:** 0.5–1 mg at bedtime.

MONITORING YOUR USE   Time to effectiveness: 30–60 minutes. **A full trial is:** A few doses, which are generally enough to establish whether it will be helpful. **Half-life of drug and active metabolites:** 10–24 hours with no active metabolites. **How to monitor dosage:** The optimal dose is determined by its effectiveness in alleviating the target symptoms. **If you miss a dose:** Do *not* try to make up for a missed dose, just continue with your regular dosing schedule. **How to monitor safety:** No specific medical tests are needed to monitor safety.

SIDE EFFECTS   Common (10–50%): Daytime fatigue, memory impairment, poor muscle coordination (causing a higher rate of falls in the elderly and a higher risk of motor vehicle accidents in all adults). **Infrequent (less than 1%):** Paradoxical agitation, anxiety, and insomnia. **Those requiring attention from your physician:** Any physical or emotional changes not described here. **Side effects associated with use longer than four weeks:** Use of estazolam longer than four weeks may cause physical and psychological dependence, and you may notice the desire for another dose as each one wears off. Ongoing anxiety, reduced effectiveness of each dose, depression, emotional blunting, and impairment of memory and cognition may occur with use longer than one year.

WHAT TO EXPECT WHEN YOU STOP   You may notice a return of your symptoms if estazolam is tapered gradually. Other withdrawal symptoms include anxiety, insomnia, irritability, headaches, tremors, nausea, diarrhea, sweating, and confusion. **If stopped abruptly:** *Seizures* can occur if estazolam is stopped abruptly, although this is extremely unlikely with routine use at recommended doses. Seizures are potentially life-threatening. As a result you should always consult with your physician about how to stop it safely.

Eszopiclone

GENERAL   Preparations: Brand name Lunesta only. **Class:** Hypnotic (sleeping aid). **Used in:** Insomnia. **Mechanism of action:** Interacts with gamma-aminobutyric acid (GABA) receptors.

PRECAUTIONS   Warnings: It may be habit-forming. **Use extra caution if you have:** *Liver problems,* as the breakdown of eszopiclone may be impaired leading to a more intense effect. **Tests needed before starting:** None. **Alcohol:** Alcohol should be avoided entirely, as the combination with eszopiclone may cause you to stop breathing. **The elderly** are especially sensitive to the effects of hypnotics and may experience pronounced side effects at low doses (see chapter 4).

DRUG INTERACTIONS   **Use with extra caution if you take:** *Clarithromicin (Biaxin), itraconozole (Sporonox), ketoconazole (Nizoril), nefazodone (Serzone), nelfinavir (Viracept), ritonavir (Norvir), or troleandomycin (Tao)* because the breakdown of eszopiclone may be impaired, leading to a more intense effect; *anticonvulsants, antidepressants, antihistamines, antipsychotics, barbiturates, benzodiazepines,* or any drug that causes sedation or central nervous system depression, because the combination with eszopiclone can cause pronounced sedation.

DOSING   **Adults:** The usual starting dose is 2 mg at bedtime, up to a maximum of 3 mg. **Children:** Not FDA-approved for under 18. **The elderly:** The usual starting dose is 1 mg at bedtime.

MONITORING YOUR USE   **Time to effectiveness:** 30–60 minutes. **Half-life of drug and active metabolites:** 6 hours with one minimally active metabolite. **How to monitor dosage:** The optimal dose is determined by its effectiveness in alleviating insomnia.

SIDE EFFECTS   **Common (10–50%):** Dry mouth, daytime fatigue, headache, hallucinations, impaired coordination, light-headedness, memory impairment. **Less common (1–10%):** Dizziness. **Those requiring attention by your physician:** Physical or emotional changes not listed.

WHAT TO EXPECT WHEN YOU STOP   You may notice anxiety, abnormal dreams, insomnia, or upset stomach.

Fluoxetine

GENERAL   **Preparations:** Generic, brand names Prozac, Sarafem, and, in combiniation with olanzapine, Symbyax. **Class:** SSRI (selective serotonin reuptake inhibitor). **Used in:** Bulimia, depression, obsessive-compulsive disorder, panic disorder, and other anxiety disorders (ADHD, developmental disorders). **Mechanism of action:** Blocks the reuptake of serotonin by presynaptic neurons.

PRECAUTIONS   **Warnings:** When taken with other serotonin reuptake inhibitors, fluoxetine can cause the *serotonin syndrome,* which consists of potentially dangerous alterations in pulse, blood pressure, hyperactivity, and mental status changes (see chapter 19). Rarely, fluoxetine can cause hyponatremia, or low sodium in your blood. **Use extra caution if you have:** *Bipolar disorder,* as fluoxetine can cause a manic episode; *diabetes,* as fluoxetine may alter control of sugar; *epilepsy,* as fluoxetine may increase the frequency of seizures; a *psychotic disorder,* as fluoxetine can worsen psychotic symptoms. **Tests needed before starting:** None. **Alcohol:** The simultaneous use of fluoxetine and alcohol causes no specific adverse consequences, but alcohol should be avoided because it worsens anxiety and depression. **Use in pregnancy:** There is a higher rate of miscarriages, heart defects, and intestinal defects in the babies of women who take fluoxetine during pregnancy.

DRUG INTERACTIONS   Don't use if you take: *Other SSRIs, St. John's wort,* or *tryptophan* as their use with fluoxetine can cause the *serotonin syndrome; MAOI antidepressants,* as their use with fluoxetine can cause a serious, sometimes fatal, reaction of agitation, fever, cardiovascular changes, and mental status changes.

DOSING   Adults: The usual starting dose is 10–20 mg once daily with increases after one month of 10–20 mg/day every one to two weeks, up to a maximum of 80 mg/day. **Children:** Not FDA-approved for under 18.

MONITORING YOUR USE   Time to effectiveness: You may notice some side effects within one to two days, but any improvement in symptoms generally takes two to four weeks. **A full trial is:** Four weeks at the maximum dose. **Half-life of drug and active metabolites:** One to three days. The half-life of a major active metabolite is 7–15 days. **How to monitor dosage:** The optimal dose is determined by its effectiveness in alleviating the target symptoms. **How to monitor safety:** No specific tests are needed to monitor your health while on fluoxetine. **If you miss a dose:** Take a missed dose if it's the same day. Do not try to make up for a missed dose the next day by doubling your dose; just continue with your regular dosing schedule.

SIDE EFFECTS   Common (10–50%): Fatigue, nausea, weakness, sweating, decreased appetite, rash, sexual dysfunction. **Less common (1–10%):** Agitation, insomnia, anxiety, tremor. **Those requiring attention from your physician:** Hyperactivity, mental status changes, or alterations in your pulse or blood pressure, which suggest the serotonin syndrome. Any physical or emotional changes not listed, such as suicidal thoughts or behavior.

WHAT TO EXPECT WHEN YOU STOP   You may notice a return of your symptoms if fluoxetine is tapered gradually. **If stopped abruptly: You may notice a flulike syndrome of nausea, vomiting, diarrhea, dizziness, as well as anxiety and depression. Fluoxetine should not be stopped abruptly, but needs to be gradually tapered in consultation with your physician.

Fluphenazine

GENERAL **Preparations:** Generic and brand name Prolixin in pills and liquid form; brand name only in long-acting injectable concentrate. **Class:** Standard antipsychotic of the phenothiazine group. **Used in:** Bipolar disorder, psychotic disorders (Alzheimer's disease, severe anxiety). **Mechanism of action:** Blocks postsynaptic dopamine receptors.

PRECAUTIONS **Warnings:** All antipsychotics can cause *neuroleptic malignant syndrome,* a rare, but severe and potentially fatal reaction consisting of fever, muscle rigidity, mental status changes, and alterations in pulse and blood pressure. They can also cause *tardive dyskinesia,* a potentially irreversible disorder of rhythmical, involuntary muscle movements (see chapter 19 for details of both conditions). **Use extra caution if you have:** *Breast cancer,* as fluphenazine can elevate prolactin, a hormone released by the pituitary that may cause breast cancer to grow faster; *epilepsy,* as fluphenazine may increase the frequency of seizures; *glaucoma, low blood pressure, prostatic hypertrophy,* or *urinary retention* as the symptoms of these disorders may worsen. **Tests before starting:** None. **Alcohol:** Should be avoided, as the simultaneous use of fluphenazine and alcohol can lower blood pressure significantly and cause confusion. Also, alcohol worsens anxiety and depression, and impairs insight and judgment. **Use in pregnancy:** Phenothiazines have been linked with the "floppy infant syndrome," in which the baby has poor muscle tone. The fetus may experience pseudoparkinsonism and dystonia, muscular side effects that may cause fetal distress before, during, and shortly after birth. **Sunlight:** Severe sunburns can occur on fluphenazine. Avoid sunbathing entirely and avoid casual exposure to the sun for more than thirty minutes. Use a sunblock with sun protection factor (SPF) of 15 or more if exposure to the sun cannot be avoided.

DRUG INTERACTIONS **Use with extra caution if you take:** *Tricyclic antidepressants,* as the combination may cause irregular heart rhythms that are potentially fatal; *anticonvulsants, antidepressants, antihistamines, antipsychotics, barbiturates, benzodiazepines,* or any drug that causes sedation or central nervous system depression, because the combination can cause pronounced sedation; *antihypertensive medication,* as fluphenazine may combine to lower blood pressure excessively; *antihistamines,* or *antiparkinsonian agents,* as they may combine to produce pronounced dry mouth, blurry vision, constipation, low blood pressure, rapid heart rate, and mental confusion.

DOSING **Adults:** The starting dose is 2–10 mg a day, with weekly increases of 5 mg/day up to a maximum of 10–30 mg/day. Fluphenazine decanoate and fluphenazine enanthenate preparations are given by injection intramuscularly with dosages of 12.5–50 mg every one to four weeks. **Children:** Not FDA-approved for under 16. Some child psychiatrists recommend doses of 2.5–10 mg/day.

MONITORING YOUR USE **Time to effectiveness:** Calming effects are often noticed within one to three hours of a dose, but several days may be needed to notice any effect on psychotic symptoms. A pronounced effect may take one to two weeks. Many months may be needed to derive full benefit. The long-acting forms take two days to begin effectiveness. **A full trial is:** Four weeks at no less than 10 mg/day. **Half-life of drug and active metabolites:** 20–40 hours with many active metabolites. The half-life of the enanthenate preparation is 2–3 days, that of the decanoate 7–10 days. **How to monitor dosage:** The optimal dose is determined by its effectiveness in alleviating the target symptoms. **How to monitor safety:** Examination for the presence of tardive dyskinesia (see below) should be performed twice yearly. **If you miss a dose:** Take a missed dose if it's the same day. Do not try to make up for a missed dose the next day by doubling your dose; just continue with your regular dosing schedule.

SIDE EFFECTS **Usual (50–100%):** Dry mouth, constipation, blurry vision. **Common (10–50%):** Low blood pressure (light-headedness, dizziness), fatigue, ataraxia (zombielike feeling), weight gain, menstrual irregularities, akathisia (restlessness), sexual dysfunction, pseudoparkinsonism (muscular tremor, rigidity, akinesia), and tardive dyskinesia, a form of involuntary muscle movements (see chapter 19 for further details). **Less common (1–10%):** Dystonia (muscle spasms, usually of the head and neck, face, and jaw), galactorrhea (milk leaking from breasts) sexual dysfunction. **Infrequent (less than 1%):** Cataracts, urinary difficulty; jaundice (yellow skin or eyes). **Those requiring attention from your physician:** Symptoms of fever, muscular rigidity, and mental status changes, as you may have neuroleptic malignant syndrome, a potentially severe reaction; any abnormal involuntary movements that suggest tardive dyskinesia; any other physical or emotional changes not described here.

WHAT TO EXPECT WHEN YOU STOP You may notice a return of your symptoms if fluphenazine is tapered gradually. **If stopped abruptly:** There is no acute withdrawal syndrome.

Flurazepam

GENERAL **Preparations:** Generic and brand name Dalmane. **Class:** Benzodiazepine. **Mechanism of action:** Intensifies the effects of gamma-aminobutyric acid (GABA). **Used in:** Insomnia.

PRECAUTIONS **Warnings:** *It is habit-forming.* Flurazepam, like all benzodiazepines, is physically and psychologically habit-forming. People who have experienced traumatic events in their lives and have chronic anxiety are especially prone to developing dependence. Prolonged use is associated with a range of problems. Use for more than four weeks is *not* recommended. If you

stop flurazepam after more than four weeks of daily use you will probably experience withdrawal symptoms (see below). **Tests needed before starting:**
None. **Alcohol:** Alcohol must be avoided entirely. The simultaneous use of flurazepam and alcohol is extremely dangerous because it can cause you to stop
breathing. The combination can cause death. **Use in pregnancy:** There is a
higher rate of babies born with a cleft palate to mothers who took benzodiazepines during pregnancy. **The elderly** are especially sensitive to the effects
of benzodiazepines and may experience pronounced side effects at low doses
(see chapter 4).

DRUG INTERACTIONS   **Use with extra caution if you take:** *Anticonvul-*
sants, antidepressants, antihistamines, antipsychotics, barbiturates, benzodi-
azepines, or any drug that causes sedation or central nervous system depression,
because the combination with flurazepam can cause pronounced sedation.

DOSING   **Adults:** The usual starting dose is 15–30 mg at bedtime. **Children:**
Not FDA-approved for under 15. Some child psychiatrists recommend the same
dosages as adults.

MONITORING YOUR USE   **Time to effectiveness:** 30–60 minutes. **A full**
trial is: A few doses, which are generally enough to establish whether it will be
helpful. **Half-life of drug and active metabolites:** Two hours, with active
metabolites with half-lives from 2–100 hours. **How to monitor dosage:** The optimal dose is determined by its effectiveness in helping you sleep. **If you miss a**
dose: Do *not* try to make up for a missed dose; just continue with your regular dosing schedule. **How to monitor safety:** No specific medical tests are needed to
monitor safety.

SIDE EFFECTS   **Common (10–50%):** Daytime fatigue, memory impairment, poor muscle coordination (causing a higher rate of falls in the elderly and a
higher rate of motor vehicle accidents in all adults). **Infrequent (less than 1%):**
Paradoxical agitation and insomnia. **Those requiring attention from your**
physician: Any physical or emotional changes not described here. **Side effects as-**
sociated with use longer than four weeks: Use of flurazepam longer than four
weeks may cause physical and psychological dependence, and you may notice the
desire for another dose as each one wears off. Ongoing anxiety, reduced effectiveness of each dose, depression, emotional blunting, and impairment of memory and
cognition may occur with use for longer than one year.

WHAT TO EXPECT WHEN YOU STOP   You may notice insomnia if flurazepam is tapered gradually. Other withdrawal symptoms include anxiety, irritability, headaches, tremors, nausea, diarrhea, sweating, and confusion. **If**
stopped abruptly: *Seizures* can occur if flurazepam is stopped abruptly, although
this is extremely unlikely with routine use at the recommended dose. Seizures are

potentially life-threatening. You should always consult with your physician how to stop it safely.

Fluvoxamine

GENERAL   Preparations: Generic and brand name Luvox. **Class:** SSRI (selective serotonin reuptake inhibitor). **Used in:** Bulimia, depression, obsessive-compulsive disorder (panic disorder, other anxiety disorders, developmental disorders). **Mechanism of action:** Blocks the reuptake of serotonin by presynaptic neurons.

PRECAUTIONS   Warnings: When taken with other serotonin reuptake inhibitors, fluvoxamine can cause the *serotonin syndrome,* which consists of potentially dangerous alterations in pulse, blood pressure, hyperactivity, and mental status changes (see chapter 19). Rarely, fluvoxamine can cause hyponatremia, or low sodium in your blood. **Use extra caution if you have:** *Bipolar disorder,* as fluvoxamine can cause a manic episode; *epilepsy,* as fluvoxamine may increase the frequency of seizures; a *psychotic disorder,* as fluvoxamine can worsen psychotic symptoms. **Tests needed before starting:** None. **Alcohol:** The simultaneous use of fluvoxamine and alcohol causes no specific adverse consequences, but alcohol should be avoided because it worsens anxiety and depression. **Use in pregnancy:** There is a higher rate of miscarriages, heart defects, and intestinal defects in the babies of women who take fluvoxamine during pregnancy.

DRUG INTERACTIONS   Don't use if you take: *Other SSRIs, Saint John's wort,* or *tryptophan,* as their use with fluvoxamine can cause the *serotonin syndrome; MAOI antidepressants,* as their use with fluvoxamine can cause a serious, sometimes fatal, reaction of agitation, fever, cardiovascular changes, and mental status changes.

DOSING   Adults: The usual starting dose is 50 mg once daily with increases of 50 mg/day every four to seven days up to a maximum of 300 mg/day. **Children:** Not FDA-approved for under 18.

MONITORING YOUR USE   Time to effectiveness: You may notice some side effects within one to two days, but any improvement in symptoms generally takes two to four weeks. **A full trial is:** Four weeks at the maximum dose. **Half-life of drug and active metabolites:** 15 hours. Metabolites are essentially inactive. **How to monitor dosage:** The optimal dose is determined by its effectiveness in alleviating the target symptoms. **How to monitor safety:** No specific tests are needed to monitor your health while on fluvoxamine. **If you miss a dose:** Take a missed dose if it's the same day. Do not try to make up for a missed dose the next day by doubling your dose; just continue with your regular dosing schedule.

SIDE EFFECTS **Common (10–50%):** Anxiety, decreased appetite, constipation, diarrhea, dizziness, dry mouth, fatigue, headache, insomnia, nausea (generally goes away after one to two weeks), rash, sexual dysfunction, sweating, weakness. **Less common (1–10%):** Sweating, tremor. **Those requiring attention from your physician:** Hyperactivity, mental status changes, or alterations in your pulse or blood pressure, which suggest the serotonin syndrome. Physical or emotional changes not listed, such as suicidal thoughts or behavior.

WHAT TO EXPECT WHEN YOU STOP You may notice a return of your symptoms if fluvoxamine is tapered gradually. **If stopped abruptly:** You may notice a flulike syndrome of nausea, vomiting, diarrhea, dizziness, as well as anxiety and depression. Fluvoxamine should not be stopped abruptly, but needs to be gradually tapered in consultation with your physician.

Gabapentin

GENERAL **Preparations:** Brand name Neurontin only. **Class:** Mood stabilizer. **Mechanism of action:** Unknown. **Used in:** Bipolar disorder; anxiety disorders.

PRECAUTIONS **Use extra caution if you have:** *Kidney disease,* as gabapentin will be more slowly excreted. **Tests needed before starting:** None. **Alcohol:** Should be avoided as it may impair the effectiveness of gabapentin. Alcohol should also be avoided because it can worsen depression and anxiety.

DRUG INTERACTIONS **Use with extra caution if you take:** *Anticonvulsants, antidepressants, antihistamines, antipsychotics, barbiturates, benzodiazepines,* or any drug that causes sedation or central nervous system depression, because the combination can cause pronounced sedation.

DOSING **Adults:** The usual starting dose is 100–300 mg on the first day, 100–300 mg twice on the second day, and 100–300 mg three times daily thereafter, with increases up to 2400 mg/day. **Children:** Not FDA-approved for under 12.

MONITORING YOUR USE **Time to effectiveness:** You may notice some side effects within one to two days, but any improvement in symptoms generally takes one to two weeks if you are manic. **A full trial is:** Three weeks at the maximum therapeutic level if you are manic. There is no set period of time with which to determine effectiveness if you start gabapentin when your mood is stable, as manic symptoms are often absent for extended periods of time. Essentially, you stay on the drug and watch for any symptoms of mania. If none appear, or if they are milder than usual, then gabapentin is at least partially effective. **Half-life of drug and active metabolites:** 5–7 hours, with no active metabolites. **How to monitor dosage:** The optimal dose is determined by its effectiveness in alleviating the target symptoms. **How to monitor safety:** No specific tests are needed to monitor your health while on gabapentin. **If you miss a dose:** Take a missed dose if it's within an hour or two. Do not try to make up for a missed dose by doubling your next dose; just continue with your regular dosing schedule.

SIDE EFFECTS   Usual (50–100%): Sedation. **Common (10–50%):** Impaired muscular coordination, gait unsteadiness. **Less common (1–10%):** Anxiety, visual changes, stuttering, memory impairment, tremor. **Those requiring attention from your physician:** Any physical or emotional changes not listed.

WHAT TO EXPECT WHEN YOU STOP   You may notice a return of your symptoms if gabapentin is tapered gradually. **If stopped abruptly:** You may develop withdrawal seizures. Gabapentin should not be stopped abruptly, but needs to be gradually tapered in consultation with your physician.

Galantamine

GENERAL   **Preparations:** Brand name Reminyl only in tablets and liquid. **Class:** Cognitive enhancer. **Used in:** Alzheimer's disease. **Mechanism of action:** Inhibits the enzyme cholinesterase, which breaks down acetylcholine.

PRECAUTIONS   Use extra caution if you have: *Asthma,* as galantamine may worsen breathing problems; *heart problems* in which the heart beats too slowly, such as bradycardia, the "sick sinus syndrome," or certain forms of heart block, as galantamine may cause your heart to beat too slowly; *kidney or liver problems,* as galantamine may build up too high; *seizures,* as galantamine increases the potential for causing seizures; *ulcers,* as galantamine may increase gastric acid secretion and worsen ulcers. **Tests needed before starting:** The diagnosis of Alzheimer's needs to be established through a neurological and physical exam, neuropsychological testing, or a brain imaging study. A complete physical examination should be done to ensure that there are no active medical problems that would preclude the use of galantamine. **Alcohol:** Although there are no specific adverse consequences when alcohol and galantamine are combined, the use of alcohol should be avoided, since it impairs thinking and judgment.

DRUG INTERACTIONS   Use with extra caution if you take: *Nonsteroidal inflammatory drugs such as aspirin, ibuprofen (Advil, Motrin), or naproxen (Aleve),* as the combination may cause stomach bleeding.

DOSING Adults: The starting and maintenance dose is 4 mg twice daily, with dosage increases of 4 mg twice daily every two weeks up to a maximum of 16 mg twice daily (32 mg total daily dose). It should be taken with food to minimize nausea.

MONITORING YOUR USE   **Time to effectiveness:** As there is no immediate obvious effect, there is no objective way to assess whether it is having a positive effect. It is reasonable to begin it as soon as the diagnosis is clear and as long as any memory function remains. **A full trial:** This lasts until there is minimal memory function remaining. **Half-life of drug and active metabolites:** 7 hours, with no active metabolites. **How to monitor dosage:** The optimal dose is determined by the absence of side effects. **If you miss a dose:** Do *not* try to make up for a missed dose; just continue with your regular dosing schedule. **How to monitor safety:** Monitor weight.

SIDE EFFECTS   **Common (10–50%):** Diarrhea, nausea, and vomiting. **Less common (1–10%):** Decreased appetite, dizziness, fatigue, fainting, headaches, indigestion, insomnia, weight loss. **Those requiring attention by your physician:** Any physical, cognitive, or emotional change not noted here.

WHAT TO EXPECT WHEN YOU STOP   There may be a further impairment in memory. **If stopped abruptly:** There is no specific withdrawal syndrome beyond the loss of effectiveness.

Guanfacine

GENERAL   **Preparations:** Generic and brand name Tenex. **Class:** A centrally acting alpha-agonist. **Used in:** ADHD. **Mechanism of action:** It stimulates postsynaptic alpha adrenergic receptors in the brain, causing lower blood pressure and heart rate.

PRECAUTIONS   **Tests needed before starting:** Measure pulse and blood pressure. **Alcohol:** The simultaneous use of guanfacine and alcohol should be avoided because guanfacine can cause excessive sedation.

DRUG INTERACTIONS   **Use with extra caution if you take:** Tricyclic antidepressants, as the combination may lower blood pressure excessively; *diltiazem, digitalis, verapamil,* and *beta-blockers,* as the combination with guanfacine may slow the heart rate excessively.

DOSING   **Adults:** The usual starting dose is 1.0 mg twice a day, with an increase up to 2 mg/day after three to four weeks. **Children:** Not FDA-approved for under 12. Some child psychiatrists recommend a starting dose of 0.5 mg/day, with increases of 0.5 mg/day every few days up to a maximum of 4.0 mg/day for those under 12.

MONITORING YOUR USE   **Time to effectiveness:** The effects on pulse and blood pressure are immediate, but the calming effect sought in ADHD may take a few days until the dose has built up. **A full trial:** Four weeks at the maximum dose. **Half-life of drug and active metabolites:** The half-life in children is

13–14 hours with no active metabolites. The half-life in adults is 17 hours. **How to monitor dosage:** The optimal dose is determined by its effectiveness in alleviating the target symptoms. **How to monitor safety:** Pulse and blood pressure should be monitored regularly. **If you miss a dose:** Do *not* try to make up for a missed dose; just continue with the regular dosing schedule.

SIDE EFFECTS Usual (50–100%): Dizziness, dry mouth, sedation. **Common (10–50%):** Constipation, weakness. **Less common (1–10%):** Headaches. **Those requiring attention from your physician:** Any physical or emotional changes not described here.

WHAT TO EXPECT WHEN YOU STOP You may notice a return of your symptoms if guanfacine is tapered gradually. **If stopped abruptly:** You can develop agitation, anxiety, headaches, and tremor. Most important, your pulse and blood pressure can rise rapidly, putting you at risk for a stroke. Guanfacine should always be tapered gradually in consultation with your doctor.

Haloperidol

GENERAL **Preparations:** Generic in pills. Brand name Haldol in liquid and long-acting injectable concentrate. **Class:** Standard antipsychotic. **Used in:** Bipolar disorder, developmental disorders, psychotic disorders (Alzheimer's disease, severe anxiety, severe ADHD). **Mechanism of action:** Blocks postsynaptic dopamine receptors.

PRECAUTIONS **Warnings:** All antipsychotics can cause *neuroleptic malignant syndrome,* a rare but severe and potentially fatal reaction consisting of fever, muscle rigidity, mental status changes, and alterations in pulse and blood pressure. They can also cause *tardive dyskinesia,* a potentially irreversible disorder of rhythmical, involuntary muscle movements (see chapter 19 for details of both conditions.) **Use extra caution if you have:** *Breast cancer,* as haloperidol can elevate prolactin, a hormone released by the pituitary that may cause breast cancer to grow faster; *epilepsy,* as haloperidol may increase the frequency of seizures; *glaucoma, low blood pressure, prostatic hypertrophy* or *urinary retention,* as the symptoms of these disorders may worsen. **Tests before starting:** None. **Alcohol:** Should be avoided, as the simultaneous use of haloperidol and alcohol can lower blood pressure significantly and cause confusion. Also, alcohol worsens anxiety and depression and impairs insight and judgment. **Use in pregnancy:** Some antipsychotics have been linked with the "floppy infant syndrome," in which the baby has poor muscle tone. The fetus may experience pseudoparkinsonism and dystonia, muscular side effects that may cause fetal distress before, during, and shortly after birth. **Sunlight:** Severe sunburns can occur on haloperidol. Avoid sunbathing entirely and avoid casual exposure to the sun for more than 30 minutes. Use a sunblock of a sun protection factor (SPF) of 15 or more if exposure to the sun cannot be avoided.

DRUG INTERACTIONS   **Use with extra caution if you take:** *Anticonvulsants, antidepressants, antihistamines, antipsychotics, barbiturates, benzodiazepines,* or any drug that causes sedation or central nervous system depression, because the combination can cause pronounced sedation; *antihypertensive medication,* as haloperidol may combine to lower blood pressure excessively; *antihistamines* or *antiparkinsonian agents* as they may combine to produce pronounced dry mouth, blurry vision, constipation, low blood pressure, rapid heart rate, and mental confusion; *lithium,* as there have been reports of confusion, weakness, and brain damage associated with their combined use.

DOSING   **Adults:** The starting dose is 2–10 mg a day. Higher doses are sometimes used for acute agitation. Doses of up to 100 mg/day have been safely used, but are rarely necessary. Haloperidol decanoate is given by injection intramuscularly with dosages of 10–100 mg every one to four weeks. **Children:** Ages 3–12: 0.5 mg/day with increases of 0.5 mg every five to seven days. There is no maximum dosage, but there is generally little improvement beyond 6 mg/day. **The elderly:** 0.5–2.0 mg one to three times daily.

MONITORING YOUR USE   **Time to effectiveness:** Calming effects are often noticed within one to three hours of a dose, but several days may be needed to notice any effect on psychotic symptoms. A pronounced effect may take one to two weeks. Many months may be needed to derive full benefit. The long-acting forms take two days to begin effectiveness. **A full trial is:** Four weeks at no less than 10 mg/day. **Half-life of drug and active metabolites:** 24 hours with one active metabolite. The half-life of the decanoate preparation is 21 days. **How to monitor dosage:** The optimal dose is determined by its effectiveness in alleviating the target symptoms. **How to monitor safety:** Examination for the presence of tardive dyskinesia (see below) should be performed twice yearly. **If you miss a dose:** Take a missed dose if it's the same day. Do not try to make up for a missed dose the next day by doubling your dose; just continue with your regular dosing schedule.

SIDE EFFECTS   **Usual (50–100%):** Sedation, dry mouth, constipation, blurry vision. **Common (10–50%):** Low blood pressure (light-headedness, dizziness), fatigue, ataraxia (zombielike feeling), weight gain, menstrual irregularities, akathisia (restlessness), sexual dysfunction, pseudoparkinsonism (muscular tremor, rigidity, akinesia), and tardive dyskinesia, a form of involuntary muscle movements (see chapter 19 for further details). **Less common (1–10%):** Dystonia (muscle spasms, usually of the head and neck, face, and jaw), galactorrhea (milk leaking from breasts), sexual dysfunction. **Infrequent (less than 1%):** Urinary difficulty; cataracts. **Those requiring attention from**

your physician: Symptoms of fever, muscular rigidity, and mental status changes, as you may have neuroleptic malignant syndrome, a potentially severe reaction; any abnormal involuntary movements that suggest tardive dyskinesia; any other physical or emotional changes not described here.

WHAT TO EXPECT WHEN YOU STOP   You may notice a return of your symptoms if haloperidol is tapered gradually. **If stopped abruptly:** There is no acute withdrawal syndrome.

Hydroxyzine

GENERAL   **Preparations:** Generic and brand name Atarax and Vistaril in pills and liquid form. **Class:** Antihistamine. **Used in:** Anxiety. **Mechanism of action:** Blocks postsynaptic histamine receptors.

PRECAUTIONS   **Use extra caution if you have:** *Asthma, low blood pressure, congestive heart failure, edema, epilepsy, glaucoma, heart disease, hyperthyroidism, enlarged prostate* or *urinary retention,* as hydroxazine can worsen the symptoms of these disorders. **Tests needed before starting:** None. **Alcohol:** Should be avoided as the simultaneous use of hydroxyzine and alcohol can lower blood pressure significantly and cause confusion. Also, alcohol worsens anxiety and depression and impairs insight and judgment.

DRUG INTERACTIONS   **Use with extra caution if you take:** *Antihypertensives,* as hydroxazine may lower blood pressure excessively; *antihistamines, phenothiazines,* or *tricyclic antidepressants,* as they may combine to produce pronounced dry mouth, blurry vision, constipation, low blood pressure, rapid heart rate, and even mental confusion; *MAOI antidepressants,* as they can intensify the side effects of hydroxazine; *anticonvulsants, antidepressants, antihistamines, antipsychotics, barbiturates, benzodiazepines,* or any drug that causes sedation or central nervous system depression, because the combination can cause pronounced sedation.

DOSING   **Adults:** 50–100 mg one to four times daily. **Children:** Under 6: 50 mg/day in divided doses. Over 6: 50–100 mg/day in divided doses.

MONITORING YOUR USE   **Time to effectiveness:** 15–30 minutes. **A full trial is:** A few days at the maximum dose. **Half-life of drug and active metabolites:** 3–20 hours, with no active metabolites. **How to monitor dosage:** The optimal dose is determined by its effectiveness in alleviating the target symptoms. **How to monitor safety:** No special medical tests are needed. **If you miss a dose:** Take a missed dose if it's within an hour or two. Do not try to make up for a missed dose by doubling your next dose; just continue with your regular dosing schedule.

SIDE EFFECTS **Usual (50–100%):** Dry mouth, sedation. **Less common (1–10%):** Blurry vision, constipation, dizziness, headache, low blood pressure, nausea. **Infrequent:** Agitation, urinary retention, visual changes. **Those requiring attention from your physician:** Any physical or emotional changes not listed.

WHAT TO EXPECT WHEN YOU STOP You may notice a return of your symptoms if it is stopped.

Imipramine

GENERAL **Preparations:** Generic and brand name Tofranil. **Class:** Tricyclic antidepressant. **Used in:** ADHD, bulimia, depression, panic disorder, other anxiety disorders. **Mechanism of action:** Blocks the reuptake of norepinephrine and serotonin into presynaptic neurons.

PRECAUTIONS **Don't use if you have:** *Heart block* (an abnormal heart rhythm) or if you recently had a *heart attack,* as imipramine may worsen heart block and dangerously affect heart function. **Use extra caution if you have:** *Bipolar disorder,* as imipramine may cause a manic episode; *epilepsy,* as imipramine may increase the frequency of seizures; *glaucoma,* as imipramine can worsen the symptoms of untreated angle closure glaucoma; *low blood pressure;* as imipramine may lower blood pressure further; a *psychotic disorder,* as imipramine may make psychotic symptoms worse; *hyperthyroidism,* as imipramine may cause irregular heart rhythms; *prostatic hypertrophy* or *urinary retention,* as imipramine may worsen urinary retention. **Tests needed before starting:** An electrocardiogram (EKG) if you are over 35, to ensure that you do not have any form of heart block. **Alcohol:** Should be avoided, as the simultaneous use of imipramine and alcohol can lower blood pressure significantly and cause confusion. Also, alcohol worsens anxiety and depression and impairs insight and judgment. **Use in pregnancy:** There is a higher rate of miscarriages born to women who take tricyclics, but no specific defect is associated with their use.

DRUG INTERACTIONS **Do not use if you take:** *MAOI antidepressants,* as their use with imipramine can cause pronounced hypertension and the potential for strokes. **Use with extra caution if you take:** *Phenothiazines,* as the combination may cause irregular heart rhythms which are potentially fatal; *antihypertensives:* as they may combine to lower blood pressure excessively; *antihistamines, phenothiazines,* and *antiparkinsonian agents,* as they may combine to produce pronounced dry mouth, blurry vision, constipation, low blood pressure, rapid heart rate, and even mental confusion; *guanethadine* to lower blood pressure, as imipramine may block its effects.

DOSING   **Adults:** The usual starting dose is 25 mg at bedtime with increases every other day up to 150 mg. Some people begin at 75 mg/day in divided doses. The maximum recommended dose is 300 mg/day. **Children:** Not FDA-approved for under 12, and several deaths have been associated with the use of desipramine, its main metabolite. Some child psychiatrists recommend a starting dose of 25 mg at bedtime with weekly increases of 25 mg/day up to a maximum dose of 100 mg/day for those over 12. **The elderly:** The usual starting dose is 10 mg at bedtime with increases every few days up to 50–100 mg/day.

MONITORING YOUR USE   **Time to effectiveness:** Side effects are generally noticeable within a few doses, but the therapeutic effect may take two to four weeks. **A full trial is:** Four weeks at the maximum tolerated dosage. **Half-life of drug and active metabolites:** 7–34 hours. The primary active metabolite is desipramine, whose half-life is 7–60 hours. **How to monitor dosage:** The optimal dose is determined by its effectiveness in alleviating the target symptoms. The therapeutic effect of imipramine is more likely when the concentration in the blood is between 150 and 300 micrograms. A blood level may be useful to assist in determining the best dosage if you do not respond or if your side effects are more pronounced than expected. **How to monitor safety:** A blood level should be obtained if doses go over 150 mg/day. An EKG may be useful to ensure that heart function is not impaired. **If you miss a dose:** Take a missed dose if it's within an hour or two. Do not try to make up for a missed dose by doubling your next dose; just continue with your regular dosing schedule.

SIDE EFFECTS   **Usual (50–100%):** Blurry vision, constipation, dizziness, dry mouth, fatigue, increased heart rate, low blood pressure. **Common (10–50%):** Agitation, sweating, weight gain. **Less common (1–10%):** Insomnia, sexual dysfunction, urinary retention. **Those requiring attention from your physician:** Any physical or emotional changes not listed, such as suicidal thoughts or behavior.

WHAT TO EXPECT WHEN YOU STOP   You may notice a return of your symptoms if imipramine is stopped. **If stopped abruptly:** You may experience agitation, headaches, insomnia, and nausea, as well as depression. Imipramine should be slowly tapered if you decide to stop it. The rate of discontinuation is different for each person and is determined by the clinical situation necessitating the change, your age, severity of symptoms, dosage size, and your duration of use.

Isocarboxazid

GENERAL   **Preparations:** Brand name Marplan only. **Class:** MAOI. **Used in:** Bulimia, depression, panic disorder (other anxiety disorders). **Mechanism of action:** Inhibits monoamine oxidase, the protein enzyme responsible for the breakdown of dopamine, epinephrine, norepinephrine, and serotonin, resulting in elevated levels of these neurotransmitters.

PRECAUTIONS **Warnings:** Isocarboxazid can cause a *hypertensive crisis* in which your blood pressure rises to a dangerously high level, putting you at risk for a brain stroke, brain damage, and death. This reaction is unlikely to occur on its own, but is possible if used in combination with foods or medicines that contain tyramine or substances similar to epinephrine. **The following medications must be avoided while you are on isocarboxazid and for two weeks following its cessation in order to avoid a hypertensive crisis:** Prescription medications: *antiasthmatics* that contain *epinephrine* or epinephrine-like compounds, most *antidepressants, antihypertensives, antiparkinsonian agents, barbiturates, buspirone (Buspar), carbamazepine (Tegretol), disulfiram, diuretics, narcotics, stimulants;* over-the-counter medications: *decongestants, dextromethorphan, tryptophan, hay fever medications, sinus medications, appetite suppressants;* recreational drugs: *amphetamines, cocaine, hallucinogenics, heroin or other narcotics.* **The following foods must be avoided while you are on isocarboxazid and for two weeks following its cessation in order to avoid a hypertensive crisis:** Aged or fermented foods; all cheese or foods containing cheese such as pizza, fondue, many Italian dishes and salad dressings (cottage cheese and cream cheese are allowed); cream, sour cream, and yogurt; foods fermented with yeast (although foods baked with yeast, such as bread, are safe), brewer's yeast; liver, processed meats, such as bologna, corned beef, hot dogs, liverwurst, pepperoni, salami, sausage; broad bean pods (fava beans); sauerkraut; pickles; soy sauce; licorice, caviar, anchovies, dried fruits (raisins, prunes), figs, raspberries, chocolate; bananas, pickled herring; excessive amounts of caffeine-containing beverages (more than one or two, although some people are more sensitive than others) like coffee, tea, sodas, and hot chocolate. **Don't use if you have:** *Congestive heart failure,* as it may make the symptoms worse; *high blood pressure,* as isocarboxazid may make the symptoms worse; *pheochromocytoma,* as it may cause a hypertensive crisis. **Use extra caution if you have:** *Bipolar disorder,* as isocarboxazid can cause a manic episode; *epilepsy,* as isocarboxazid may increase seizure frequency; *low blood pressure,* as isocarboxazid may make symptoms worse; a *psychotic disorder,* as isocarboxazid can worsen psychotic symptoms. **Tests needed before starting:** None. **Alcohol:** Beer, wine, Chianti, sherry, and liqueurs, whether they contain alcohol or not, can cause a hypertensive crisis. Hard liquor has no specific adverse consequences, but should be avoided because it can worsen anxiety, depression, and low blood pressure.

DRUG INTERACTIONS *Antihypertensives,* as isocarboxazid can lower blood pressure further; *narcotics,* as the combination can produce coma, fever, and high blood pressure.

DOSING **Adults:** 30 mg/day in single or divided doses. Once improvement is noted, a reduction to 10–20 mg may minimize some side effects. Dosages over 30 mg/day are unlikely to be more helpful. **Children:** Not FDA-approved for children under 16.

MONITORING YOUR USE   Time to effectiveness: Side effects may be noted with a few days, but the therapeutic effect may take two to six weeks. **A full trial is:** Four weeks at the maximum tolerated dose. **Half-life of drug and active metabolites:** Unknown. The effect can last for two weeks after the last dose. **How to monitor dosage:** The optimal dose is determined by its effectiveness in alleviating the target symptoms. **How to monitor safety:** Monitor blood pressure. **If you miss a dose:** Take a missed dose if it's within an hour or two. Do not try to make up for a missed dose the next day by doubling your dose; just continue with your regular dosing schedule.

SIDE EFFECTS   Common (10–50%): Agitation, constipation, dizziness, headaches, insomnia, sedation, sexual dysfunction, tremor, muscle twitching, weight gain. **Those requiring attention from your physician:** A sudden headache, palpitations, rapid heart rate, sweating, throat constriction, neck stiffness, nausea or vomiting can be a sign that you are having a hypertensive crisis: you should consult your physician immediately and go to the emergency room for treatment of any elevation of blood pressure; physical or emotional changes not listed, such as suicidal thoughts or behavior.

WHAT TO EXPECT WHEN YOU STOP   You may notice a return of your symptoms if you taper and stop isocarboxazid. **If stopped abruptly: An uncommon withdrawal syndrome starting one to three days after cessation of isocarboxazid in which agitation, nightmares, seizures, and psychotic thinking may occur.

Lamotrigine

GENERAL   Preparations: Brand name Lamictal only. **Class:** Mood stabilizer. **Used in:** Bipolar disorder. **Mechanism of action:** Unknown.

PRECAUTIONS   Lamotrigine causes a severe *rash* in 1/1000 adults and 1/50–100 in children under 16. These rashes generally occur in the first two to eight weeks, but have occurred as late as six months of treatment. Those on valproate or taking a large dose may be more likely to develop a rash. The rash may be permanently disfiguring and is potentially life-threatening. A separate concern is death from *liver failure,* which occurred in 5/7000 people who had serious medical disorders such as overwhelming infection and status epilepticus. **Tests needed before starting: Kidney and liver function blood tests. **Alcohol:** Should be avoided as it may impair the effectiveness of lamotrigine. Alcohol should also be avoided because it can worsen depression in bipolar disorder.

DRUG INTERACTIONS Use with extra caution if you take: *Anticonvulsants, antidepressants, antihistamines, antipsychotics, barbiturates, benzodiazepines,* or any drug that causes sedation or central nervous system depression, because the combination can cause pronounced sedation.

DOSING **Adults:** The usual starting dose is 50 mg/day for two weeks, then twice daily for two weeks, with further increases of 100 mg/day every one to two weeks up to a maximum dose of 500 mg/day. If you are on valproate, use half these doses. **Children:** Not FDA-approved for under 16.

MONITORING YOUR USE **Time to effectiveness:** You may notice some side effects within one to two days, but any improvement in symptoms generally takes one to two weeks. **A full trial is:** Three weeks at the maximum therapeutic level if you are manic. There is no set period of time with which to determine effectiveness if you start lamotrigine when your mood is stable, as manic symptoms are often absent for extended periods of time. Essentially, you stay on the drug and watch for any symptoms of mania. If none appear, or if they are milder than usual, then lamotrigine is at least partially effective. **Half-life of drug and active metabolites:** 14–59 hours. With steady use, half-life decreases by 25 percent. There are no active metabolites. **How to monitor dosage:** The optimal dose is determined by its effectiveness in alleviating the target symptoms. **How to monitor safety:** No specific tests are needed to monitor safety. **If you miss a dose:** Take a missed dose if it's within a few hours. Do not try to make up for a missed dose by doubling your next dose; just continue with your regular dosing schedule.

SIDE EFFECTS **Common (10–50%):** Mild sedation, impaired muscular coordination, an unsteady gait, and nausea are common when you first start, but tend to go away within the first week. Others include headaches, nasal congestion, blurry or double vision. **Those requiring attention from your physician:** You should consult your physician immediately if you notice the first sign of a rash; you should also consult your physician immediately if you notice yellow eyes or skin, signs of liver failure; any physical or emotional changes not listed.

WHAT TO EXPECT WHEN YOU STOP You may notice a return of your symptoms if lamotrigine is tapered gradually. **If stopped abruptly:** You may develop withdrawal seizures. Lamotrigine should not be stopped abruptly, but needs to be gradually tapered in consultation with your physician.

Lithium

GENERAL **Preparations:** Generic and brand name Lithonate, Lithotabs, Eskalith, and Lithobid in pills, and Lithium Citrate in liquid. **Class:** Mood stabilizer. **Used in:** Bipolar disorder (depression). **Mechanism of action:** Unknown.

PRECAUTIONS   Warnings: *Lithium toxicity* can occur if the level of lithium is too high. Symptoms include tremor, nausea, vomiting, mental confusion, slurred speech, lack of coordination, and muscular weakness. Consult your physician and obtain a blood lithium level immediately if you suspect your lithium level is too high. Avoid *dehydration,* as lithium may rise to toxic levels. **Use extra caution if you have:** *Kidney* or *thyroid disease,* as lithium can worsen disorders of either organ. **Tests needed before starting:** Kidney and thyroid function tests. Some doctors recommend an EKG because lithium can cause changes in the EKG. Although this is insignificant to your health, it may impair the interpretation of the EKG if heart problems arise at a later date. **Alcohol:** Should be avoided because it can worsen depression. **Use in pregnancy:** When taken during the first trimester, lithium can cause a heart defect.

DRUG INTERACTIONS   Use with extra caution if you take: *Anti-inflammatory agents (aspirin, ibuprofen, naproxen),* or *diuretics,* as they can increase lithium to toxic levels; *haloperidol,* as the combination has been (rarely) associated with weakness, confusion, fever, and tremor and even brain damage.

DOSING   Adults: The usual starting dose is 300 mg one to two times daily with increases every three to seven days up to a maximum of 1800 mg/day. Rarely, higher doses are used. **Children:** Over 12: the same as adults. Not FDA-approved for under 12. Some child psychiatrists recommend approximately the same dosages as adults to children under 12.

MONITORING YOUR USE   Time to effectiveness: One to two weeks for acute mania. **A full trial is:** During an acute episode, three weeks at the maximum therapeutic blood level with no response. There is no set period of time with which to determine effectiveness if you start lithium when your mood is stable, as manic symptoms are often absent for extended periods of time. Essentially, you stay on the drug and watch for any symptoms of mania. If none appear, or if they are milder than usual, then lithium is thought to be at least partially effective. **Half-life of drug and active metabolites:** 20–24 hours with no active metabolites. **How to monitor dosage:** The optimal dose is determined by a blood level of 0.5–1.2 milliequivalents/ml of blood, obtained 12 hours after your last dose. Improved effectiveness can sometimes be achieved by maintaining the level at the higher end of the therapeutic range. **How to monitor safety:** Check your levels until a dose has been established that will maintain a therapeutic level. Routine levels every six months thereafter is sufficient. Kidney and thyroid function tests should be done every six months to screen for any impairment of functioning caused by lithium. Serum calcium should be checked yearly, as lithium can lead to elevated levels of calcium. **If you miss a dose:** Take a missed dose if it's within a few hours. Do not try to make up for a missed dose by doubling your next dose, just continue with your regular dosing schedule.

SIDE EFFECTS **Common (10–50%):** Diarrhea, increased appetite, increased thirst and urination, thyroid dysfunction, tremor, weight gain. **Less common (1–10%):** Acne, dry mouth, kidney impairment. **Those requiring attention from your physician:** Physical or emotional changes not listed.

WHAT TO EXPECT WHEN YOU STOP You may notice a return of your symptoms if lithium is tapered gradually. **If stopped abruptly:** There is no acute withdrawal syndrome. Lithium should not be stopped abruptly or you may experience pronounced mood swings. It needs to be gradually tapered in consultation with your physician.

Lorazepam

GENERAL **Preparations:** Generic and brand name Ativan. **Class:** Benzodiazepine. **Used in:** Anxiety disorders, bipolar disorder, insomnia (alcohol withdrawal, Alzheimer's disease, antipsychotic-induced akathisia [restlessness]). **Mechanism of action:** Intensifies the effects of gamma-aminobutyric acid (GABA).

PRECAUTIONS **Warnings:** *It is habit-forming.* Lorazepam, like all benzodiazepines, is physically and psychologically habit-forming. People who have experienced traumatic events in their lives and have chronic anxiety are especially prone to developing dependence. Prolonged use is associated with a range of problems. Use for more than four weeks is *not* recommended. If you stop lorazepam after more than four weeks of daily use you will probably experience withdrawal symptoms (see below). *Seizures can occur if it is stopped abruptly,* so consultation with your physician is essential if you wish to stop. **Tests needed before starting:** None. **Alcohol:** Alcohol must be avoided entirely. The simultaneous use of lorazepam and alcohol is extremely dangerous because it can cause you to stop breathing. The combination can cause death. **Use in pregnancy:** There is a higher rate of babies born with a cleft palate to mothers who took benzodiazepines during pregnancy. **The elderly** are especially sensitive to the effects of benzodiazepines and may experience pronounced side effects at low doses (see chapter 4).

DRUG INTERACTIONS **Use with extra caution if you take:** *Anticonvulsants, antidepressants, antihistamines, antipsychotics, barbiturates, benzodiazepines,* or any drug that causes sedation or central nervous system depression, because the combination with lorazepam can cause pronounced sedation.

DOSING **Adults:** The usual starting dose is 0.5–2 mg one to three times a day depending on the severity of the symptoms, up to a maximum of 8 mg/day. **Children:** Not FDA-approved for under 12. Some child psychiatrists recommend 1–6 mg day.

MONITORING YOUR USE   **Time to effectiveness:** 15–30 minutes. **A full trial is:** A few doses, which are generally enough to establish whether it will be helpful. **Half-life of drug and active metabolites:** 12 hours with no active metabolites. **How to monitor dosage:** The optimal dose is determined by its effectiveness in alleviating the target symptoms. **If you miss a dose:** Do *not* try to make up for a missed dose; just continue with your regular dosing schedule. **How to monitor safety:** No specific medical tests are needed to monitor safety.

SIDE EFFECTS   **Common (10–50%):** Sedation, memory impairment, poor muscle coordination (causing a higher rate of falls in the elderly and a higher risk of motor vehicle accidents in all adults). **Infrequent (less than 1%):** Paradoxical agitation and insomnia. **Those requiring attention from your physician:** Any physical or emotional changes not described here. **Side effects associated with use longer than four weeks:** Use of lorazepam longer than four weeks may cause physical and psychological dependence, and you may notice the desire for another dose as each one wears off. Ongoing anxiety, reduced effectiveness of each dose, depression, emotional blunting, and impairment of memory and cognition may occur with use longer than one year.

WHAT TO EXPECT WHEN YOU STOP   You may notice a return of your symptoms if lorazepam is tapered gradually. Other withdrawal symptoms include anxiety, insomnia, irritability, headaches, tremors, nausea, diarrhea, sweating, and confusion. The rate at which you should taper is affected by the duration of your use and the size of your dose, but may take months if you have been on it for an extended period of time. **If stopped abruptly:** *Seizures* can occur if lorazepam is stopped abruptly. They are potentially life-threatening. You should never stop lorazepam abruptly and you should always work with your physician to taper it gradually.

Loxapine

GENERAL   **Preparations:** Generic in pills, brand name Loxitane in pills and liquid form. **Class:** Standard antipsychotic. **Used in:** Bipolar disorder, psychotic disorders (Alzheimer's disease, severe anxiety). **Mechanism of action:** Blocks postsynaptic dopamine receptors.

PRECAUTIONS   **Warnings:** All antipsychotics can cause *neuroleptic malignant syndrome,* a rare but severe and potentially fatal reaction consisting of fever, muscle rigidity, mental status changes, and alterations in pulse and blood pressure. They can also cause *tardive dyskinesia,* a potentially irreversible disorder of rhythmical, involuntary muscle movements (see chapter 19 for details of both conditions). **Use extra caution if you have:** *Breast cancer,* as loxapine can elevate prolactin, a hormone released by the pituitary that may cause breast cancer to grow faster; *epilepsy,* as loxapine may increase the frequency of seizures; *glaucoma,* *low blood pressure, prostatic hypertrophy* or *urinary retention,* as the symptoms may worsen. **Tests before starting:** None. **Alcohol:** Should be avoided, as the simultaneous use of loxapine and alcohol can lower blood pressure significantly and cause confusion. Also, alcohol worsens anxiety and depression and impairs insight and judgment. **Use in pregnancy:** Some antipsychotics have been linked with the "floppy infant syndrome," in which the baby has poor muscle tone. The fetus may also experience pseudoparkinsonism and dystonia, muscular side effects that may cause fetal distress before, during, and shortly after birth. **Sunlight:** Severe sunburns can occur on loxapine. Avoid sunbathing entirely and avoid casual exposure to the sun for more than 30 minutes. Use a sunblock of a sun protection factor (SPF) of 15 or more if exposure to the sun cannot be avoided.

DRUG INTERACTIONS **Use with extra caution if you take:** *Anticonvulsants, antidepressants, antihistamines, antipsychotics, barbiturates, benzodiazepines,* or any drug that causes sedation or central nervous system depression, because the combination can cause pronounced sedation; *antihypertensive medication,* as loxapine may combine to lower blood pressure excessively; *antihistamines,* or *antiparkinsonian agents,* as they may combine to produce pronounced dry mouth, blurry vision, constipation, low blood pressure, rapid heart rate, and mental confusion.

DOSING **Adults:** The starting dose is 10–25 mg one to two times a day with weekly increases of 25–50 mg/day up to maximum of 250 mg/day. **Children:** Not FDA-approved for under 16.

MONITORING YOUR USE **Time to effectiveness:** Calming effects are often noticed within one to three hours of a dose, but several days may be needed to notice any effect on psychotic symptoms. A pronounced effect may take one to two weeks. Many months may be needed to derive full benefit. **A full trial is:** Four weeks at no less than 100 mg/day. **Half-life of drug and active metabolites:** Four hours with several active metabolites. **How to monitor dosage:** The optimal dose is determined by its effectiveness in alleviating the target symptoms. **How to monitor safety:** Examination for the presence of tardive dyskinesia (see below) should be performed twice yearly. **If you miss a dose:** Take a missed dose if it's the same day. Do not try to make up for a missed dose the next day by doubling your dose; just continue with your regular dosing schedule.

SIDE EFFECTS **Usual (50–100%):** Dry mouth, constipation, blurry vision. **Common (10–50%):** Low blood pressure (light-headedness, dizziness), fatigue, ataraxia (zombielike feeling), weight gain, menstrual irregularities, akathisia (restlessness), sexual dysfunction, pseudoparkinsonism (muscular tremor, rigidity, akinesia), and tardive dyskinesia, a form of involuntary muscle movements (see chapter 19 for further details). **Less common (1–10%):** Dystonia (muscle spasms, usually of the head and neck, face, and jaw), galactorrhea (milk leaking from breasts), sedation, sexual dysfunction. **Infrequent (less than 1%):**

Cataracts, urinary difficulty. **Those requiring attention from your physician:** Symptoms of fever, muscular rigidity, and mental status changes, as you may have neuroleptic malignant syndrome, a potentially severe reaction; any abnormal involuntary movements that suggest tardive dyskinesia; any other physical or emotional changes not described here.

WHAT TO EXPECT WHEN YOU STOP   You may notice a return of your symptoms if loxapine is tapered gradually. **If stopped abruptly:** There is no acute withdrawal syndrome.

Maprotiline

GENERAL   **Preparations:** Generic and brand name Ludiomil. **Class:** Antidepressant. **Used in:** Depression. **Mechanism of action:** Blocks the reuptake of norepinephrine into presynaptic neurons.

PRECAUTIONS   **Warnings:** *Seizures* can occur with the use of maprotiline. They are more likely if you also use phenothiazines, exceed the usual dosage, or rapidly taper a benzodiazepine. **Use extra caution if you have:** *Bipolar disorder,* as maprotiline may cause a manic episode; *heart disease* or if you recently had a *heart attack,* as maprotiline may dangerously affect heart function; *hyperthyroidism,* as maprotiline may cause irregular heart rhythms; *asthma, low blood pressure, congestive heart failure, edema, epilepsy, glaucoma, enlarged prostate,* or *urinary retention,* as maprotiline may worsen the symptoms; a *psychotic disorder,* as maprotiline may make psychotic symptoms worse. **Tests needed before starting:** None. **Alcohol:** Should be avoided as the simultaneous use of maprotiline and alcohol can increase the risk of seizures, lower blood pressure significantly, and cause confusion. Also, alcohol worsens anxiety and depression and impairs insight and judgment.

DRUG INTERACTIONS   **Don't use if you take:** *MAOI antidepressants,* as their use with maprotiline can cause pronounced hypertension and the potential for strokes. **Use with extra caution if you take:** *Antihypertensives,* as maprotiline may lower blood pressure excessively; *antihistamines, phenothiazines,* or *tricyclic antidepressants,* as they may combine to produce pronounced dry mouth, blurry vision, constipation, low blood pressure, rapid heart rate, and even mental confusion; *anticonvulsants, antidepressants, antihistamines, antipsychotics, barbiturates, benzodiazepines,* or any drug that causes sedation or central nervous system depression, because the combination can cause pronounced sedation; *benzodiazepines,* because the risk of seizures is elevated if you taper the benzodiazepine quickly; *phenothiazines,* as the combination puts you at a higher risk of developing seizures.

DOSING **Adults:** The usual starting dose is 75 mg daily, with increases every two weeks of 25 mg up to a maximum of 225 mg/day. **Children:** Not FDA-approved for under 18. **The elderly:** The starting dose is 25 mg/day with increases every two weeks up to a maximum of 75 mg/day.

MONITORING YOUR USE **Time to effectiveness:** Side effects are generally noticeable within a few doses, but the therapeutic effect may take one to four weeks. **A full trial is:** Four weeks at the maximum tolerated dosage. **Half-life of drug and active metabolites:** 27–58 hours with at least one active metabolite. **How to monitor dosage:** The optimal dose is determined by its effectiveness in alleviating the target symptoms. **How to monitor safety:** No specific tests needed. **If you miss a dose:** Take a missed dose if it's within an hour or two. Do not try to make up for a missed dose by doubling your next dose, just continue with your regular dosing schedule.

SIDE EFFECTS **Common (10–50%):** Blurry vision, constipation, dizziness, dry mouth, fatigue, headache, insomnia, nausea, sweating, tremor. **Less common (1–10%):** Agitation, anxiety, sexual dysfunction. **Infrequent (less than 1%):** Confusion, memory impairment, urinary difficulty, weight gain. **Those requiring attention from your physician:** Any physical or emotional changes not listed, such as suicidal thoughts or behavior.

WHAT TO EXPECT WHEN YOU STOP You may notice a return of your symptoms if maprotiline is stopped. **If stopped abruptly:** There is no specific withdrawal syndrome.

Mesoridazine

GENERAL **Preparations:** Brand name Serentil only in pills and liquid form. **Class:** Standard antipsychotic of the phenothiazine group. **Used in:** Bipolar disorder, psychotic disorders (Alzheimer's disease, severe anxiety). **Mechanism of action:** Blocks postsynaptic dopamine receptors.

PRECAUTIONS **Warnings:** All antipsychotics can cause *neuroleptic malignant syndrome,* a rare, but severe and potentially fatal reaction consisting of fever, muscle rigidity, mental status changes, and alterations in pulse and blood pressure. They can also cause *tardive dyskinesia,* a potentially irreversible disorder of rhythmical, involuntary muscle movements (see chapter 19 for details of both conditions). **Don't use if you have:** Known prolongation of QT interval on your EKG, or if you take other drugs that can prolong the QT interval (such as quinidine, pimozide, and others), as mesoridazine causes QTc prolongation and can result in irregular heart rhythms and death. **Use extra caution if you have:** *Breast cancer,* as mesoridazine can elevate prolactin, a hormone released by the pituitary that may cause breast cancer to grow faster; *epilepsy,* as mesoridazine may increase the frequency of seizures; *glaucoma, low blood pressure, prostatic hypertrophy* or *urinary retention,* as the symptoms may worsen. **Tests before starting:** None. **Alcohol:** Should be avoided, as the simultaneous use of mesoridazine and alcohol can lower blood pressure significantly and cause confusion. Also, alcohol worsens anxiety and depression and impairs insight and judgment. **Use in pregnancy:** Some antipsychotics have been linked with the "floppy infant syndrome," in which the baby has poor muscle tone. The fetus may also experience pseudoparkinsonism and dystonia, muscular side effects that may cause fetal distress before, during, and shortly after birth. **Sunlight:** Severe sunburns can occur on mesoridazine. Avoid sunbathing entirely and avoid casual exposure to the sun for more than thirty minutes. Use a sunblock of a sun protection factor (SPF) of 15 or more if exposure to the sun cannot be avoided.

DRUG INTERACTIONS   Use with extra caution if you take: *Tricyclic antidepressants,* as the combination may cause irregular heart rhythms that are potentially fatal; *anticonvulsants, antidepressants, antihistamines, antipsychotics, barbiturates, benzodiazepines,* or any drug that causes sedation or central nervous system depression, because the combination can cause pronounced sedation; *antihypertensive medication,* as mesoridazine may combine to lower blood pressure excessively; *antihistamines,* or *antiparkinsonian agents,* as they may combine to produce pronounced dry mouth, blurry vision, constipation, low blood pressure, rapid heart rate, and mental confusion.

DOSING   Adults: The starting dose is 25–50 mg one to three times a day with weekly increases of 25–50 mg/day up to maximum of 400 mg/day. **Children:** Not FDA-approved for under 12. Some child psychiatrists recommend adult doses for those over 12.

MONITORING YOUR USE   Time to effectiveness: Calming effects are often noticed within one to three hours of a dose, but several days may be needed to notice any effect on psychotic symptoms. A pronounced effect may take one to two weeks. Many months may be needed to derive full benefit. **A full trial is:** Four weeks at no less than 100 mg/day. **Half-life of drug and active metabolites:** 20–40 hours with active metabolites. **How to monitor dosage:** The optimal dose is determined by its effectiveness in alleviating the target symptoms. **How to monitor safety:** Examination for the presence of tardive dyskinesia (see below) should be performed twice yearly. **If you miss a dose:** Take a missed dose if it's the same day. Do not try to make up for a missed dose the next day by doubling your dose; just continue with your regular dosing schedule.

SIDE EFFECTS   Usual (50–100%): Sedation, dry mouth, constipation, blurry vision. **Common (10–50%):** Low blood pressure (light-headedness, dizziness), fatigue, ataraxia (zombielike feeling), weight gain, menstrual irregularities, akathisia (restlessness), sexual dysfunction, pseudoparkinsonism (muscular tremor, rigidity, akinesia), and tardive dyskinesia, a form of involuntary muscle movements (see chapter 19 for further details). **Less common (1–10%):** Dystonia (muscle spasms, usually of the head and neck, face, and jaw), galactorrhea (milk leaking from breasts), sexual dysfunction. **Infrequent (less than 1%):** Cataracts, urinary difficulty. **Those requiring attention from your physician:** Symptoms of fever, muscular rigidity, and mental status changes, as you may have neuroleptic malignant syndrome, a potentially severe reaction; any abnormal involuntary movements that suggest tardive dyskinesia; any irregular heartbeats, as you need an EKG to determine if you are having a dangerous heart rhythm; any other physical or emotional changes not described here.

WHAT TO EXPECT WHEN YOU STOP You may notice a return of your symptoms if mesoridazine is tapered gradually. **If stopped abruptly:** There is no acute withdrawal syndrome.

Methadone

GENERAL **Preparations:** Generic and brand name Dolophine in pills and liquid form. **Class:** Narcotic. **Used in:** Methadone is a narcotic available by regular prescription to the general public as a pain reliever. It is used to minimize withdrawal symptoms in people dependent on narcotics who are undergoing detoxification. It is also used as a long-term maintenance treatment of narcotic addiction in combination with medical and psychological treatment through FDA-approved facilities. **Mechanism of action:** Stimulates postsynaptic opiate receptors.

PRECAUTIONS **Warnings:** Methadone is addictive in its own right. It produces euphoria when first begun, although much less than heroin. **Use extra caution if you have:** *Asthma or other breathing problems,* as methadone may impair breathing further; *kidney or liver impairment,* as the metabolism of methadone will be impaired and lead to more intense effects and side effects; *low blood pressure,* as methadone may lower blood pressure further; *urinary retention* or *prostatic hypertrophy,* as methadone may worsen urinary retention. **Tests needed before starting:** None. **Alcohol:** Alcohol should be avoided, as alcohol will lower blood pressure and may impair breathing, as well as worsen anxiety and depression and cause confusion. **Use in pregnancy:** Babies born to mothers on methadone go through a withdrawal syndrome.

DRUG INTERACTIONS **Don't use if you take:** *MAOI antidepressants,* as the combination of narcotics and MAOIs can impair breathing, lower blood pressure, and impair your level of consciousness. On occasion, it has been fatal. **Use**

with extra caution if you take: *Pentazocine, phenytoin,* or *rifampin,* as the combination may cause withdrawal symptoms; *anticonvulsants, antidepressants, antihistamines, antipsychotics, barbiturates, benzodiazepines,* or any drug that causes sedation or central nervous system depression, because the combination with methadone can cause pronounced sedation.

DOSING   Adults: The usual starting dose is 15–40 mg/day with increases up to 120 mg/day.

MONITORING YOUR USE   Time to effectiveness: 30–60 minutes. **A full trial is:** Determined by adherence to the treatment program and abstinence from other substance use. **Half-life of drug:** 13–47 hours. **How to monitor dosage:** Dosage size is determined by the ability to suppress withdrawal symptoms. **How to monitor safety:** No specific medical tests are needed. Monitoring compliance with the treatment program is performed through FDA-regulated clinics only. **If you miss a dose:** Don't double up on the next dose; continue with the regular dosing schedule.

SIDE EFFECTS   Usual (50–100%): Constipation, decreased appetite, dry mouth, euphoria, sexual dysfunction, urinary difficulty. **Less common (1–10%):** Agitation, fainting, headache, insomnia, low heart rate, rash. **Those requiring attention from your physician:** Any emotional, cognitive, and physical changes not listed here.

WHAT TO EXPECT WHEN YOU STOP   You will experience narcotic withdrawal symptoms: runny nose, sneezing, sweating, goose bumps, fever, chills, restlessness, irritability, weakness, anxiety, depression, dilated pupils, rapid heart beat, abdominal cramps, body aches, twitching, decreased appetite, nausea, vomiting, diarrhea, and weight loss. The severity of these symptoms depends on the length of time you have taken methadone, how much you took each day, whether you also take other drugs, and the rate of tapering. There may be psychological dependence and a craving for narcotics long after the last dose is taken. **If stopped abruptly:** The withdrawal symptoms will be pronounced.

Methamphetamine

GENERAL   Preparations: Generic and brand name Desoxyn Gradumet (long-release) tablets. **Class:** Amphetamine stimulant. **Used in:** ADD (developmental disorders). **Mechanism of action:** Releases dopamine and norepinephrine from presynaptic neurons.

PRECAUTIONS   Warnings: *Abuse potential:* Amphetamines have been extensively abused for their stimulant effects of euphoria and increased energy. Extreme psychological dependence has occurred in some individuals, who may exhibit insomnia, irritability, hyperactivity, and personality changes. **Do not use if you have:** *Heart disease,* as amphetamines can cause an elevated heart rate; *hypertension,* as amphetamines can elevate blood pressure; *hyperthyroidism,* as amphetamines can cause a further elevation of heart rate; *glaucoma,* as amphetamines can worsen the symptoms; *Tourette's disorder* or *tics,* as amphetamines can worsen tics. **Use extra caution if you have:** *Bipolar disorder,* as amphetamines can cause a manic episode; *epilepsy,* as amphetamines may increase the frequency of seizures; a *psychotic disorder,* as amphetamines can worsen psychotic symptoms. **Tests needed before starting:** None. **Alcohol:** The simultaneous use of amphetamines and alcohol causes no specific adverse consequences, but alcohol should be avoided because it worsens anxiety and depression and impairs judgment and thinking. **Use in pregnancy:** Infants born to mothers dependent on amphetamines have an increased risk of premature delivery and low birth weight.

DRUG INTERACTIONS **Don't use if you take:** *MAOI antidepressants,* as their use with amphetamines can cause pronounced hypertension and the potential for strokes.

DOSING **Adults:** The usual starting dose is 5 mg once or twice daily with weekly increases of 5 mg up to a maximum of 25 mg/day. **Children:** Not recommended for under 6. For children over 6 the doses are the same as for adults.

MONITORING YOUR USE **Time to effectiveness:** Some effects are noticeable within a few doses. **A full trial is:** Four weeks at the maximum dose. **Half-life of drug and active metabolites:** 4–5 hours. **How to monitor dosage:** The optimal dose is determined by its effectiveness in alleviating the target symptoms. **How to monitor safety:** Weight and height should be monitored regularly, as amphetamines may slow growth. Examination for tics should occur regularly. **If you miss a dose:** Take a missed dose if it's within an hour or two. Do not try to make up for a missed dose by doubling your next dose; just continue with your regular dosing schedule.

SIDE EFFECTS **Common (10–50%):** Abdominal pain, insomnia, tremor, headaches, dry mouth, decreased appetite with weight loss, palpitations, blood pressure increase. **Less common (1–10%):** Tics, growth suppression, psychosis with prolonged excessive use. **Those requiring attention from your physician:** Any physical or emotional changes not listed.

WHAT TO EXPECT WHEN YOU STOP You may notice a return of your symptoms if amphetamines are stopped. **If stopped abruptly:** After prolonged use at a high dose, abrupt cessation can cause fatigue and depression.

Methylphenidate

GENERAL   **Preparations:** Generic and brand names Concerta, Focalin, Metadate CD, Metadate ER, Ritalin, Ritalin LA, and Ritalin SR. **Class:** Stimulant. **Used in:** ADHD (depression, developmental disorders). **Mechanism of action:** Blocks the reuptake of dopamine into presynaptic neurons.

PRECAUTIONS   **Warnings:** *Abuse potential:* Methylphenidate has been extensively abused for its stimulant effects of euphoria and increased energy. Extreme psychological dependence has occurred in some individuals, who may exhibit insomnia, irritability, hyperactivity, and personality changes. **Don't use if you have:** *Glaucoma,* as methylphenidate can worsen the symptoms; *heart disease,* as methylphenidate can cause an elevated heart rate; *hypertension,* as methylphenidate can elevate blood pressure; *hyperthyroidism,* as methylphenidate can cause a further elevation of heart rate; *Tourette's disorder* or *tics,* as methylphenidate can worsen tics. **Use extra caution if you have:** *Bipolar disorder,* as methylphenidate can cause a manic episode; *epilepsy,* as methylphenidate may increase the frequency of seizures; a *psychotic disorder,* as methylphenidate can worsen psychotic symptoms. **Tests needed before starting:** None. **Alcohol:** The simultaneous use of methylphenidate and alcohol causes no specific adverse consequences, but alcohol should be avoided because it worsens anxiety and depression, and impairs judgment and thinking.

DRUG INTERACTIONS   **Use with extra caution if you take:** *MAOI antidepressants,* as there is a potential for hypertensive crises.

DOSING   **Adults:** The usual starting dose is 5–10 mg twice daily with weekly increases of 10–20 mg up to a maximum of 1 mg/kilogram of body weight. **Children:** The usual starting dose for children over age five is 5 mg once or twice daily, with increases of 5 mg/week up to a maximum of 60 mg/day.

MONITORING YOUR USE   **Time to effectiveness:** Improvement of attention span is noticeable within 20–30 minutes of an effective dose. An improvement in depression generally takes weeks. **A full trial is:** Four weeks at the maximum dose. **Half-life of drug and active metabolites:** 2–3 hours with no active metabolites. **How to monitor dosage:** The optimal dose is determined by its effectiveness in alleviating the target symptoms. **How to monitor safety:** Weight and height should be monitored regularly, as methylphenidate may slow growth. Examination for tics should occur regularly. **If you miss a dose:** Take a missed dose if it's within an hour or two. Do not try to make up for a missed dose by doubling your next dose; just continue with your regular dosing schedule.

SIDE EFFECTS   **Common (10–50%):** Abdominal pain, insomnia, tremor, headaches, dry mouth, decreased appetite with weight loss, palpitations, blood pressure increase. **Less common (1–10%):** Tics, growth suppression, psychosis with prolonged excessive use. **Those requiring attention from your physician:** Any physical or emotional changes not listed.

WHAT TO EXPECT WHEN YOU STOP You may notice a return of your symptoms if methylphenidate is stopped. **If stopped abruptly:** After prolonged use at a high dose, abrupt cessation can cause fatigue and depression.

Mirtazapine

GENERAL **Preparations:** Generic and brand name Remeron. **Class:** Antidepressant. **Used in:** Depression (insomnia). **Mechanism of action:** Blocks presynaptic receptors leading to increased norepinephrine and serotonin.

PRECAUTIONS **Warnings:** Mirtazapine can cause *agranulocytosis*, a severe reaction that is potentially fatal (see chapter 19). **Use extra caution if you have:** *Bipolar disorder*, as mirtazapine may cause a manic episode; *epilepsy*, as mirtazapine may increase the frequency of seizures; *low blood pressure*, as mirtazapine may lower it further; a *psychotic disorder*, as mirtazapine may make psychotic symptoms worse. **Tests needed before starting:** An electrocardiogram (EKG) if you are over 35, to ensure you do not have any form of heart block. **Alcohol:** Should be avoided because it may cause excessive sedation and low blood pressure and cause confusion. Alcohol also worsens anxiety and depression.

DRUG INTERACTIONS **Don't use if you take:** *MAOI antidepressants*, as their use with mirtazapine can cause pronounced high blood pressure and the potential for strokes. **Use with extra caution if you take:** *Anticonvulsants, antidepressants, antihistamines, antipsychotics, barbiturates, benzodiazepines,* or any drug that causes sedation or central nervous system depression, because the combination can cause pronounced sedation. **Use with extra caution if you take:** *Antihypertensives*, as mirtazapine may lower blood pressure excessively.

DOSING **Adults:** The usual starting dose is 15 mg at bedtime with increases of 15 mg/day every week up to 45 mg/day. **Children:** Not FDA-approved for under 18.

MONITORING YOUR USE **Time to effectiveness:** Side effects are generally noticeable within a few doses. The antidepressant effect takes two to four weeks. **A full trial is:** Four weeks at the maximum tolerated dosage. **Half-life of drug and active metabolites:** 20–40 hours. Metabolites possess minimal activity. **How to monitor dosage:** The optimal dose is determined by its effectiveness in alleviating the target symptoms. **How to monitor safety:** No specific tests are needed. **If you miss a dose:** Take a missed dose if it's within an hour or two. Do not try to make up for a missed dose by doubling your next dose; just continue with your regular dosing schedule.

SIDE EFFECTS   Usual (50–100%): Fatigue. **Common (10–50%):** Increased appetite, constipation, dizziness, dry mouth, weight gain. **Those requiring attention from your physician:** Any sign of infection, such as lethargy, fever, or sore throat, which may be due to agranulocytosis; any physical or emotional changes not listed, such as suicidal thoughts or behavior.

WHAT TO EXPECT WHEN YOU STOP   You may notice a return of your symptoms if mirtazapine is stopped.

Molindone

GENERAL   Preparations: Generic and brand name Moban. **Class:** Standard antipsychotic. **Used in:** Bipolar disorder, psychotic disorders (Alzheimer's disease, severe anxiety). **Mechanism of action:** Blocks postsynaptic dopamine receptors.

PRECAUTIONS   Warnings: All antipsychotics can cause *neuroleptic malignant syndrome,* a rare but severe and potentially fatal reaction consisting of fever, muscle rigidity, mental status changes, and alterations in pulse and blood pressure. They can also cause *tardive dyskinesia,* a potentially irreversible disorder of rhythmical, involuntary muscle movements (see chapter 19 for details of both conditions). **Use extra caution if you have:** *Breast cancer:* as molindone can elevate prolactin, a hormone released by the pituitary that may cause breast cancer to grow faster; *epilepsy,* as molindone may increase the frequency of seizures; *glaucoma, low blood pressure, prostatic hypertrophy* or *urinary retention,* as the symptoms may worsen. **Tests before starting:** None. **Alcohol:** Should be avoided, as the simultaneous use of molindone and alcohol can lower blood pressure significantly and cause confusion. Also, alcohol worsens anxiety and depression and impairs insight and judgment. **Use in pregnancy:** Some neuroleptics have been linked with the "floppy infant syndrome," in which the baby has poor muscle tone. The fetus may experience pseudoparkinsonism and dystonia, muscular side effects which may cause fetal distress before, during, and shortly after birth. **Sunlight:** Severe sunburns can occur on molindone. Avoid sunbathing entirely and avoid casual exposure to the sun for more than thirty minutes. Use a sunblock of a sun protection factor (SPF) of 15 or more if exposure to the sun cannot be avoided.

DRUG INTERACTIONS   Use with extra caution if you take: *Anticonvulsants, antidepressants, antihistamines, antipsychotics, barbiturates, benzodiazepines,* or any drug that causes sedation or central nervous system depression, because the combination can cause pronounced sedation; *antihypertensives,* as molindone may combine to lower blood pressure excessively; *antihistamines,* or *antiparkinsonian agents,* as they may combine to produce pronounced dry mouth, blurry vision, constipation, low blood pressure, rapid heart rate, and mental confusion.

DOSING **Adults:** The starting dose is 50–75 mg/day with weekly increases of 25–50 mg/day up to a maximum of 225 mg/day. **Children:** Not FDA-approved for under 12. Some child psychiatrists recommend the same dosages as adults for those over 12.

MONITORING YOUR USE **Time to effectiveness:** Calming effects are often noticed within one to three hours of a dose, but several days may be needed to notice any effect on psychotic symptoms. A pronounced effect may take one to two weeks. Many months may be needed to derive full benefit. **A full trial is:** Four weeks at no less than 100 mg/day. **Half-life of drug and active metabolites:** 12 hours with many active metabolites. **How to monitor dosage:** The optimal dose is determined by its effectiveness in alleviating the target symptoms. **How to monitor safety:** Examination for the presence of tardive dyskinesia (see below) should be performed twice yearly. **If you miss a dose:** Take a missed dose if it's the same day. Do not try to make up for a missed dose the next day by doubling your dose; just continue with your regular dosing schedule.

SIDE EFFECTS **Usual (50–100%):** Sedation. **Common (10–50%):** Blurry vision, constipation, dry mouth, depression, fatigue, ataraxia (zombielike feeling), weight gain, menstrual irregularities, akathisia (restlessness), pseudoparkinsonism (muscular tremor, rigidity, akinesia), and tardive dyskinesia, a form of involuntary muscle movements (see chapter 19 for further details). **Less common (1–10%):** Dystonia (muscle spasms, usually of the head and neck, face, and jaw), galactorrhea (milk leaking from breasts), sexual dysfunction. **Infrequent (less than 1%):** Urinary difficulty, cataracts. **Those requiring attention from your physician:** Any other physical or emotional changes not described here.

WHAT TO EXPECT WHEN YOU STOP You may notice a return of your symptoms if molindone is tapered gradually. **If stopped abruptly:** There is no acute withdrawal syndrome.

Nadolol

GENERAL **Preparations:** Generic and brand name Corgard. **Class:** Beta-blocker. **Used in:** Antipsychotic-induced akathisia, lithium-induced tremor (developmental disorders). **Mechanism of action:** Blocks the beta-adrenergic receptors on muscle and brain cells.

PRECAUTIONS **Don't use if you have:** *Asthma,* as nadolol may worsen breathing; *heart block* (an abnormal heart rhythm), *heart failure,* or a *slow heart rate,* as nadolol may worsen heart block and dangerously affect heart function. **Use extra caution if you have:** *Diabetes,* as nadolol may block the signs of hypoglycemia, thereby delaying needed treatment with glucose; *thyroid dysfunction,* as nadolol may mask symptoms of excessive thyroid hormone production, thereby delaying needed treatment. **Tests needed before starting:** None. **Alcohol:** Should be avoided. The simultaneous use of nadolol and alcohol may cause dizziness, confusion, and low blood pressure. **Use in pregnancy:** Beta-blocker use by pregnant mothers is associated with babies who were born small for their gestational age.

DRUG INTERACTIONS   Use with extra caution if you take: *Verapamil (Calan)* or *diltiazem (Cardizem),* as the combination may cause heart block and impair heart function; *reserpine,* as the combination may cause excessively low blood pressure.

DOSING   Adults: The usual starting dose is 40 mg one to two times a day, with weekly increases of 40–80 mg/day up to a maximum of 240 mg/day. **Children:** Not FDA-approved for under 18.

MONITORING YOUR USE   Time to effectiveness: Improvement in akathisia or tremor is generally noticed within a couple of doses. **A full trial is:** One week at the maximum dose. **Half-life of drug and active metabolites:** 10–24 hours with no active metabolites. **How to monitor dosage:** The optimal dose is determined by its effectiveness in alleviating the target symptoms. Some psychiatrists recommend that you reduce your dose if your pulse goes below 60 beats per minute. **How to monitor safety:** Monitor pulse and blood pressure. It is generally wise to avoid doses that lower your pulse below sixty beats a minute. **If you miss a dose:** Take a missed dose if it's within an hour or two. Do not try to make up for a missed dose by doubling your next dose; just continue with your regular dosing schedule.

SIDE EFFECTS   Less common (1–10%): Low blood pressure, slowed heart rate, fatigue. **Those requiring attention from your physician:** Physical or emotional changes not listed.

WHAT TO EXPECT WHEN YOU STOP   ** You may notice a return of your symptoms when nadolol is stopped. **If stopped abruptly: You may notice a withdrawal syndrome with symptoms of headache, malaise, palpitations, sweating, and tremor. People with heart disease may notice chest pain or angina upon withdrawal. Nadolol should always be tapered gradually in consultation with your physician.

Naltrexone

GENERAL   Preparations: Generic and brand names Depade, ReVia, Trexan. **Class:** Opioid blocker. **Used in:** Alcohol dependence, narcotic addiction (developmental disorders). **Mechanism of action:** Binds to postsynaptic opiate receptors. It is unknown how this effect influences alcohol consumption.

PRECAUTIONS **Do not use if you have:** Used any opiates within the previous 10 days, as naltrexone may cause symptoms of narcotic withdrawal; don't attempt to overcome the effect of naltrexone by taking a large amount of an opiate, as this can cause impaired breathing and a fatal overdose; *liver disease,* as naltrexone can cause further liver impairment. **Tests needed before starting:** Liver function tests. **Alcohol:** Though not dangerous, the use of alcohol should be avoided.

DRUG INTERACTIONS **Use with extra caution if you take:** *Disulfiram,* as the combination may cause liver damage.

DOSING **Adults:** The usual starting dose is 25 mg daily. If no withdrawal symptoms appear, the dose can be raised to the maintenance dose of 50 mg daily. 100 mg every other day may be as effective but may be more likely to cause liver damage. **Children:** Not FDA-approved for under 18.

MONITORING YOUR USE **Time to effectiveness:** 30–60 minutes. **A full trial is:** Determined by the effectiveness in maintaining abstinence. **Half-life of drug and active metabolites:** Four hours; one active metabolite with a half-life of 13 hours. **How to monitor dosage:** The optimal dose is determined by its effectiveness in maintaining abstinence. **How to monitor safety:** Blood tests to measure liver function. **If you miss a dose:** Don't double your next dose; just continue with your regular dosing schedule.

SIDE EFFECTS **Common (10–50%):** Nausea, indigestion. **Less common (1–10%):** Anxiety, dizziness, fatigue, headache, insomnia, nausea. **Those requiring attention from your physician:** Any physical changes not noted here.

WHAT TO EXPECT WHEN YOU STOP There may be a withdrawal syndrome with symptoms of tearfulness, nausea, abdominal cramps, restlessness, bone or joint pain, muscle aches, and nasal congestion. You may experience a craving for alcohol or opiates.

Nefazodone

GENERAL **Preparations:** Brand name Serzone only. **Class:** Antidepressant. **Used in:** Depression. **Mechanism of action:** Blocks the reuptake of norepinephrine and serotonin into presynaptic neurons.

PRECAUTIONS **Warnings:** Rarely, nefazodone has caused liver failure and death. **Use extra caution if you have:** *Asthma, low blood pressure, congestive heart failure, edema, epilepsy, glaucoma, heart disease, hyperthyroidism, enlarged prostate* or *urinary retention,* as nefazodone can worsen the symptoms of these disorders; *bipolar disorder,* as nefazodone may cause a manic episode; a *psychotic disorder,* as nefazodone may make psychotic symptoms worse. **Tests needed before starting:** None. **Alcohol:** Should be avoided as the simultaneous use of nefazodone and alcohol can lower blood pressure significantly and cause confusion. Also, alcohol worsens anxiety and depression and impairs insight and judgment.

DRUG INTERACTIONS   **Don't use if you take:** *MAOI antidepressants,* as their use with nefazodone can cause pronounced hypertension and the potential for strokes; *terfenadine (Seldane), astemizole (Hismanal),* or *cisapride (Propulsid),* as the combination with nefazodone can cause irregular heart rhythms that are potentially life threatening; *alprazolam (Xanax)* and *triazolam (Halcion),* as nefazodone may intensify their effects and significantly impair your thinking and coordination. **Use with extra caution if you take:** *Antihypertensives,* as nefazodone may lower blood pressure excessively; *antihistamines, phenothiazines,* or *tricyclic antidepressants,* as they may combine to produce pronounced dry mouth, blurry vision, constipation, low blood pressure, rapid heart rate, and even mental confusion; *anticonvulsants, antidepressants, antihistamines, antipsychotics, barbiturates, benzodiazepines,* or any drug that causes sedation or central nervous system depression, because the combination can cause pronounced sedation.

DOSING   **Adults:** The usual starting dose is 100 mg twice daily, with weekly increases of 100 mg/day up to 300–600 mg/day. **Children:** Not FDA-approved for under 18.

MONITORING YOUR USE   **Time to effectiveness:** Side effects are generally noticeable within a few doses but the therapeutic effect may take two to four weeks. **A full trial is:** Four weeks at the maximum tolerated dosage. **Half-life of drug and active metabolites:** 2–4 hours with many active metabolites with half-lives of 4–33 hours. **How to monitor dosage:** The optimal dose is determined by its effectiveness in alleviating the target symptoms. **How to monitor safety:** No specific tests needed. **If you miss a dose:** Take a missed dose if it's within an hour or two. Do not try to make up for a missed dose by doubling your next dose; just continue with your regular dosing schedule.

SIDE EFFECTS   **Common (10–50%):** Blurry vision, constipation, dizziness, dry mouth, fatigue, headache, insomnia, nausea, sweating, weight gain. **Less common (1–10%):** Confusion, memory impairment, sexual dysfunction. **Infrequent (less than 1%):** Urinary difficulty. **Those requiring attention from your physician:** Abdominal pain, yellow eyes or skin, or any sign of liver impairment. Any physical or emotional changes not listed, such as suicidal thoughts or behavior.

WHAT TO EXPECT WHEN YOU STOP   You may notice a return of your symptoms if nefazodone is stopped. **If stopped abruptly:** There is no specific withdrawal syndrome.

Nortriptyline

GENERAL   **Preparations:** Generic and brand names Aventyl and Pamelor in pills and liquid form. **Class:** Tricyclic antidepressant. **Used in:** ADHD, bulimia, depression, panic disorder, other anxiety disorders. **Mechanism of action:** Blocks the reuptake of norepinephrine and serotonin into presynaptic neurons.

PRECAUTIONS   **Don't use if you have:** *Heart block* (an abnormal heart rhythm) or if you recently had a *heart attack,* as nortriptyline may worsen heart block and dangerously affect heart function. **Use extra caution if you have:** *Bipolar disorder,* as nortriptyline may cause a manic episode; *epilepsy,* as nortriptyline may increase the frequency of seizures; *glaucoma,* as nortriptyline can worsen the symptoms of untreated angle closure glaucoma; *low blood pressure;* as nortriptyline may lower blood pressure further; a *psychotic disorder,* as nortriptyline may make psychotic symptoms worse; *hyperthyroidism,* as nortriptyline may cause irregular heart rhythms; *prostatic hypertrophy* or *urinary retention,* as nortriptyline may worsen urinary retention. **Tests needed before starting:** An electrocardiogram (EKG) if you are over 35, to ensure that you do not have any form of heart block. **Alcohol:** Should be avoided, as the simultaneous use of nortripyline and alcohol can lower blood pressure significantly and cause confusion. Also, alcohol worsens anxiety and depression, and impairs insight and judgment. **Use in pregnancy:** There is a higher rate of miscarriages born to women who take tricyclics, but no specific defect is associated with their use.

DRUG INTERACTIONS   **Don't use if you take:** *MAOI antidepressants,* as their use with nortriptyline can cause pronounced hypertension and the potential for strokes. **Use with extra caution if you take:** *Phenothiazines,* as the combination may cause irregular heart rhythms which are potentially fatal; *antihypertensives,* as they may combine to lower blood pressure excessively; *antihistamines, phenothiazines,* and *antiparkinsonian agents,* as they may combine to produce pronounced dry mouth, blurry vision, constipation, low blood pressure, rapid heart rate, and even mental confusion; *guanethadine* to lower blood pressure, as nortriptyline may block its effects.

DOSING   **Adults:** The usual starting dose is 25 mg at bedtime with increases every other day up to 150 mg/day. Doses up to 300 mg/day are sometimes used. **Children:** Not FDA-approved for under 12. Some child psychiatrists recommend a starting dose of 25 mg/day with weekly increases of 25 mg/day up to a maximum of 75 mg/day for those over 12. **The elderly:** The usual starting dose is 10 mg at bedtime with weekly increases of 10 mg/day every few days up to 50–100 mg/day.

MONITORING YOUR USE   **Time to effectiveness:** Side effects are generally noticeable within a few doses, but the therapeutic effect may take weeks. **A full trial is:** Four weeks at the maximum tolerated dosage. **Half-life of drug and active metabolites:** 22–58 hours, with no active metabolites. **How to monitor dosage:** The optimal dose is determined by its effectiveness in alleviating the target symptoms. The therapeutic effect of nortriptyline is more likely when the concentration in the blood is between 50 and 150 micrograms. A blood level may be useful to assist in determining the best dosage if you do not respond or if your side effects are more pronounced than expected. **How to monitor safety:** A blood level should be obtained if doses go over 150 mg/day. An EKG may be useful to ensure that heart function is not impaired. **If you miss a dose:** Take a missed dose if it's within an hour or two. Do not try to make up for a missed dose by doubling your next dose; just continue with your regular dosing schedule.

SIDE EFFECTS   **Usual (50–100%):** Blurry vision, constipation, dry mouth, fatigue, increased heart rate, low blood pressure. **Common (10–50%):** Sweating, weight gain. **Less common (1–10%):** Sexual dysfunction, urinary retention. **Those requiring attention from your physician:** Physical or emotional changes not listed, such as suicidal thoughts or behavior.

WHAT TO EXPECT WHEN YOU STOP   You may notice a return of your symptoms if nortriptyline is stopped. **If stopped abruptly:** You may experience agitation, headaches, insomnia, and nausea, as well as depression. Nortriptyline should be slowly tapered if you decide to stop it. The rate of discontinuation is different for each person and is determined by the clinical situation necessitating the change, your age, severity of symptoms, dosage size, and your duration of use.

Olanzapine

GENERAL   **Preparations:** Brand name Zyprexa and orally disintegrating Zyprexa Zydis. **Class:** Atypical antipsychotic. **Used in:** Bipolar disorder, psychotic disorders (Alzheimer's disease, severe anxiety, developmental disorders). **Mechanism of action:** Blocks a subset of dopamine and serotonin receptors.

PRECAUTIONS   **Warnings:** All antipsychotics can cause *neuroleptic malignant syndrome,* a rare, but severe and potentially fatal reaction consisting of fever, muscle rigidity, mental status changes, and alterations in pulse and blood pressure. They can also cause *tardive dyskinesia,* a potentially irreversible disorder of rhythmical, involuntary muscle movements (see chapter 19 for details of both conditions). Olanzapine and other atypical antipsychotics are associated with the development of *weight gain, high cholesterol, and diabetes mellitus*. Olanzapine and other atypical antipsychotics are also associated with a higher incidence of *strokes* and *sudden death* in elderly people with dementia. **Use extra caution if you have:** *Breast cancer,* as olanzapine can elevate prolactin, a hormone released by the pituitary which may cause breast cancer to grow faster; *epilepsy:* as olanzapine may increase the frequency of seizures; *liver disease,* as olanzapine may worsen impairment of liver functioning; *low blood pressure,* as olanzapine can lower blood pressure even further. **Tests before starting:** None. **Alcohol:** Should be avoided, as the simultaneous use of olanzapine and alcohol can lower blood pressure significantly and cause confusion. Also, alcohol worsens anxiety and depression and impairs insight and judgment.

DRUG INTERACTIONS **Use with extra caution if you take:** *Anticonvulsants, antidepressants, antihistamines, antipsychotics, barbiturates, benzodiazepines,* or any drug that causes sedation or central nervous system depression, because the combination can cause pronounced sedation; *antihypertensive medication,* as olanzapine may combine to lower blood pressure excessively; *antihistamines* or *antiparkinsonian agents,* as they may combine to produce pronounced dry mouth, blurry vision, constipation, low blood pressure, rapid heart rate, and mental confusion.

DOSING **Adults:** The starting dose is 10 mg/day with weekly increases of 10 mg/day up to a maximum of 30 mg/day. **Children:** Not FDA-approved for under 18. Some child psychiatrists begin older adolescents on 5–10 mg/day, with weekly increases of 5 mg/day up to a maximum of 20 mg/day.

MONITORING YOUR USE **Time to effectiveness:** The first effects may be noticed within some days, but it may take one to three weeks to notice a pronounced change. It may take several months to derive full benefit. **A full trial is:** Four weeks at no less than 20 mg/day. **Half-life of drug and active metabolites:** 21–54 hours with no active metabolites. **How to monitor dosage:** The optimal dose is determined by its effectiveness in alleviating the target symptoms. **How to monitor safety:** Pretreatment and periodic weight measurements should be performed to assess weight gain; blood glucose, cholesterol, and lipid profiles should be obtained after three months and yearly thereafter to check for diabetes and elevations in cholesterol or triglycerides. A physical examination for the presence of tardive dyskinesia (see below) should be done twice yearly. **If you miss a dose:** Take a missed dose if it's the same day. Do not try to make up for a missed dose the next day by doubling your dose; just continue with your regular dosing schedule.

SIDE EFFECTS **Common (10–50%):** Low blood pressure (light-headedness, dizziness), cholesterol elevations, constipation, fatigue, weight gain, menstrual irregularities, akathisia (restlessness), sexual dysfunction. **Less common (1–10%):**

Cognitive changes (memory impairment, stuttering), tardive dyskinesia. **Those requiring attention from your physician:** Symptoms of fever, muscular rigidity, and mental status changes, as you may have neuroleptic malignant syndrome, a potentially severe reaction; any abnormal involuntary movements which suggest tardive dyskinesia; Any other physical or emotional changes not described here.

WHAT TO EXPECT IF YOU STOP   You may notice a return of your symptoms if olanzapine is tapered gradually. **If stopped abruptly:** There is no acute withdrawal syndrome, but symptoms may return quickly.

Oxcarbazepine

GENERAL   **Preparations:** Brand name Trileptal only in pills and liquid. **Class:** Mood stabilizer. **Used in:** Bipolar disorder. **Mechanism of action:** Oxcarbazepine has many actions in the brain on receptors, neurotransmitter concentrations, ion channels, and second messenger systems, but it is unknown which effect stabilizes mood.

PRECAUTIONS   **Warnings:** Oxcarbazepine can cause serious skin reactions that are potentially fatal, though quite rare. Oxcarbazepine causes *hyponatremia* in about 1 percent of people who take it. Hyponatremia means a low sodium level in the blood. It is a serious abnormality that requires immediate medical attention. **Use extra caution if you have:** *Kidney* or *liver disease,* as they may slow the rate of metabolism; *glaucoma,* as oxcarbazepine can worsen the symptoms. **Tests needed before starting:** Blood electrolytes. **Alcohol:** It should be avoided, as it may impair the effectiveness of oxcarbazepine. Alcohol should also be avoided because it can worsen depression and cause confusion in bipolar disorder. **Use in pregnancy:** Similar drugs (e.g., carbamazepine) are known to cause birth defects, so use in pregnancy is not recommended.

DRUG INTERACTIONS   **Don't use if you take:** *MAOI antidepressants,* as their use with oxcarbazepine can cause a dangerous elevation of blood pressure and a stroke. **Use with extra caution if you take:** *Anticonvulsants, antidepressants, antihistamines, antipsychotics, barbiturates, benzodiazepines,* or any drug that causes sedation or central nervous system depression, because the combination can cause pronounced sedation; *oral or subdermal implant contraceptives,* as their reliability may be affected and pregnancy result.

DOSING Adults: The usual starting dose is 300 mg twice daily, with weekly increases of 300 mg/day up to a maximum of 1200 mg/day. Doses up to 2400 mg/day may be more effective, but many people experience pronounced side effects at doses higher than 1200/day. **Children:** Ages 4–16: the usual starting dose is 8–10 mg/day, divided into two doses, with increases over two weeks to reach a dose of

900 mg/day if the child weighs 20–29 kg, 1200 mg/day if the child weighs 29–39 kg, and 1800 mg/day if the child weighs more than 39 kg.

MONITORING YOUR USE   **Time to effectiveness:** You may notice some side effects within one to two days, but any improvement in symptoms generally takes one to two weeks if you are manic. **A full trial is:** Three weeks at the maximum therapeutic level if you are manic. There is no set period of time with which to determine effectiveness if you start carbamazepine when your mood is stable, as manic symptoms are often absent for extended periods of time. Essentially, you stay on the drug and watch for any symptoms of mania. If none appear, or if they are milder than usual, then oxcarbazepine is at least partially effective. **Half-life of drug and active metabolites:** The half-life of oxcarbazepine is 2 hours, but that of its active metabolite is 9 hours. **How to monitor dosage:** The optimal dose is determined by its effectiveness in managing symptoms. Improved effectiveness can sometimes be achieved by maintaining the level at the higher end of the dosage range. **How to monitor safety:** Serum sodium should be monitored regularly. **If you miss a dose:** Take a missed dose if it's within a few hours. Do not try to make up for a missed dose by doubling your next dose; just continue with your regular dosing schedule.

SIDE EFFECTS   **Common (10–50%):** Abdominal pain, dizziness, fatigue, headache, nausea and vomiting, sedation, tremor, vertigo, double vision, an unsteady gait. **Less common: (1–10%):** Constipation, diarrhea, indigestion, rash. **Those requiring attention from your physician:** Any rash should be immediately reported, as it may progress to a life-threatening reaction. Nausea, fatigue, headache, lethargy, and confusion may be due to hyponatremia and need immediate medical evaluation.

WHAT TO EXPECT WHEN YOU STOP   You may notice a return of your symptoms if oxcarbazepine is tapered gradually. **If stopped abruptly:** You may develop withdrawal seizures. Oxcarbazepine should not be stopped abruptly, but needs to be gradually tapered in consultation with your physician.

Oxazepam

GENERAL   **Preparations:** Generic and brand name Serax. **Class:** Benzodiazepine. **Used in:** Alcohol withdrawal, anxiety disorders, bipolar disorder (Alzheimer's disease, antipsychotic-induced akathisia ([restlessness]), insomnia). **Mechanism of action:** Intensifies the effects of gamma-aminobutyric acid (GABA).

PRECAUTIONS   **Warnings:** *It is habit-forming.* Oxazepam, like all benzodiazepines, is physically and psychologically habit-forming. People who have experienced traumatic events in their lives and have chronic anxiety are especially prone to developing dependence. Prolonged use is associated with a range of problems. Use for more than four weeks is *not* recommended. If you stop oxazepam after more than four weeks of daily use you will probably experience withdrawal symptoms (see below). *Seizures can occur if it is stopped abruptly,* so consultation with your physician is essential if you wish to stop. **Tests needed before starting:** None. **Alcohol:** Alcohol must be avoided entirely. The simultaneous use of oxazepam and alcohol is extremely dangerous because it can cause you to stop breathing. The combination can cause death. **Use in pregnancy:** There is a higher rate of babies born with a cleft palate to mothers who took benzodiazepines during pregnancy. **The elderly** are especially sensitive to the effects of benzodiazepines and may experience pronounced side effects at low doses (see chapter 4).

DRUG INTERACTIONS   **Use with extra caution and notify your physician if you take:** *Anticonvulsants, antidepressants, antihistamines, antipsychotics, barbiturates, benzodiazepines,* or any drug that causes sedation or central nervous system depression, because the combination with oxazepam can cause pronounced sedation.

DOSING   **Adults:** The usual starting dose is 10–30 mg one to four times a day with a maximum dose of 120 mg/day. **Children:** Not FDA-approved for under 12. Some child psychiatrists recommend adult dosages.

MONITORING YOUR USE   **Time to effectiveness:** 60–120 minutes. **A full trial is:** A few doses are generally enough to establish whether it will be helpful. **Half-life of drug and active metabolites:** 5–15 hours, with no active metabolites. **How to monitor dosage:** The optimal dose is determined by its effectiveness in alleviating the target symptoms. **If you miss a dose:** Do *not* try to make up for a missed dose; just continue with your regular dosing schedule. **How to monitor safety:** No specific medical tests are needed to monitor safety.

SIDE EFFECTS   **Common (10–50%):** Sedation, memory impairment, poor muscle coordination (causing a higher rate of falls in the elderly and a higher risk of motor vehicle accidents in all adults). **Infrequent (less than 1%):** Paradoxical agitation and insomnia. **Those requiring attention from your physician:** Any physical or emotional changes not described here. **Side effects associated with use longer than four weeks:** Use of oxazepam longer than four weeks may cause physical and psychological dependence, and you may notice the desire for another dose as each one wears off. Ongoing anxiety, reduced effectiveness of each dose, depression, emotional blunting, and impairment of memory and cognition may occur with use longer than one year.

WHAT TO EXPECT WHEN YOU STOP   You may notice a return of your symptoms if oxazepam is tapered gradually. Other withdrawal symptoms include anxiety, insomnia, irritability, headaches, tremors, nausea, diarrhea, sweating, and confusion. The rate at which you should taper is affected by the duration of your use and the size of your dose, but may take months if you have been on it for an extended period of time. **If stopped abruptly:** *Seizures* can occur if oxazepam is stopped abruptly. They are potentially life-threatening. As a result you should never stop oxazepam abruptly and you should always work with your physician to taper it gradually.

Paroxetine

GENERAL **Preparations:** Generic and brand name Paxil. **Class:** SSRI (selective serotonin reuptake inhibitor). **Used in:** Bulimia, depression, obsessive-compulsive disorder, panic disorder (other anxiety disorders, developmental disorders). **Mechanism of action:** Blocks the reuptake of serotonin by presynaptic neurons.

PRECAUTIONS **Warnings:** When taken with other serotonin reuptake inhibitors, paroxetine can cause the *serotonin syndrome,* which consists of potentially dangerous alterations in pulse, blood pressure, hyperactivity, and mental status changes (see chapter 19). Rarely, paroxetine can cause hyponatremia, or low sodium in your blood. **Use extra caution if you have:** *Bipolar disorder,* as paroxetine can cause a manic episode; *epilepsy,* as paroxetine may increase the frequency of seizures; a *psychotic disorder,* as paroxetine can worsen psychotic symptoms. **Tests needed before starting:** None. **Alcohol:** The simultaneous use of paroxetine and alcohol causes no specific adverse consequences, but alcohol should be avoided because it worsens anxiety and depression. **Use in pregnancy:** There is a higher rate of miscarriage, heart defects, and intestinal defects in the babies of women who take paroxetine during pregnancy.

DRUG INTERACTIONS **Don't use if you take:** *Other SSRIs, St. John's wort,* or *tryptophan* as their use with paroxetine can cause the *serotonin syndrome; MAOI antidepressants,* as their use with paroxetine can cause a serious, sometimes fatal, reaction of agitation, fever, cardiovascular changes, and mental status changes.

DOSING **Adults:** The usual starting dose is 10–20 mg once daily with weekly increases of 10 mg/day up to a maximum of 60 mg/day. **Children:** Not FDA-approved for under 18. Some child psychiatrists start with 5 mg/day with increases of 5–10 mg/day every one to four weeks.

MONITORING YOUR USE **Time to effectiveness:** You may notice some side effects within one to two days, but any improvement in symptoms generally takes two to four weeks. **A full trial is:** Four weeks at the maximum dose. **Half-life of drug and active metabolites:** 20 hours with no active metabolites. **How to monitor dosage:** The optimal dose is determined by its effectiveness in alleviating the target symptoms. **How to monitor safety:** No specific tests are needed to monitor your health while on paroxetine. **If you miss a dose:** Take a missed dose if it's the same day. Do not try to make up for a missed dose the next day by doubling your dose; just continue with your regular dosing schedule.

SIDE EFFECTS   **Common (10–50%):** Nausea, fatigue, weakness, sweating, decreased appetite, and sexual dysfunction. **Less common (1–10%):** Insomnia, anxiety, tremor. **Those requiring attention from your physician:** Hyperactivity, mental status changes, or alterations in your pulse or blood pressure, which suggest the serotonin syndrome; any physical or emotional changes not listed, such as suicidal thoughts and behavior.

WHAT TO EXPECT WHEN YOU STOP   You may notice a return of your symptoms if paroxetine is tapered gradually. **If stopped abruptly:** You may notice a flulike syndrome of nausea, vomiting, diarrhea, dizziness, as well as anxiety and depression. Paroxetine should not be stopped abruptly but needs to be gradually tapered in consultation with your physician.

Pemoline

GENERAL   **Preparations:** Generic and brand name Cylert. **Class:** Stimulant. **Used in:** ADHD. **Mechanism of action:** Blocks the reuptake of dopamine into presynaptic neurons.

PRECAUTIONS   **Warnings:** *Abuse potential:* Pemoline can be abused for its stimulant effects of euphoria and increased energy. Dependence can occur in some individuals, who may exhibit insomnia, irritability, hyperactivity, and personality changes. *Liver damage and failure* has occurred in 13 people since pemoline was introduced in 1975. **Don't use if you have:** *Heart disease,* as pemoline can cause an elevated heart rate; *hypertension,* as pemoline can elevate blood pressure; *hyperthyroidism,* as pemoline can cause a further elevation of heart rate; *liver disease,* as pemoline may further damage the liver; *Tourette's disorder* or *tics,* as pemoline can worsen tics. **Use extra caution if you have:** *Bipolar disorder,* as pemoline can cause a manic episode; *epilepsy,* as pemoline may increase the frequency of seizures; a *psychotic disorder,* as pemoline can worsen psychotic symptoms. **Tests needed before starting:** None. **Alcohol:** The simultaneous use of pemoline and alcohol causes no specific adverse consequences, but alcohol should be avoided because it worsens anxiety and depression, and impairs judgment and thinking.

DRUG INTERACTIONS   **Use with extra caution if you take:** *MAOI antide-pressants,* as there is a potential for a hypertensive crisis.

DOSING   **Adults and children over 6:** The usual starting dose is 37.5 mg once in the morning with weekly increases of 18.75 mg/day up to a maximum of 112.5 mg/day.

MONITORING YOUR USE   **Time to effectiveness:** Improvement is gradual and may take weeks. **A full trial is:** Four weeks at the maximum dose. **Half-life of drug and active metabolites:** 9–14 hours in adults, 2–12 hours in children. At least one metabolite has mild activity similar to pemoline. **How to monitor dosage:** The optimal dose is determined by its effectiveness in alleviating the target symptoms. **How to monitor safety:** Liver function tests should be obtained prior to starting and followed periodically thereafter to screen for the emergence of liver damage. Weight and height should be monitored regularly, as pemoline may slow growth. Examination for tics should occur regularly. **If you miss a dose:** Take a missed dose if it's within an hour or two. Do not try to make up for a missed dose by doubling your next dose; just continue with your regular dosing schedule.

SIDE EFFECTS   **Common (10–50%):** Abdominal pain, insomnia, tremor, headaches, dry mouth, decreased appetite, transient weight loss, which usually reverses itself in three to six months. **Less common (1–10%):** Nausea, psychosis with prolonged excessive use, tics. **Infrequent (less than 1%):** Rash. **Those requiring attention from your physician:** Abdominal pain, yellow skin or eyes, or any sign of liver impairment; any physical or emotional changes not listed.

WHAT TO EXPECT WHEN YOU STOP   You may notice a return of your symptoms if pemoline is stopped. **If stopped abruptly:** After prolonged use at a high dose, abrupt cessation can cause fatigue and depression.

Perphenazine

GENERAL   **Preparations:** Generic and brand name Trilafon in pills and liquid form. **Class:** Standard antipsychotic of the phenothiazine group. **Used in:** Bipolar disorder, psychotic disorders (Alzheimer's disease, severe anxiety). **Mechanism of action:** Blocks postsynaptic dopamine receptors.

PRECAUTIONS   **Warnings:** All antipsychotics can cause *neuroleptic malignant syndrome,* a rare but severe and potentially fatal reaction consisting of fever, muscle rigidity, mental status changes, and alterations in pulse and blood pressure. They can also cause *tardive dyskinesia,* a potentially irreversible disorder of rhythmical, involuntary muscle movements (see chapter 19 for details of both conditions). **Use extra caution if you have:** *Breast cancer,* as perphenazine can elevate prolactin, a hormone released by the pituitary that may cause breast cancer to grow faster; *epilepsy,* as perphenazine may increase the frequency of seizures; *glaucoma, low blood pressure, prostatic hypertrophy* or *urinary retention,* as the symptoms may worsen. **Tests before starting:** None. **Alcohol:** Should be avoided, as the simultaneous use of perphenazine and alcohol can lower blood pressure significantly and cause confusion. Also, alcohol worsens anxiety and depression, and impairs insight and judgment. **Use in pregnancy:** Phenothiazines have been linked with the "floppy infant syndrome," in which the baby has poor muscle tone. The fetus may experience pseudoparkinsonism and dystonia, muscular side effects that may cause fetal distress before, during, and shortly after birth. **Sunlight:** Severe sunburns can occur on perphenazine. Avoid sunbathing entirely and avoid casual exposure to the sun for more than thirty minutes. Use a sunblock of a sun protection factor (SPF) of 15 or more if exposure to the sun cannot be avoided.

DRUG INTERACTIONS **Use with extra caution if you take:** *Tricyclic antidepressants,* as the combination may cause irregular heart rhythms that are potentially fatal; *anticonvulsants, antidepressants, antihistamines, antipsychotics, barbiturates, benzodiazepines,* or any drug that causes sedation or central nervous system depression, because the combination can cause pronounced sedation; *antihypertensive medication,* as perphenazine may combine to lower blood pressure excessively; *antihistamines* or *antiparkinsonian agents,* as they may combine to produce pronounced dry mouth, blurry vision, constipation, low blood pressure, rapid heart rate, and mental confusion.

DOSING **Adults:** The starting dose is 4–8 mg three times a day with weekly increases of 8 mg/day up to a maximum of 64 mg/day **Children:** Not FDA-approved for under 12.

MONITORING YOUR USE **Time to effectiveness:** Calming effects are often noticed within one to three hours of a dose, but several days may be needed to notice any effect on psychotic symptoms. A pronounced effect may take one to two weeks. Many months may be needed to derive full benefit. **A full trial is:** Four weeks at no less than 16 mg/day. **Half-life of drug and active metabolites:** 20–40 hours with active metabolites. **How to monitor dosage:** The optimal dose is determined by its effectiveness in alleviating the target symptoms. **How to monitor safety:** Examination for the presence of tardive dyskinesia (see below) should be performed twice yearly. **If you miss a dose:** Take a missed dose if it's the same day. Do not try to make up for a missed dose the next day by doubling your dose; just continue with your regular dosing schedule.

SIDE EFFECTS **Usual (50–100%):** Dry mouth, constipation, blurry vision. **Common (10–50%):** Low blood pressure (light-headedness, dizziness), fatigue, ataraxia (zombielike feeling), weight gain, menstrual irregularities, akathisia (restlessness), pseudoparkinsonism (muscular tremor, rigidity, akinesia), and tardive dyskinesia, a form of involuntary muscle movements (see chapter 19 for further details). **Less common (1–10%):** Dystonia (muscle spasms, usually of the head and neck, face, and jaw), galactorrhea (milk leaking from breasts), sedation, sexual dysfunction. **Infrequent (less than 1%):** Cataracts. **Those requiring attention from your physician:** Jaundice (yellow eyes or skin); neuroleptic malignant syndrome, a rare but severe and potentially fatal reaction consisting of fever, muscle rigidity, mental status changes, and alterations in pulse and blood pressure (see chapter 19 for further details); any other physical or emotional changes not described here.

WHAT TO EXPECT WHEN YOU STOP You may notice a return of your symptoms if perphenazine is tapered gradually. **If stopped abruptly:** There is no acute withdrawal syndrome.

Phenelzine

GENERAL **Preparations:** Brand name Nardil only. **Class:** MAOI. **Used in:** Bulimia, depression, panic disorder (other anxiety disorders). **Mechanism of action:** Inhibits monoamine oxidase, the protein enzyme responsible for the breakdown of dopamine, epinephrine, norepinephrine, and serotonin, resulting in elevated levels of these neurotransmitters.

PRECAUTIONS **Warnings:** Phenelzine can cause a *hypertensive crisis* in which your blood pressure rises dangerously high, putting you at risk for a brain stroke, brain damage, and death. This reaction is unlikely to occur on its own, but is possible if used in combination with foods or medicines that contain tyramine or substances similar to epinephrine. **The following medications must be avoided while you are on phenelzine and for two weeks following its cessation in order to avoid a hypertensive crisis:** Prescription medications: *Antiasthmatics* that contain *epinephrine* or epinephrine-like compounds, most *antidepressants, antihypertensives, antiparkinsonian agents, barbiturates, buspirone (Buspar), carbamazepine (Tegretol), disulfiram, diuretics, narcotics, stimulants;* over-the-counter medications: *decongestants, dextromethorphan, tryptophan, hay fever medications, sinus medications, appetite suppressants;* recreational drugs: *amphetamines, cocaine, hallucinogenics, heroin, or other narcotics.* **The following foods must be avoided while you are on phenelzine and for two weeks following its cessation in order to avoid a hypertensive crisis:** Aged or fermented foods; all cheese or foods containing cheese such as pizza, fondue, many Italian dishes and salad dressings (cottage cheese and cream cheese are allowed); cream, sour cream, and yogurt; foods fermented with yeast (although foods baked with yeast, such as bread, are safe), brewer's yeast; liver, processed meats, such as bologna, corned beef, hot dogs, liverwurst, pepperoni, salami, sausage; broad bean pods (fava beans); sauerkraut; pickles; soy sauce; licorice, caviar, anchovies, dried fruits (raisins, prunes), figs, raspberries, chocolate; bananas, pickled herring; excessive amounts of caffeine-containing beverages (more than one or two, although some people are more sensitive than others) like coffee, tea, sodas, and hot chocolate. **Don't use if you have:** *Congestive heart failure,* as it may make the symptoms worse; *high blood pressure,* as phenelzine may make the symptoms worse; *pheochromocytoma,* as it may cause a hypertensive crisis. **Use extra caution if you have:** *Bipolar disorder,* as phenelzine can cause a manic episode; *epilepsy,* as phenelzine may increase seizure frequency; *low blood pressure,* as phenelzine may make symptoms worse; a *psychotic disorder,* as phenelzine can worsen psychotic symptoms. **Tests needed before starting:** None. **Alcohol:** Beer, wine, Chianti, sherry, and liqueurs, whether they contain alcohol or not, can cause a hypertensive crisis. Hard liquor has no specific adverse consequences, but should be avoided because it can worsen anxiety, depression, and low blood pressure.

DRUG INTERACTIONS   *Antihypertensives,* as phenelzine can lower blood pressure further; *narcotics,* as the combination can produce coma, fever, and high blood pressure.

DOSING   **Adults:** 15 mg two to three times a day with weekly increases of 15 mg/day up to a maximum of 45 mg twice a day. **Children:** Not FDA-approved for under 16.

MONITORING YOUR USE   **Time to effectiveness:** Side effects may be noted within a few days, but the therapeutic effect may take two to six weeks. **A full trial is:** Four weeks at the maximum tolerated dose. **Half-life of drug and active metabolites:** The specific half-life is unknown but is believed to be fairly short. The effect can last for two weeks after the last dose. **How to monitor dosage:** The optimal dose is determined by its effectiveness in alleviating the target symptoms. **How to monitor safety:** Monitor blood pressure. **If you miss a dose:** Take a missed dose if it's within an hour or two. Do not try to make up for a missed dose the next day by doubling your dose; just continue with your regular dosing schedule.

SIDE EFFECTS   **Common (10–50%):** Agitation, constipation, dizziness, headaches, insomnia, sedation, sexual dysfunction, tremor, muscle twitching, weight gain. **Those requiring attention from your physician:** A sudden headache, palpitations, rapid heart rate, sweating, throat constriction, neck stiffness, nausea, or vomiting can be a sign that you are having a hypertensive crisis; You should consult your physician immediately and go to the emergency room for treatment of any elevation of blood pressure; physical and emotional changes not listed, such as suicidal thoughts or behavior.

WHAT TO EXPECT WHEN YOU STOP   You may notice a return of your symptoms if you taper and stop phenelzine. **If stopped abruptly:** An uncommon withdrawal syndrome starting one to three days after cessation of phenelzine, with agitation, nightmares, seizures, and psychotic thinking, may occur.

Pimozide

GENERAL   **Preparations:** Generic and brand name Orap. **Class:** Standard antipsychotic. **Used in:** Psychotic disorders. **Mechanism of action:** Blocks postsynaptic dopamine receptors.

PRECAUTIONS   **Warnings:** Pimozide can cause *irregular heart rhythms.* Sudden unexpected deaths have occurred in people on pimozide and it is possible that this is the cause. The manufacturer does not provide information about the frequency of this occurrence. All antipsychotics can cause *neuroleptic malignant syndrome,* a rare, but severe and potentially fatal reaction consisting of fever, muscle rigidity, mental status changes, and alterations in pulse and blood pressure. They can also cause *tardive dyskinesia,* a potentially irreversible disorder of rhythmical, involuntary muscle movements (see chapter 19 for details of both conditions). **Use extra caution if you have:** *Breast cancer,* as pimozide can elevate prolactin, a hormone released by the pituitary which may cause breast cancer to grow faster; *epilepsy,* as pimozide may increase the frequency of seizures; *glaucoma, low blood pressure, prostatic hypertrophy* or *urinary retention,* as the symptoms of these disorders may worsen. **Tests before starting:** An EKG. **Alcohol:** Should be avoided, as the simultaneous use of pimozide and alcohol can lower blood pressure significantly and cause confusion. Also, alcohol worsens anxiety and depression, and impairs insight and judgment. **Use in pregnancy:** Some antipsychotics have been linked with the "floppy infant syndrome," in which the baby has poor muscle tone. The fetus may experience pseudoparkinsonism and dystonia, muscular side effects which may cause fetal distress before, during, and shortly after birth. **Sunlight:** Severe sunburns can occur on pimozide. Avoid sunbathing entirely and avoid casual exposure to the sun for more than thirty minutes. Use a sunblock of a sun protection factor (SPF) of 15 or more if exposure to the sun cannot be avoided.

DRUG INTERACTIONS   **Do not use if you take:** Antibiotics *erythromycin, azithromycin, clarithromycin,* or *dirithromycin;* antifungal agents *itraconazole* or *ketoconazole;* or protease inhibitors *indinavir, nelfanavir, ritonavir,* or *saquinavir* as the combination can cause irregular heart rhythms that are potentially fatal. **Use with extra caution if you take:** *Phenothiazines* or *tricyclic antidepressants,* as the combination may cause irregular heart rhythms that are potentially fatal; *anticonvulsants, antidepressants, antihistamines, antipsychotics, barbiturates, benzodiazepines,* or any drug that causes sedation or central nervous system depression, because the combination can cause pronounced sedation; *antihypertensive medication,* as pimozide may combine to lower blood pressure excessively; *antihistamines* or *antiparkinsonian agents,* as they may combine to produce pronounced dry mouth, blurry vision, constipation, low blood pressure, rapid heart rate, and mental confusion.

DOSING   **Adults:** The starting dose is 1–2 mg one to two times a day with weekly increases of 1–2 mg twice daily up to a maximum of 10 mg/day. **Children:** There is limited experience with ages 2–12. As a result some child psychiatrists recommend a starting dose of 0.5 mg one to two times daily with increases of 0.5 mg/day one to two times a week up to a maximum of 0.2 mg/kg/day or 10 mg daily, whichever is less.

MONITORING YOUR USE   **Time to effectiveness:** Calming effects are often noticed within one to three hours of a dose, but several days may be needed to notice any effect on psychotic symptoms. A pronounced effect may take one to two weeks. Many months may be needed to derive full benefit. **A full trial is:** Four weeks at the maximum tolerated dose, but no higher than 10 mg/day. **Half-life of drug and active metabolites:** 55 hours with metabolites of unknown activity. **How to monitor dosage:** The optimal dose is determined by its effectiveness in alleviating the target symptoms. **How to monitor safety:** An EKG should be obtained before starting and after any upward dosage adjustments. Examination for the presence of tardive dyskinesia (see below) should be performed twice yearly. **If you miss a dose:** Take a missed dose if it's the same day. Do not try to make up for a missed dose the next day by doubling your dose, just continue with your regular dosing schedule.

SIDE EFFECTS   **Usual (50–100%):** Sedation, dry mouth, constipation, blurry vision. **Common (10–50%):** Headache, low blood pressure (light-headedness, dizziness), fatigue, ataraxia (zombielike feeling), weight gain, menstrual irregularities, akathisia (restlessness), sexual dysfunction, pseudoparkinsonism (muscular tremor, rigidity, akinesia), and tardive dyskinesia, a form of involuntary muscle movements (see chapter 19 for further details). **Less common (1–10%):** Dystonia (muscle spasms, usually of the head and neck, face, and jaw), galactorrhea (milk leaking from breasts), sexual dysfunction. **Infrequent (less than 1%):** Urinary difficulty; cataracts. **Those requiring attention from your physician:** Symptoms of fever, muscular rigidity, and mental status changes, as you may have neuroleptic malignant syndrome, a potentially severe reaction; any abnormal involuntary movements that suggest tardive dyskinesia; any other physical or emotional changes not described here.

WHAT TO EXPECT WHEN YOU STOP   You may notice a return of your symptoms if pimozide is tapered gradually. **If stopped abruptly:** There is no acute withdrawal syndrome.

Procyclidine

GENERAL   **Preparations:** Generic and brand name Kemadrin in pills and liquid form. **Class:** Antiparkinsonian agent. **Used in:** The treatment of side effects induced by antipsychotics: akathisia, dystonia, and pseudoparkinsonism (tremor, rigidity, akinesia). **Mechanism of action:** Blocks postsynaptic acetylcholine receptors.

PRECAUTIONS   **Use extra caution if you have:** *Congestive heart failure, edema, epilepsy, glaucoma, low blood pressure, prostatic hypertrophy* or *urinary retention,* as procyclidine may worsen the symptoms of the disorder. **Tests needed before starting:** None. **Alcohol:** Should be avoided, as the simultaneous use of procyclidine and alcohol can lower blood pressure significantly and cause confusion. Also, alcohol worsens anxiety and depression and impairs insight and judgment.

DRUG INTERACTIONS   *Antihypertensives,* as they may combine to lower blood pressure excessively; *antihistamines, phenothiazines,* or *tricyclic antidepressants,* as they may combine to produce pronounced dry mouth, blurry vision, constipation, low blood pressure, rapid heart rate, and even mental confusion.

DOSING   **Adults:** The usual starting dose is 2.5 mg three times daily, with daily increases of 2.5 mg/day up to 20 mg/day. **Children:** Not FDA-approved for under 18.

MONITORING YOUR USE   **Time to effectiveness:** One to two hours, but the full effect may take two to three days. **A full trial is:** A few days at the maximum recommended dose. **Half-life of drug and active metabolites:** The half-life and metabolism of procyclidine are unknown, but the effects generally last for 6–12 hours. **How to monitor dosage:** The optimal dose is determined by its effectiveness in alleviating the target symptoms. **How to monitor safety:** No special medical tests are needed. **If you miss a dose:** Take a missed dose if it's within an hour or two. Do not try to make up for a missed dose by doubling your next dose; just continue with your regular dosing schedule.

SIDE EFFECTS   **Usual (50–100%):** Blurry vision, constipation, dry mouth. **Less common (1–10%):** Heart rate elevation, low blood pressure, nausea, vomiting. **Infrequent (less than 1%):** Rash, urinary difficulty. **Those requiring attention from your physician:** Physical or emotional changes not listed.

WHAT TO EXPECT WHEN YOU STOP   You may notice a return of your symptoms if procyclidine is stopped. **If stopped abruptly:** There are no acute withdrawal effects.

Propranolol

GENERAL   **Preparations:** Generic and brand name Inderal in regular and long-acting tablets. **Class:** Beta-blocker. **Used in:** Antipsychotic-induced akathisia, performance anxiety, lithium-induced tremor (developmental disorders). **Mechanism of action:** Blocks postsynaptic beta-adrenergic receptors in muscle and brain cells.

PRECAUTIONS   **Don't use if you have:** *Asthma,* as propranolol may worsen breathing; *heart block* (an abnormal heart rhythm), *heart failure,* or a *slow heart rate,* as propranolol may worsen heart block and dangerously affect heart function. **Use extra caution if you have:** *Diabetes,* as propranolol may block the signs of hypoglycemia, thereby delaying needed treatment with glucose; *thyroid dysfunction,* as propranolol may mask symptoms of excessive thyroid hormone production, thereby delaying needed treatment. **Tests needed before starting:** None. **Alcohol:** Should be avoided. The simultaneous use of propranolol and alcohol may cause dizziness, confusion, and low blood pressure. **Use in pregnancy:** Propranolol use by pregnant mothers is associated with babies who were born small for their gestational age. It is passed in the breast milk and may slow the heart rate of the infant.

DRUG INTERACTIONS   **Use with extra caution if you take:** *Verapamil (Calan)* or *diltiazem (Cardizem),* as the combination may cause heart block and impair heart function; *reserpine,* as the combination may cause excessively low blood pressure.

DOSING   **Adults:** *Performance anxiety:* A single dose of 40–80 mg one hour prior to the performance; *akathisia:* The usual starting dose is 10–40 mg two to three times daily, with weekly increases of 10–20 mg/day up to a maximum of 160 mg/day; *developmental disorders:* A starting dose of 40 mg twice daily with weekly increases of 40 mg/day up to a maximum of 160 mg/day; *tremor:* The usual starting dose is 10 mg two times daily, with weekly increases of 10–20 mg/day up to a maximum of 80 mg/day. **Children:** Not FDA-approved for under 18.

MONITORING YOUR USE   **Time to effectiveness:** 30–90 minutes. **A full trial is:** One week at the maximum dose. **Half-life of drug and active metabolites:** 4 hours for the regular preparation and 10 hours for the long-acting form. **How to monitor dosage:** The optimal dose is determined by its effectiveness in alleviating the target symptoms. **How to monitor safety:** Monitor pulse and blood pressure. It is generally wise to avoid doses which lower your pulse below 60 beats per minute. **If you miss a dose:** Take a missed dose if it's within an hour or two. Do not try to make up for a missed dose by doubling your next dose; just continue with your regular dosing schedule.

SIDE EFFECTS   **Less common (1–10%):** Low blood pressure, slow heart rate, fatigue. **Those requiring attention from your physician:** Any physical or emotional changes not listed.

WHAT TO EXPECT WHEN YOU STOP   You may notice a return of your symptoms when propranolol is stopped.

Protriptyline

GENERAL   **Preparations:** Generic and brand name Vivactil. **Class:** Tricyclic antidepressant. **Used in:** Anxiety disorders, bulimia, and depression. **Mechanism of action:** Blocks the reuptake of norepinephrine and serotonin into presynaptic neurons.

PRECAUTIONS   **Don't use if you have:** *Heart block* (an abnormal heart rhythm) or if you recently had a *heart attack,* as protriptyline may worsen heart block and dangerously affect heart function. **Use extra caution if you have:** *Bipolar disorder,* as protriptyline may cause a manic episode; *epilepsy,* as protriptyline may increase the frequency of seizures; *glaucoma,* as protriptyline can worsen the symptoms of untreated angle closure glaucoma; *low blood pressure,* as protriptyline may lower blood pressure further; a *psychotic disorder,* as protriptyline may make psychotic symptoms worse; *hyperthyroidism,* as protriptyline may cause irregular heart rhythms; *prostatic hypertrophy* or *urinary retention,* as protriptyline may worsen urinary retention. **Tests needed before starting:** An electrocardiogram (EKG) if you are over 35, to ensure that you do not have any form of heart block. **Alcohol:** Should be avoided, as the simultaneous use of protriptyline and alcohol can lower blood pressure significantly and cause confusion. Also, alcohol worsens anxiety and depression and impairs insight and judgment. **Use in pregnancy:** There is a higher rate of miscarriages born to women who take tricyclics, but no specific defect is associated with their use.

DRUG INTERACTIONS   **Do not use if you take:** *MAOI antidepressants,* as their use with protriptyline can cause pronounced hypertension and the potential for strokes. **Use with extra caution if you take:** *Phenothiazines,* as the combination may cause irregular heart rhythms which are potentially fatal; *antihypertensives,* as they may combine to lower blood pressure excessively; *antihistamines, phenothiazines,* and *antiparkinsonian agents,* as they may combine to produce pronounced dry mouth, blurry vision, constipation, low blood pressure, rapid heart rate, and even mental confusion; *guanethadine* to lower blood pressure, as protriptyline may block its effects.

DOSING   **Adults:** The usual starting dose is 15–40 mg/day at bedtime with increases every few days of 5–10 mg up to a maximum dose of 60 mg/day. **Children:** Not FDA-approved for under 12. **The elderly:** The usual starting dose is 15 mg/day with a maximum dose of 20 mg/day.

MONITORING YOUR USE   **Time to effectiveness:** Side effects are generally noticeable within a few doses, but the therapeutic effect may take two to four weeks. **A full trial is:** Four weeks at the maximum tolerated dosage. **Half-life of drug and active metabolites:** 54–92 hours with active metabolites. **How to monitor dosage:** The optimal dose is determined by its effectiveness in alleviating the target symptoms. **How to monitor safety:** An EKG may be useful to ensure that heart function is not impaired. **If you miss a dose:** Take a missed dose if it's within an hour or two. Do not try to make up for a missed dose by doubling your next dose; just continue with your regular dosing schedule.

SIDE EFFECTS   Usual (50–100%): Blurry vision, constipation, dry mouth, fatigue, increased heart rate, low blood pressure. **Common (10–50%):** Sweating, weight gain. **Less common (1–10%):** Sexual dysfunction, urinary retention. **Those requiring attention from your physician:** Any physical or emotional changes not listed, such as suicidal thoughts or behavior.

WHAT TO EXPECT WHEN YOU STOP   You may notice a return of your symptoms if protriptyline is stopped. **If stopped abruptly:** You may experience agitation, headaches, insomnia, and nausea, as well as depression. Protriptyline should be slowly tapered if you decide to stop it. The rate of discontinuation is different for each person and is determined by the clinical situation necessitating the change, your age, severity of symptoms, dosage size, and your duration of use.

Quazepam

GENERAL   Preparations: Generic and brand name Doral. **Class:** Benzodiazepine. **Used in:** Insomnia. **Mechanism of action:** Intensifies the effects of gamma-aminobutyric acid (GABA).

PRECAUTIONS   Warnings: *It is habit-forming.* Quazepam, like all benzodiazepines, is physically and psychologically habit-forming. People who have experienced traumatic events in their lives and have chronic anxiety are especially prone to developing dependence. Prolonged use is associated with a range of problems. Use for more than four weeks is *not* recommended. If you stop quazepam after more than four weeks of daily use, you will probably experience withdrawal symptoms (see below). **Tests needed before starting:** None. **Alcohol:** Alcohol must be avoided entirely. The simultaneous use of quazepam and alcohol is extremely dangerous because it can cause you to stop breathing. The combination can cause death. **Use in pregnancy:** There is a higher rate of babies born with a cleft palate to mothers who took benzodiazepines during pregnancy. **The elderly** are especially sensitive to the effects of benzodiazepines and may experience pronounced side effects at low doses (see chapter 4).

DRUG INTERACTIONS   **Use with extra caution if you take:** *Anticonvulsants, antidepressants, antihistamines, antipsychotics, barbiturates, benzodiazepines,* or any drug that causes sedation or central nervous system depression, because the combination with quazepam can cause pronounced sedation.

DOSING   **Adults:** The usual dose is 7.5–15 mg at bedtime. **Children:** Not FDA-approved for under 18. **The elderly:** the usual starting dose is 7.5 mg at bedtime.

MONITORING YOUR USE   **Time to effectiveness:** 30–60 minutes. **A full trial is:** A few doses are generally enough to establish whether it will be helpful. **Half-life of drug and active metabolites:** 39 hours with two active metabolites with half-lives of 39 and 73 hours. **How to monitor dosage:** The optimal dose is determined by its effectiveness in helping you to sleep. **If you miss a dose:** Do *not* try to make up for a missed dose; just continue with your regular dosing schedule. **How to monitor safety:** No specific medical tests are needed to monitor safety.

SIDE EFFECTS   **Common (10–50%):** Daytime fatigue, memory impairment, poor muscle coordination (causing a higher rate of falls in the elderly and a higher risk of motor vehicle accidents in all adults). **Less common (1–10%):** Headache. **Infrequent (less than 1%):** Paradoxical agitation and insomnia. **Those requiring attention from your physician:** Any physical or emotional changes not described here. **Side effects associated with use longer than four weeks:** Use of quazepam for longer than four weeks may cause physical and psychological dependence, and you may notice the desire for another dose as each one wears off. Ongoing anxiety, reduced effectiveness of each dose, depression, emotional blunting, and impairment of memory and cognition may occur with use longer than one year.

WHAT TO EXPECT WHEN YOU STOP   You may notice insomnia if quazepam is tapered gradually. Other withdrawal symptoms include anxiety, insomnia, irritability, headaches, tremors, nausea, diarrhea, sweating, and confusion. **If stopped abruptly:** *Seizures* can occur if quazepam is stopped abruptly, although this is extremely unlikely with routine use at recommended dosages. Seizures are potentially life-threatening. You should always consult with your physician as to how to stop it safely.

Quetiapine

GENERAL   **Preparations:** Brand name Seroquel only. **Class:** Atypical antipsychotic. **Used in:** Psychotic disorders (severe anxiety, Alzheimer's disease, bipolar disorder, developmental disorders, insomnia). **Mechanism of action:** Blocks a subset of dopamine and serotonin receptors.

PRECAUTIONS   Warnings: All antipsychotics can cause *neuroleptic malignant syndrome,* a rare but severe and potentially fatal reaction consisting of fever, muscle rigidity, mental status changes, and alterations in pulse and blood pressure. They can also cause *tardive dyskinesia,* a potentially irreversible disorder of rhythmical, involuntary muscle movements. (see chapter 19 for details of both conditions). Quetiapine and other atypical antipsychotics are associated with the development of *weight gain, high cholesterol, and diabetes mellitus.* Quetiapine and other atypical antipsychotics are also associated with a higher incidence of *strokes* and *sudden death* in elderly people with dementia. **Use extra caution if you have:** *Breast cancer,* as quetiapine may elevate prolactin, a hormone released by the pituitary that may cause breast cancer to grow faster; *cataracts,* as quetiapine may cause cataracts or worsen existing ones; *epilepsy,* as quetiapine may increase the frequency of seizures; *liver disease,* as quetiapine may worsen impairment of liver functioning; *low blood pressure,* as quetiapine can lower blood pressure even further; *hypothyroidism,* as quetiapine may impair thyroid function further. **Tests before starting:** None. **Alcohol:** Should be avoided, as the simultaneous use of quetiapine and alcohol can lower blood pressure significantly and cause confusion. Also, alcohol worsens anxiety and depression and impairs insight and judgment.

DRUG INTERACTIONS   Use with extra caution if you take: *Anticonvulsants, antidepressants, antihistamines, antipsychotics, barbiturates, benzodiazepines,* or any drug that causes sedation or central nervous system depression, because the combination can cause pronounced sedation; *antihypertensives,* as quetiapine may combine to lower blood pressure excessively; *antihistamines* or *antiparkinsonian agents,* as they may combine to produce pronounced dry mouth, blurry vision, constipation, low blood pressure, rapid heart rate, and mental confusion.

DOSING   Adults: The starting dose is 25 mg twice daily, with increases every few days of 25–50 mg/twice a day up to a maximum of 750 mg/day. **Children:** Not FDA-approved for under 18.

MONITORING YOUR USE   Time to effectiveness: The first effects may be noticed within some days, but it may be one to three weeks to notice a pronounced change. It may take several months to derive full benefit. **A full trial is:** Four weeks at no less than 300 mg/day. **Half-life of drug and active metabolites:** Six hours with no active metabolites. **How to monitor dosage:** The optimal dose is determined by its effectiveness in alleviating the target symptoms. **How to monitor safety:** Pretreatment and periodic weight measurements should be performed to assess weight gain; blood glucose, cholesterol, and lipid profiles should be obtained after three months and yearly thereafter to check for diabetes and elevations in cholesterol or triglycerides; a physical examination for the presence of tardive dyskinesia (see below) should be done twice yearly; periodic eye evaluation to screen for cataracts. **If you miss a dose:** Take a missed dose if it's within an hour or two. Do not try to make up for a missed dose the next day by doubling your dose; just continue with your regular dosing schedule.

SIDE EFFECTS   **Common (10–50%):** Low blood pressure (light-headedness, dizziness), elevations in cholesterol, diabetes, headaches, weight gain. **Less common (1–10%):** Constipation, fatigue, menstrual irregularities, akathisia (restlessness), sexual dysfunction, indigestion, tardive dyskinesia. **Those requiring attention from your physician:** Symptoms of fever, muscular rigidity, and mental status changes, as you may have neuroleptic malignant syndrome, a potentially severe reaction; any abnormal involuntary movements that suggest tardive dyskinesia; any other physical or emotional changes not described here.

WHAT TO EXPECT IF YOU STOP   You may notice a return of your symptoms if quetiapine is tapered gradually. **If stopped abruptly:** There is no acute withdrawal syndrome, but symptoms may return quickly.

Ramelteon

GENERAL   **Preparations:** Brand name Rozerem only. **Class:** Hypnotic (sleeping aid). **Used in:** Insomnia. **Mechanism of action:** Interacts with melatonin receptors.

PRECAUTIONS   **Don't use if your have:** *Liver problems,* as the breakdown of ramelteon may be impaired leading to a more intense effect. **Tests needed before starting:** None. **Alcohol:** Alcohol should be avoided entirely as the combination with ramelteon may cause excessive sedation. **The elderly** may be more sensitive to the effects of ramelteon and may experience a more intense effect at the same dose as other adults. **Use in pregnancy:** Ramelteon causes birth defects in rats and rabbits. No studies have confirmed its safety in humans.

DRUG INTERACTIONS   **Do not use if you take:** *Fluvoxamine (Luvox)* because the breakdown of ramelteon may be impaired, leading to a more intense effect. **Use with extra caution if you take:** *Itraconozole (Sporonox)* or *ketoconozole (Nizoril),* because the breakdown of ramelteon may be impaired, leading to a more intense effect; *Anticonvulsants, antidepressants, antihistamines, antipsychotics, barbiturates, benzodiazepines, other hypnotics,* or any drug that causes sedation or central nervous system depression, because the combination with ramelteon can cause pronounced sedation.

DOSING   **Adults:** 8 mg at bedtime. It should not be taken after a high-fat meal because it will not be absorbed as well, impairing its effectiveness. **Children:** Not FDA-approved for under 18. **The elderly:** 8 mg at bedtime.

MONITORING YOUR USE   Time to effectiveness: 30–60 minutes. **Half-life of drug and active metabolites:** 1–2.6 hours with one active metabolite with a half-life of 2–5 hours. **How to monitor dosage:** The optimal dose is determined by its effectiveness in alleviating insomnia.

SIDE EFFECTS   Common (10–50%): With use over four weeks, ramelteon can cause elevations in prolactin and decreases in testosterone, two hormones involved in reproductive functioning. Alterations in prolactin can cause cessation of menses, galactorrhea, decreased libido, and problems with fertility. **Less common (1–10%):** Dizziness, fatigue, headaches, nausea. **Those requiring attention from your physician:** Cessation of menses or galactorrhea in females; decreased libido or problems with fertility. Physical or emotional changes not listed.

WHAT TO EXPECT WHEN YOUR STOP   There is no recognized withdrawal syndrome.

Risperidone

GENERAL   Preparations: Brand name Risperdal in pills and liquid form, long-acting injectable Risperdal Consta, and orally disintegrating Risperdal M-tabs. **Class:** Atypical antipsychotic. **Used in:** Bipolar disorder, psychotic disorders (Alzheimer's disease, severe anxiety, developmental disorders). **Mechanism of action:** Blocks a subset of dopamine and serotonin receptors.

PRECAUTIONS   Warnings: All antipsychotics can cause *neuroleptic malignant syndrome,* a rare but severe and potentially fatal reaction consisting of fever, muscle rigidity, mental status changes, alterations in pulse and blood pressure, and *strokes* and *sudden death.* They can also cause *tardive dyskinesia,* a potentially irreversible disorder of rhythmical, involuntary muscle movements (see chapter 19 for details of both conditions). Risperidone and other atypical antipsychotics are associated with the development of *weight gain, high cholesterol, and diabetes mellitus.* Risperidone and other atypical antipsychotics are also associated with a higher incidence of *strokes* and *sudden death* in elderly people with dementia. **Use extra caution if you have:** *Breast cancer,* as risperidone may elevate prolactin, a hormone released by the pituitary that may cause breast cancer to grow faster; *epilepsy,* as risperidone may increase the frequency of seizures; *heart problems,* as risperidone can worsen heart function further; *low blood pressure,* as risperidone can lower blood pressure even further. **Tests before starting:** None. **Alcohol:** Should be avoided, as the simultaneous use of risperidone and alcohol can lower blood pressure significantly and cause confusion. Also, alcohol worsens anxiety and depression, and impairs insight and judgment.

DRUG INTERACTIONS   **Use with extra caution if you take:** *Anticonvulsants, antidepressants, antihistamines, antipsychotics, barbiturates, benzodiazepines,* or any drug that causes sedation or central nervous system depression, because the combination can cause pronounced sedation; *antihypertensives,* as risperidone may combine to lower blood pressure excessively; *antihistamines* or *antiparkinsonian agents,* as they may combine to produce pronounced dry mouth, blurry vision, constipation, low blood pressure, rapid heart rate, and mental confusion.

DOSING   Adults: The starting dose is 1 mg one to two times a day with increases every week of 1–2 mg up to a maximum of 8 mg/day. Risperdal Consta is started with a dose of 25 mg injected every other week. The dose can be increased to 37.5 or 50 mg every other week. **Children:** Not FDA-approved for under 16.

MONITORING YOUR USE   Time to effectiveness: The first effects may be noticed within some days, but it may take one to three weeks to notice a pronounced change. It may take several months to derive full benefit. Risperdal Consta injections take three weeks to begin to work, and stabilization may take several months. **A full trial is:** Four weeks at no less than 6 mg/day. **Half-life of drug and active metabolites:** 3–20 hours with active metabolites. **How to monitor dosage:** The optimal dose is determined by its effectiveness in alleviating the target symptoms. **How to monitor safety:** Pretreatment and periodic weight measurements should be performed to assess weight gain; blood glucose, cholesterol, and lipid profiles should be obtained after three months and yearly thereafter to check for diabetes and elevations in cholesterol or triglycerides; a physical examination for the presence of tardive dyskinesia (see below) should be done twice yearly. **If you miss a dose:** Take a missed dose if it's within an hour or two. Do not try to make up for a missed dose the next day by doubling your dose; just continue with your regular dosing schedule.

SIDE EFFECTS   Common (10–50%): Low blood pressure (light-headedness, dizziness), elevations in cholesterol, diabetes, headaches, weight gain. **Less common (1–10%):** Agitation, akathisia (restlessness), constipation, fatigue, menstrual irregularities, nausea, sedation, sexual dysfunction, pseudoparkinsonism (muscular tremor, rigidity, akinesia), tardive dyskinesia. **Those requiring attention from your physician:** Symptoms of fever, muscular rigidity, and mental status changes, as you may have neuroleptic malignant syndrome, a potentially severe reaction; any abnormal involuntary movements that suggest tardive dyskinesia; any other physical or emotional changes not described here.

WHAT TO EXPECT IF YOU STOP   You may notice a return of your symptoms if risperidone is tapered gradually. **If stopped abruptly:** There is no acute withdrawal syndrome, but symptoms may return quickly.

Rivastigmine

GENERAL   **Preparations:** Brand name Exelon only in tablets. **Class:** Cognitive enhancer. **Used in:** Alzheimer's disease. **Mechanism of action:** Inhibits the enzyme cholinesterase, which breaks down acetylcholine.

PRECAUTIONS   **Use extra caution if you have:** *Asthma,* as rivastigmine may worsen breathing problems; *heart problems* in which the heart beats too slowly, such as bradycardia, the "sick sinus syndrome," or certain forms of heart block, as rivastigmine may cause your heart to beat too slowly; *seizures,* as rivastigmine increases the potential for causing seizures; *ulcers,* as rivastigmine may increase gastric acid secretion and worsen ulcers. **Tests needed before starting:** The diagnosis of Alzheimer's needs to be established through a neurological and physical exam, neuropsychological testing, or a brain imaging study. A complete physical examination should be done to ensure that there are no active medical problems that would preclude the use of rivastigmine. **Alcohol:** Although there are no specific adverse consequences when alcohol and rivastigmine are combined, the use of alcohol should be avoided, since it impairs thinking and judgment.

DRUG INTERACTIONS   **Use with extra caution if you take:** *Nonsteroidal inflammatory drugs such as aspirin, ibuprofen (Advil, Motrin), or naproxen (Aleve),* as the combination may cause stomach bleeding.

DOSING   **Adults:** The starting and maintenance dose is 1.5 mg twice daily, with dosage increases of 1.5 mg twice daily every two weeks up to a maximum of 6 mg twice daily (12 mg total daily dose). It should be taken with food.

MONITORING YOUR USE   **Time to effectiveness:** As there is no immediate obvious effect, there is no objective way to assess whether it is having a positive effect. It is reasonable to begin it as soon as the diagnosis is clear and as long as any memory function remains. **A full trial:** This lasts until there is minimal memory function remaining. **Half-life of drug and active metabolites:** 1.5 hours, with no active metabolites. **How to monitor dosage:** The optimal dose is determined by the absence of side effects. **If you miss a dose:** Do *not* try to make up for a missed dose; just continue with your regular dosing schedule. **How to monitor safety:** Monitor weight.

SIDE EFFECTS   **Common (10–50%):** Abdominal pain, decreased appetite, diarrhea, dizziness, fatigue, headaches, nausea and vomiting, weight loss. **Less common (1–10%):** Fainting, indigestion, insomnia. **Those requiring attention by your physician:** Any physical, cognitive, or emotional change not noted here.

WHAT TO EXPECT WHEN YOU STOP   There may be a further impairment in memory. **If stopped abruptly:** There is no specific withdrawal syndrome beyond the loss of effectiveness.

Selegiline

GENERAL   **Preparations:** Brand name Eldepryl only. **Class:** Selective MAOI (type B inhibitor). **Used in:** Bulimia, depression, panic disorder (other anxiety disorders). **Mechanism of action:** Inhibits monoamine oxidase, the protein enzyme responsible for the breakdown of dopamine, epinephrine, norepinephrine, and serotonin, resulting in elevated levels of these neurotransmitters.

PRECAUTIONS   **Warnings:** At doses over 10 mg/day, selegiline can cause a *hypertensive crisis* in which your blood pressure rises dangerously high, putting you at risk for a brain stroke, brain damage, and death. This reaction is unlikely to occur on its own but is possible if used in combination with foods or medicines which contain tyramine or substances similar to epinephrine. In theory, at doses below 10 mg/day, selegiline can be safely used without the dietary precautions necessary listed below. However, hypertensive crises have occurred even at this low dose. **The following medications must be avoided while you are on selegiline and for two weeks following its cessation in order to avoid a hypertensive crisis:** Prescription medications: *Antiasthmatics* that contain *epinephrine* or epinephrine-like compounds, most *antidepressants, antihypertensives, antiparkinsonian agents, barbiturates, buspirone (Buspar), carbamazepine (Tegretol), disulfiram; diuretics, narcotics, stimulants;* over-the-counter medications: *decongestants, dextromethorphan, tryptophan, hay fever medications, sinus medications, appetite suppressants;* recreational drugs: *amphetamines, cocaine, hallucinogenics, heroin, or other narcotics.* **The following foods must be avoided while you are on selegiline and for two weeks following its cessation in order to avoid a hypertensive crisis:** Aged or fermented foods; all cheese or foods containing cheese such as pizza, fondue, many Italian dishes and salad dressings (cottage cheese and cream cheese are allowed); cream, sour cream, and yogurt; foods fermented with yeast (although foods baked with yeast, such as bread, are safe), brewer's yeast; liver, processed meats, such as bologna, corned beef, hot dogs, liverwurst, pepperoni, salami, sausage; broad bean pods (fava beans); sauerkraut; pickles; soy sauce; licorice, caviar, anchovies, dried fruits (raisins, prunes), figs, raspberries, chocolate; bananas, pickled herring; excessive amounts of caffeine-containing beverages (more than one or two, although some people are more sensitive than others) like coffee, tea, sodas, and hot chocolate. **Don't use if you have:** *Congestive heart failure* and *high blood pressure,* as selegiline may make the symptoms worse; *pheochromocytoma,* as it may cause a hypertensive crisis. **Use extra caution if you have:** *Bipolar disorder,* as selegiline can cause a manic episode; *epilepsy,* as selegiline may increase seizure frequency; *low blood pressure,* as selegiline may make symptoms worse; a *psychotic disorder,* as selegiline can worsen psychotic symptoms. **Tests needed before starting:** None. **Alcohol:** Beer, wine, Chianti, sherry, and liqueurs, whether they contain alcohol or not, can cause a hypertensive crisis. Hard liquor has no specific adverse consequences, but should be avoided because it can worsen anxiety, depression, and low blood pressure.

DRUG INTERACTIONS *Antihypertensives,* as selegiline can lower blood pressure further; *narcotics,* as the combination can produce coma, fever, and high blood pressure.

DOSING **Adults:** A starting dose of 5 mg/twice daily is also the maximum dose if you want to avoid the dietary and medication restrictions described above. Doses up to 20 mg twice daily may be needed for effective relief of symptoms. **Children:** Not FDA-approved for under 18.

MONITORING YOUR USE **Time to effectiveness:** Side effects may be noted with a few days, but the therapeutic effect may take two to six weeks. **A full trial is:** Four weeks at the maximum tolerated dose. **Half-life of drug and active metabolites:** The specific half-life is unknown but is believed to be fairly short. There are three metabolites with half-lives from 2–20 hours. The effects can last for two weeks after the last dose. **How to monitor dosage:** The optimal dose is determined by its effectiveness in alleviating the target symptoms. **How to monitor safety:** Monitor blood pressure. **If you miss a dose:** Take a missed dose if it's within an hour or two. Do not try to make up for a missed dose the next day by doubling your dose; just continue with your regular dosing schedule.

SIDE EFFECTS **Common (10–50%):** Insomnia, nausea, sedation, sexual dysfunction, tremor, weight gain. **Less common (1–10%):** Agitation, confusion, dry mouth, hallucinations, headaches, light-headedness. **Those requiring attention from your physician:** A sudden headache, palpitations, rapid heart rate, sweating, throat constriction, neck stiffness, nausea, or vomiting can be a sign that you are having a hypertensive crisis: you should consult your physician immediately and go to the emergency room for treatment of any elevation of blood pressure; physical or emotional changes not listed, such as suicidal thoughts or behavior.

WHAT TO EXPECT WHEN YOU STOP You may notice a return of your symptoms if you taper and stop selegiline. **If stopped abruptly:** An uncommon withdrawal syndrome starting one to three days after cessation of selegiline, with agitation, confusion, hallucinations, nausea, nightmares, or seizures, may occur.

Sertraline

GENERAL   **Preparations:** Brand name Zoloft only. **Class:** SSRI (selective serotonin reuptake inhibitor). **Used in:** Depression (other anxiety disorders, developmental disorders, obsessive-compulsive disorder, panic disorder). **Mechanism of action:** Blocks the reuptake of serotonin by presynaptic neurons.

PRECAUTIONS   **Warnings:** When taken with other serotonin reuptake inhibitors, sertraline can cause the *serotonin syndrome,* which consists of potentially dangerous alterations in pulse, blood pressure, hyperactivity, and mental status changes (see chapter 19). Rarely, sertraline can cause hyponatremia, or low sodium in your blood. **Use extra caution if you have:** *Bipolar disorder,* as sertraline can cause a manic episode; *epilepsy,* as sertraline may increase the frequency of seizures; a *psychotic disorder,* as sertraline can worsen psychotic symptoms. **Tests needed before starting:** None. **Alcohol:** The simultaneous use of sertraline and alcohol causes no specific adverse consequences, but alcohol should be avoided because it worsens anxiety and depression. **Use in pregnancy:** There is a higher rate of miscarriages, heart defects, and intestinal defects in the babies of women who take sertraline during pregnancy.

DRUG INTERACTIONS   **Don't use if you take:** *Other SSRIs, St. John's wort,* or *tryptophan,* as their use with sertraline can cause the *serotonin syndrome; MAOI antidepressants,* as their use with sertraline can cause a serious, sometimes fatal, reaction of agitation, fever, cardiovascular changes, and mental status changes.

DOSING   **Adults:** The usual starting dose is 25–50 mg once daily with weekly increases of 50 mg/day up to a maximum of 200 mg/day. **Children:** The usual starting dose is 25 mg once daily, with weekly increases of 25–50 mg/day up to a maximum of 200 mg/day.

MONITORING YOUR USE   **Time to effectiveness:** You may notice some side effects within one to two days, but any improvement in symptoms generally takes two to four weeks. **A full trial is:** Four weeks at the maximum dose. **Half-life of drug and active metabolites:** 25 hours with partially active metabolites. **How to monitor dosage:** The optimal dose is determined by its effectiveness in alleviating the target symptoms. **How to monitor safety:** No specific tests are needed to monitor your health while on sertraline. **If you miss a dose:** Take a missed dose if it's the same day. Do not try to make up for a missed dose the next day by doubling your dose; just continue with your regular dosing schedule.

SIDE EFFECTS   **Common (10–50%):** Diarrhea, dizziness, dry mouth, nausea (generally goes away after one to two weeks), fatigue, headache, insomnia, weakness, decreased appetite, and sexual dysfunction. **Less common (1–10%):** Anxiety, palpitations, sweating, tremor. **Those requiring attention from your physician:** Hyperactivity, mental status changes, or alterations in your pulse or blood pressure that suggest the serotonin syndrome. Any physical or emotional changes not listed, such as suicidal thoughts and behavior.

WHAT TO EXPECT WHEN YOU STOP You may notice a return of your symptoms if sertraline is tapered gradually. **If stopped abruptly:** You may notice a flulike syndrome of nausea, vomiting, diarrhea, dizziness, as well as anxiety and depression. Sertraline should not be stopped abruptly but needs to be gradually tapered in consultation with your physician.

Sildenafil

GENERAL **Preparations:** Brand name Viagra only. **Used in:** Impotence from any etiology, including that caused by psychiatric medications. Its use in women with difficulty achieving orgasm is under investigation. **Mechanism of action:** Inhibits phosphodiesterase type 5, causing increased levels of guanosine monophosphate, relaxation of smooth muscle, and greater blood flow to the penis, enhancing erection during sexual stimulation.

PRECAUTIONS **Warnings:** Deaths have been associated with the simultaneous use of Viagra and nitrates (used both in prescription medicines for heart disease, such as nitroglycerin, Nitrobid, or Isordil, and drugs of abuse such as amyl nitrite). Decreased or a loss of vision can occur with sildenafil due to nonarteritic anterior ischemic optic neuropathy (NAION). **Don't use if you have:** *Heart disease,* as there is a degree of heart risk associated with sexual activity. **Use with extra caution if you have:** *Retinitis pigmentosa,* as there is the potential for adverse effects with the use of sildenafil. **Tests needed before starting:** None. **Alcohol:** The manufacturer describes no specific adverse consequences.

DRUG INTERACTIONS **Do not use if you take:** Any form of nitrates; *alpha-adrenergic blocking agents* (used in high blood pressure) such as *doxazosin* or *terazosin,* as blood pressure can go too low.

DOSING **Adults:** The usual starting dose is 25–50 mg one half hour to four hours before sexual activity. Subsequent doses up to a maximum of 100 mg.

MONITORING YOUR USE **Time to effectiveness:** 30–60 minutes. **A full trial is:** Two to three tries at the maximum dose. **Half-life of drug and active metabolites:** Four hours with one active metabolite. **How to monitor dosage:** The optimal dose is determined by its effectiveness in enhancing potency. **How to monitor safety:** No tests needed.

SIDE EFFECTS **Common (10–50%):** Flushing, headache. **Less common (1–10%):** Indigestion, nasal congestion, dizziness, color-tinged vision. **Those requiring attention from your physician:** Erections lasting more than four hours require immediate medical attention, as damage to the penis can result; any physical symptoms not noted here.

Tacrine

GENERAL **Preparations:** Brand name Cognex only. **Class:** Cognitive enhancer. **Used in:** Alzheimer's disease. **Mechanism of action:** Inhibits the enzyme cholinesterase, which breaks down acetylcholine.

PRECAUTIONS **Warnings:** *Liver damage* can result from the use of tacrine. Cessation of tacrine at the first sign of liver damage generally restores liver function, but some deaths have occurred in people with infections, gallstones, and cancer. Don't use if you have liver disease of any kind. **Use extra caution if you have:** *Asthma, heart block, slow heart rate,* or *irregular heart beats,* as tacrine may worsen the problem; *ulcers,* as tacrine may increase acid secretion and worsen the ulcer. **Tests needed before starting:** The diagnosis of Alzheimer's needs to be established through a neurological and physical exam, neuropsychological testing, or a brain imaging study. A complete physical examination should be done to ensure that there are no active medical problems that would preclude the use of tacrine. Liver function tests (blood tests) are absolutely necessary. **Alcohol:** Although there are no specific adverse consequences when alcohol and tacrine are combined, the use of alcohol should be avoided since it impairs thinking and judgment.

DRUG INTERACTIONS **Use with extra caution if you take:** *Nonsteroidal anti-inflammatory drugs such as aspirin, ibuprofen (Motrin),* or *naproxen (Aleve),* as the combination may cause stomach bleeding.

DOSING **Adults:** The starting and maintenance dose is 10 mg four times daily, with increases of 10 mg four times daily every four weeks up to a maximum of 40 mg four times daily (total dose of 160 mg/day). Doses should be taken one hour before meals, as food reduces the amount absorbed.

MONITORING YOUR USE **Time to effectiveness:** As the effect of tacrine is to slow memory impairment, there is no dramatic effect. There is no objective way to assess whether or not it is having a positive effect. It is reasonable to begin it as soon as the diagnosis is clear and as long as any memory function remains. **A full trial:** Lasts until there is minimal memory function remaining. **Half-life of drug and active metabolites:** Two to four hours with metabolites of unknown activity. **How to monitor dosage:** The optimal dose is determined by the absence of side effects. **If you miss a dose:** Do *not* try to make up for a missed dose; just continue with your regular dosing schedule. **How to monitor safety:** Liver function tests are needed every other week starting at week four. If there is evidence of significant liver impairment, dosage should be lowered or stopped. If liver function returns to normal, it is reasonable to consider another trial, with weekly tests of the liver. If there is a rash or fever associated with impaired liver function, dosage should be stopped immediately and not restarted.

SIDE EFFECTS   Common (10–50%): Liver impairment, diarrhea, dizziness, headache, nausea. **Less common (1–10%):** Decreased appetite, indigestion. **Those requiring attention from your physician:** Any physical, cognitive, or emotional change not noted here.

WHAT TO EXPECT WHEN YOU STOP   There may be a further impairment in memory. **If stopped abruptly:** There may be an abrupt worsening of cognitive function.

Tadalafil

GENERAL   Preparations: Brand name Cialis only. **Used in:** Impotence from any etiology, including that caused by psychiatric medications. **Mechanism of action:** Inhibits phosphodiesterase type 5, causing increased levels of guanosine monophosphate, relaxation of smooth muscle, and greater blood flow to the penis, enhancing erection during sexual stimulation.

PRECAUTIONS   Warnings: Deaths have been associated with the simultaneous use of this type of medication and nitrates (used both in prescription medicines for heart disease such as nitroglycerin, Nitrobid, or Isordil, and drugs of abuse such as amyl nitrate.) Decreased or a loss of vision can occur with tadalafil due to nonarteritic anterior ischemic optic neuropathy (NAION). **Don't use if you have:** *Heart disease,* as there is a degree of heart risk associated with sexual activity. **Use with extra caution if you have:** *Kidney or liver problems,* as tadalafil is not cleared from the body as efficiently; *retinitis pigmentosa,* as there is the potential for adverse effects with the use of tadalafil. **Tests needed before starting:** None. **Alcohol:** The combination can cause low blood pressure, elevated heart rate, headaches, and dizziness.

DRUG INTERACTIONS   Don't use if you take: *Nitrates,* as blood pressure can go too low; *alpha-adrenergic blocking agents* (used in high blood pressure) such as *doxazosin* or *terazosin,* as blood pressure can go too low. **Use with extra caution if you take:** *Erythromycin, indinavir, itraconazole, ketoconazole,* or *ritonivir,* as these drugs decrease the breakdown of tadalafil and blood pressure can go too low.

DOSING   Adults: The usual starting dose is 10 mg at least 60 minutes before sexual activity, no more than once a day. Subsequent doses up to a maximum of 20 mg/day can be used. People with significant kidney dysfunction should take no more than 5 mg in a 24-hour period; those with liver problems should take no more than 10 mg in a 24-hour period.

MONITORING YOUR USE   Time to effectiveness: 60 minutes. **A full trial is:** 2–3 tries at the maximum dose. **Half-life of drug and active metabolites:** 17.5 hours with no active metabolites. **How to monitor dosage:** The optimal dose is determined by its effectiveness in enhancing potency. **How to monitor safety:** No tests needed.

SIDE EFFECTS   Common (10–50%): Headache, indigestion. **Less common (1–10%):** Back pain, flushing, muscle aches, nasal congestion, color-tinged visual changes. **Those requiring attention by your physician:** Erections lasting more than four hours require immediate medical attention, as damage to the penis can result.

Temazepam

GENERAL   Preparations: Generic and brand name Restoril. **Class:** Benzodiazepine. **Used in:** Insomnia. **Mechanism of action:** Intensifies the effects of gamma-aminobutyric acid (GABA).

PRECAUTIONS   Warnings: *It is habit-forming.* Temazepam, like all benzodiazepines, is physically and psychologically habit-forming. People who have experienced traumatic events in their life and have chronic anxiety are especially prone to developing dependence. Prolonged use is associated with a range of problems. Use for more than four weeks is *not* recommended. If you stop temazepam after more than four weeks of daily use you will probably experience withdrawal symptoms (see below). **Tests needed before starting:** None. **Alcohol:** Alcohol must be avoided entirely. The simultaneous use of temazepam and alcohol is extremely dangerous because it can cause you to stop breathing. The combination can cause death. **Use in pregnancy:** There is a higher rate of babies born with a cleft palate to mothers who took benzodiazepines during pregnancy. **The elderly** are especially sensitive to the effects of benzodiazepines and may experience pronounced side effects at low doses (see chapter 4).

DRUG INTERACTIONS   Use with extra caution if you take: *Anticonvulsants, antidepressants, antihistamines, antipsychotics, barbiturates, benzodiazepines,* or any drug that causes sedation or central nervous system depression, because the combination with temazepam can cause pronounced sedation.

DOSING　**Adults:** The usual dose is 7.5–30 mg at bedtime. **Children:** Not FDA-approved for under 18. **The elderly:** The usual starting dose is 7.5 mg at bedtime.

MONITORING YOUR USE　**Time to effectiveness:** 30–60 minutes. **A full trial is:** A few doses, which are generally enough to establish whether it will be helpful. **Half-life of drug and active metabolites:** 8–15 hours with no active metabolites. **How to monitor dosage:** The optimal dose is determined by its effectiveness in helping you to sleep. **If you miss a dose:** Do *not* try to make up for a missed dose; just continue with your regular dosing schedule. **How to monitor safety:** No specific medical tests are needed to monitor safety.

SIDE EFFECTS　**Common (10–50%):** Daytime fatigue, memory impairment, poor muscle coordination (causing a higher rate of falls in the elderly and a higher risk of motor vehicle accidents in all adults). **Infrequent (less than 1%):** Paradoxical agitation and insomnia. **Those requiring attention from your physician:** Any physical or emotional changes not described here. **Side effects associated with use longer than four weeks:** Use of temazepam longer than four weeks may cause physical and psychological dependence, and you may notice the desire for another dose as each one wears off. Ongoing anxiety, reduced effectiveness of each dose, depression, emotional blunting, and impairment of memory and cognition may occur with use longer than one year.

WHAT TO EXPECT WHEN YOU STOP　You may notice insomnia if temazepam is tapered gradually. Other withdrawal symptoms include anxiety, irritability, headaches, tremors, nausea, diarrhea, sweating, and confusion. **If stopped abruptly:** *Seizures* can occur if temazepam is stopped abruptly, although this is extremely unlikely with routine use at recommended dosages. Seizures are potentially life-threatening. You should always consult with your physician as to how to stop it safely.

Thioridazine

GENERAL　**Preparations:** Generic and brand name Mellaril in tablets and liquid form. **Class:** Standard antipsychotic of the phenothiazine group. **Used in:** Psychotic disorders (Alzheimer's disease, severe anxiety, severe ADHD, bipolar disorder, developmental disorders, insomnia). **Mechanism of action:** Blocks postsynaptic dopamine receptors.

PRECAUTIONS　**Warnings:** All antipsychotics can cause *neuroleptic malignant syndrome,* a rare but severe and potentially fatal reaction consisting of fever, muscle rigidity, mental status changes, and alterations in pulse and blood pressure. They can also cause *tardive dyskinesia,* a potentially irreversible disorder of rhythmical, involuntary muscle movements (see chapter 19 for details of both conditions). *Eye retinal changes* can occur with use over 800 mg/day. **Don't use if you have:** Known prolongation of QT interval on your EKG, or if you take other drugs that can prolong the QT interval (such as quinidine, pimozide, and others), as thioridazine causes QTc prolongation and can result in irregular heart rhythms and death. **Use extra caution if you have:** *Breast cancer,* as thioridazine can elevate prolactin, a hormone released by the pituitary which may cause breast cancer to grow faster; *epilepsy,* as thioridazine may increase the frequency of seizures; *glaucoma, low blood pressure, prostatic hypertrophy* or *urinary retention,* as the symptoms may worsen. **Tests before starting:** None. **Alcohol:** Should be avoided, as the simultaneous use of thioridazine and alcohol can lower blood pressure significantly and cause confusion. Also, alcohol worsens anxiety and depression and impairs insight and judgment. **Use in pregnancy:** Phenothiazines have been linked with the "floppy infant syndrome," in which the baby has poor muscle tone. The fetus may experience pseudoparkinsonism and dystonia, muscular side effects which may cause fetal distress before, during, and shortly after birth. Thioridazine is passed in breast milk. **Sunlight:** Severe sunburns can occur on thioridazine. Avoid sunbathing entirely and avoid casual exposure to the sun for more than 30 minutes. Use a sunblock of a sun protection factor (SPF) of 15 or more if exposure to the sun cannot be avoided.

DRUG INTERACTIONS   **Use with extra caution if you take:** *Tricyclic antidepressants,* as the combination may cause irregular heart rhythms that are potentially fatal; *anticonvulsants, antidepressants, antihistamines, antipsychotics, barbiturates, benzodiazepines,* or any drug that causes sedation or central nervous system depression, because the combination can cause pronounced sedation. *Antihypertensive medication,* as thioridazine may combine to lower blood pressure excessively; *antihistamines* or *antiparkinsonian agents,* as they may combine to produce pronounced dry mouth, blurry vision, constipation, low blood pressure, rapid heart rate, and mental confusion.

DOSING   **Adults:** The starting dose is 25–50 mg one to three times a day, with increases of 25–50 mg/day up to a maximum of 800 mg/day. **Children:** Under 12: 0.5 mg/kg/day to a maximum of 3 mg/kg/day.

MONITORING YOUR USE   **Time to effectiveness:** Calming effects are often noticed within one to three hours of a dose, but several days may be needed to notice any effect on psychotic symptoms. A pronounced effect may take one to two weeks. Many months may be needed to derive full benefit. **A full trial is:** Four weeks at no less than 300 mg/day. **Half-life of drug and active metabolites:** 20–40 hours with many active metabolites. **How to monitor dosage:** The optimal dose is determined by its effectiveness in alleviating the target symptoms. **How to monitor safety:** Examination for the presence of tardive dyskinesia (see below) should be performed twice yearly. **If you miss a dose:** Take a missed dose if it's within an hour or two. Do not try to make up for a missed dose by doubling your next dose; just continue with your regular dosing schedule.

SIDE EFFECTS   **Usual (50–100%):** Sedation, dry mouth, constipation, blurry vision. **Common (10–50%):** Low blood pressure (light-headedness, dizziness), fatigue, ataraxia (zombielike feeling), weight gain, menstrual irregularities, akathisia (restlessness), sexual dysfunction, pseudoparkinsonism (muscular tremor, rigidity, akinesia), and tardive dyskinesia. **Less common (1–10%):** Dystonia (muscle spasms, usually of the head and neck, face, and jaw), galactorrhea (milk leaking from breasts), sexual dysfunction, cataracts. **Infrequent (less than 1%):** Jaundice (yellow eyes and skin, from liver impairment), cataracts, urinary difficulty. **Those requiring attention from your physician:** Symptoms of fever, muscular rigidity, and mental status changes, as you may have neuroleptic malignant syndrome, a potentially severe reaction; any abnormal involuntary movements that suggest tardive dyskinesia; any irregular heartbeats, as you need an EKG to determine if you are having a dangerous heart rhythm; any other physical or emotional changes not described here.

WHAT TO EXPECT WHEN YOU STOP   You may notice a return of your symptoms if thioridazine is tapered gradually. **If stopped abruptly:** You may experience nausea, vomiting, stomach upset, dizziness, and tremor. These effects are unpleasant but not dangerous.

Thiothixene

GENERAL   **Preparations:** Generic and brand name Navane in tablets and liquid form. **Class:** Standard antipsychotic. **Used in:** Psychotic disorders, bipolar disorder (Alzheimer's disease, severe anxiety). **Mechanism of action:** Blocks postsynaptic dopamine receptors.

PRECAUTIONS   **Warnings:** All antipsychotics can cause *neuroleptic malignant syndrome,* a rare, but severe and potentially fatal reaction consisting of fever, muscle rigidity, mental status changes, and alterations in pulse and blood pressure. They can also cause *tardive dyskinesia,* a potentially irreversible disorder of rhythmical, involuntary muscle movements (see chapter 19 for details of both conditions). **Use extra caution if you have:** *Breast cancer,* as thiothixene can elevate prolactin, a hormone released by the pituitary which may cause breast cancer to grow faster; *epilepsy,* as thiothixene may increase the frequency of seizures; *glaucoma, low blood pressure, prostatic hypertrophy,* or *urinary retention,* as the symptoms may worsen. **Tests before starting:** None. **Alcohol:** Should be avoided, as the simultaneous use of thiothixene and alcohol can lower blood pressure significantly and cause confusion. Also, alcohol worsens anxiety and depression and impairs insight and judgment. **Use in pregnancy:** Some neuroleptics have been linked with the "floppy infant syndrome," in which the baby has poor muscle tone. The fetus may experience pseudoparkinsonism and dystonia, muscular side effects which may cause fetal distress before, during, and shortly after birth. Thiothixene is passed in breast milk. **Sunlight:** Severe sunburns can occur on thiothixene. Avoid sunbathing entirely and avoid casual exposure to the sun for more than thirty minutes. Use a sunblock of a sun protection factor (SPF) of 15 or more if exposure to the sun cannot be avoided.

DRUG INTERACTIONS   **Use with extra caution if you take:** *Anticonvulsants, antidepressants, antihistamines, antipsychotics, barbiturates, benzodiazepines,* or any drug that causes sedation or central nervous system depression, because the combination can cause pronounced sedation; *antihypertensive medication,* as thiothixene may combine to lower blood pressure excessively; *antihistamines* or *antiparkinsonian agents,* as they may combine to produce pronounced dry mouth, blurry vision, constipation, low blood pressure, rapid heart rate, and mental confusion.

DOSING   **Adults:** The starting dose is 5–10 mg one to two times a day, with increases of 5–10 mg/day up to a maximum of 60 mg/day. **Children:** Not FDA-approved for under 12. Some child psychiatrists recommend 2 mg/ three times a day with increases every few days up to a maximum of 60 mg/day for those over 12.

MONITORING YOUR USE   **Time to effectiveness:** Calming effects are often noticed within one to three hours of a dose, but several days may be needed to notice any effect on psychotic symptoms. A pronounced effect may take one to two weeks. Many months may be needed to derive full benefit. **A full trial is:** Four weeks at no less than 30 mg/day. **Half-life of drug and active metabolites:** 20–40 hours with many active metabolites. **How to monitor dosage:** The optimal dose is determined by its effectiveness in alleviating the target symptoms. **How to monitor safety:** Examination for the presence of tardive dyskinesia (see below) should be performed twice yearly. **If you miss a dose:** Take a missed dose if it's within an hour or two. Do not try to make up for a missed dose by doubling your next dose; just continue with your regular dosing schedule.

SIDE EFFECTS   **Usual (50–100%):** Dry mouth, constipation, blurry vision. **Common (10–50%):** Low blood pressure (light-headedness, dizziness), fatigue, ataraxia (zombielike feeling), weight gain, missed menstrual periods, akathisia (restlessness), sexual dysfunction, pseudoparkinsonism (muscular tremor, rigidity, akinesia), and tardive dyskinesia. **Less common (1–10%):** Dystonia (muscle spasms, usually of the head and neck, face, and jaw), galactorrhea (milk leaking from breasts), sexual dysfunction. **Infrequent (less than 1%):** Cataracts, urinary difficulty. **Those requiring attention from your physician:** Symptoms of fever, muscular rigidity, and mental status changes, as you may have neuroleptic malignant syndrome, a potentially severe reaction; any abnormal involuntary movements that suggest tardive dyskinesia; any other physical or emotional changes not described here.

WHAT TO EXPECT WHEN YOU STOP   You may notice a return of your symptoms if thiothixene is tapered gradually. **If stopped abruptly:** You may experience nausea, vomiting, stomach upset, dizziness, and tremor. These effects are unpleasant but not dangerous.

Topiramate

GENERAL   **Preparations:** Generic and brand name Topamax. **Class:** Mood stabilizer. **Used in:** Binge-eating disorder, bipolar disorder. **Mechanism of action:** Topiramate has at least three different effects on the brain, but it is unknown precisely how it affects mood and appetite.

PRECAUTIONS   **Use with extra caution if you have:** Kidney or liver impairment, as the metabolic breakdown of topiramate will be reduced, increasing the intensity and duration of its effects; kidney stones, as topiramate may increase their frequency. **Tests before starting:** None. **Alcohol:** Should be avoided because it may impair the effectiveness of topiramate and because it can worsen depression in bipolar disorder.

DRUG INTERACTIONS   **Use with extra caution if you take:** *Anticonvulsants, antidepressants, antihistamines, antipsychotics, barbiturates, benzodiazepines,* or any drug that causes sedation or central nervous system depression, because the combination with topiramate can cause pronounced sedation; *phenytoin (Dilantin),* as the combination may require lower doses of phenytoin and higher doses of topiramate than would otherwise be expected; *oral contraceptives (birth control pills),* because topiramate may make them less effective.

DOSING   **Adults:** The usual starting dose is 50 mg daily. Increases of 50 mg daily each week up to a maximum of 200 mg twice daily is the highest dose found to be helpful for seizures, but the maximum dose useful for bipolar disorder has not been established. **Children:** Same as adults. **The elderly:** Same as adults.

MONITORING YOUR USE   **Time to effectiveness:** You may notice some side effects within the first few doses, but any substantial effect on mood may take some weeks. **A full trial is:** Four weeks at the maximum dose if you are manic. There is no set time with which to determine effectiveness if you start topiramate when your mood is stable, as manic symptoms are often absent for extended periods of time. If none appear, or if they are milder than usual, then topiramate is at least partially effective. **Half-life of drug and active metabolites:** 21 hours with no active metabolites. **How to monitor dosage:** The optimal dose is determined by its effectiveness in stabilizing your mood. **How to monitor safety:** No specific medical tests are needed to monitor safety. **If you miss a dose:** Do not try to make up for a missed dose, just continue with your regular dosing schedule.

SIDE EFFECTS   Common (10–50%): Anxiety, decreased appetite, impaired cognition, depression, dizziness, an unsteady gait, memory impairment, impaired muscular coordination, nausea, respiratory infections, sedation, speech problems, tingling in the extremities, double vision and other visual abnormalities, weight loss. These effects tend to be more pronounced at higher doses. **Less common (1–10%):** Weight increase. **Those requiring attention from your physician:** Any physical or emotional changes not described here.

WHAT TO EXPECT WHEN YOU STOP   You may notice a return of your symptoms if topiramate is tapered gradually. **If stopped abruptly:** You may develop withdrawal seizures. Topiramate should not be stopped abruptly, but needs to be tapered gradually in consultation with your physician.

Tranylcypromine

GENERAL   Preparations: Brand name Parnate only. **Class:** MAOI. **Used in:** Bulimia, depression, panic disorder (other anxiety disorders). **Mechanism of action:** Inhibits monoamine oxidase, the protein enzyme responsible for the breakdown of dopamine, epinephrine, norepinephrine, and serotonin, resulting in elevated levels of these neurotransmitters.

PRECAUTIONS   Warnings: Tranylcypromine can cause a *hypertensive crisis* in which your blood pressure rises dangerously high, putting you at risk for a brain stroke, brain damage, and death. This reaction is unlikely to occur on its own, but is possible if used in combination with foods or medicines that contain tyramine or substances similar to epinephrine. **The following medications must be avoided while you are on tranylcypromine and for two weeks following its cessation in order to avoid a hypertensive crisis:** Prescription medications: *antiasthmatics* that contain *epinephrine* or epinephrine-like compounds, most *antidepressants, antihypertensives, antiparkinsonian agents, barbiturates, buspirone (Buspar), carbamazepine (Tegretol), disulfiram, diuretics, narcotics; stimulants;* over-the-counter medications: *decongestants, dextromethorphan, tryptophan, hay fever medications, sinus medications, appetite suppressants;* recreational drugs: *amphetamines, cocaine, hallucinogenics, heroin, or other narcotics.* **The following foods must be avoided while you are on tranylcypromine and for two weeks following its cessation in order to avoid a hypertensive crisis:** Aged or fermented foods; all cheese or foods containing cheese such as pizza, fondue, many Italian dishes and salad dressings (cottage cheese and cream cheese are allowed); cream, sour cream, and yogurt; foods fermented with yeast (although foods baked with yeast, such as bread, are safe), brewer's yeast; liver, processed meats, such as bologna, corned beef, hot dogs, liverwurst, pepperoni, salami, sausage; broad bean pods (fava beans); sauerkraut; pickles; soy sauce; licorice, caviar, anchovies, dried fruits (raisins, prunes), figs, raspberries, chocolate; bananas, pickled herring; excessive amounts of caffeine-containing beverages (more than one or two, although some people are more sensitive than others) like coffee, tea, sodas, and hot chocolate. **Don't use if you have:** *Congestive heart failure,* as it may make the symptoms worse; *high blood pressure,* as tranylcypromine may make the symptoms worse; *pheochromocytoma,* as it may cause a hypertensive crisis. **Use extra caution if you have:** *Bipolar disorder,* as tranylcypromine can cause a manic episode; *epilepsy,* as tranylcypromine may increase seizure frequency; *low blood pressure,* as tranylcypromine may make symptoms worse; a *psychotic disorder,* as tranylcypromine can worsen psychotic symptoms. **Tests needed before starting:** None. **Alcohol:** Alcohol should be avoided because it worsens anxiety and depression. Beer, wine, Chianti, sherry, and liqueurs, whether they contain alcohol or not, can cause a hypertensive crisis. Hard liquor has no specific adverse consequences, but should be avoided because it can worsen anxiety, depression, and low blood pressure.

DRUG INTERACTIONS   *Antihypertensives,* as tranylcypromine can lower blood pressure further; *narcotics,* as the combination can produce coma, fever, and high blood pressure.

DOSING   **Adults:** 15 mg twice a day with weekly increases of 15 mg/day up to a maximum of 30 mg twice a day. **Children:** Not FDA-approved for under 16.

MONITORING YOUR USE   **Time to effectiveness:** Side effects may be noted within a few days, but the therapeutic effect may take two to six weeks. **A full trial is:** Four weeks at the maximum tolerated dose. **Half-life of drug and active metabolites:** 2–3 hours with active metabolites. The effect can last for two weeks after the last dose. **How to monitor dosage:** The optimal dose is determined by its effectiveness in alleviating the target symptoms. **How to monitor safety:** Monitor blood pressure. **If you miss a dose:** Take a missed dose if it's within an hour or two. Do not try to make up for a missed dose the next day by doubling your dose; just continue with your regular dosing schedule.

SIDE EFFECTS   **Common (10–50%):** Agitation, constipation, dizziness, headaches, insomnia, sedation, sexual dysfunction, tremor, muscle twitching, weight gain. **Those requiring attention from your physician:** A sudden headache, palpitations, rapid heart rate, sweating, throat constriction, neck stiffness, nausea, or vomiting can be a sign that you are having a hypertensive crisis; you should consult your physician immediately and go to the emergency room for treatment of any elevation of blood pressure; physical or emotional changes not listed, such as suicidal thoughts or behavior.

WHAT TO EXPECT WHEN YOU STOP   You may notice a return of your symptoms if you taper and stop tranylcypromine. **If stopped abruptly:** An uncommon withdrawal syndrome starting one to three days after cessation of tranylcypromine with agitation, nightmares, seizures, and psychotic thinking may occur.

Trazodone

GENERAL   **Preparations:** Generic and brand name Desyrel. **Class:** Antidepressant. **Used in:** Anxiety disorders, depression, insomnia. **Mechanism of action:** Blocks the reuptake of serotonin into presynaptic neurons.

PRECAUTIONS   **Warnings:** *Priapism,* which is a sustained erection of the penis not due to sexual arousal, can be caused by trazodone. Priapism can damage the penis and calls for immediate intervention. Treatment generally consists of an injection into the penis. Though uncomfortable, there are no long-lasting effects. Rarely, surgical intervention has been required, with the result of impotence. **Use extra caution if you have:** *Asthma, low blood pressure, congestive heart failure, edema, epilepsy, glaucoma, heart disease, hyperthyroidism, enlarged prostate,* or *urinary retention,* as trazodone can worsen the symptoms; *bipolar disorder,* as trazodone may cause a manic episode; a *psychotic disorder,* as trazodone may make psychotic symptoms worse. **Tests needed before starting:** None. **Alcohol:** Should be avoided, as the simultaneous use of trazodone and alcohol can lower blood pressure significantly and cause confusion. Also, alcohol worsens anxiety and depression and impairs insight and judgment.

DRUG INTERACTIONS   **Do not use if you take:** *MAOI antidepressants,* as their use with trazodone can cause pronounced hypertension and the potential for strokes; *terfenadine (Seldane), astemizole (Hismanal),* or *cisapride (Propulsid),* as the combination with trazodone can cause irregular heart rhythms that are potentially life-threatening; *alprazolam (Xanax)* and *triazolam (Halcion),* as trazodone may intensify their effects and significantly impair your thinking and coordination. **Use with extra caution if you take:** *Antihypertensives,* as trazodone may lower blood pressure excessively; *antihistamines, phenothiazines,* or *tricyclic antidepressants,* as they may combine to produce pronounced dry mouth, blurry vision, constipation, low blood pressure, rapid heart rate, and even mental confusion; *anticonvulsants, antidepressants, antihistamines, antipsychotics, barbiturates, benzodiazepines,* or any drug that causes sedation or central nervous system depression, because the combination can cause pronounced sedation.

DOSING   **Adults:** The usual starting dose is 50–100 mg twice daily, with weekly increases of 100 mg/day up to 300–600 mg/day. **Children:** Not FDA-approved for under 18. For those over 6, some child psychiatrists recommend a starting dose of 1.5–2 mg/kg/day with 1 mg/kg/day increases every few days up to a maximum of 6 mg/kg/day.

MONITORING YOUR USE   **Time to effectiveness:** Side effects are generally noticeable within a few doses, but the therapeutic effect may take one to four weeks. **A full trial is:** Four weeks at the maximum tolerated dosage. **Half-life of drug and active metabolites:** 4–8 hours with one active metabolite with a half-life of 4–14 hours. **How to monitor dosage:** The optimal dose is determined by its effectiveness in alleviating the target symptoms. **How to monitor safety:** No specific tests needed. **If you miss a dose:** Take a missed dose if it's within an hour or two. Do not try to make up for a missed dose by doubling your next dose; just continue with your regular dosing schedule.

SIDE EFFECTS   Common: (10–50%): Blurry vision, constipation, dizziness, dry mouth, fatigue, headache, insomnia, nausea, sweating, weight gain. **Less common (1–10%):** Confusion, memory impairment, sexual dysfunction. **Infrequent (less than 1%):** Urinary difficulty. **Those requiring attention from your physician:** Physical or emotional changes not listed, such as suicidal thoughts or behavior.

WHAT TO EXPECT WHEN YOU STOP   You may notice a return of your symptoms if trazodone is stopped. **If stopped abruptly:** There is no specific withdrawal syndrome.

Triazolam

GENERAL   Preparations: Generic and brand name Halcion. **Class:** Benzodiazepine. **Used in:** Insomnia. **Mechanism of action:** Intensifies the effects of gamma-aminobutyric acid (GABA).

PRECAUTIONS   Warnings: Confusion, bizarre behavior, agitation, and hallucinations have occurred in some people who took triazolam. *It is habit-forming.* Triazolam, like all benzodiazepines, is physically and psychologically habit-forming. People who have experienced traumatic events in their lives and have chronic anxiety are especially prone to developing dependence. Prolonged use is associated with a range of problems. Use for more than four weeks is *not* recommended. If you stop triazolam after more than four weeks of daily use you will probably experience withdrawal symptoms (see below). **Tests needed before starting:** None. **Alcohol:** Alcohol must be avoided entirely. The simultaneous use of triazolam and alcohol is extremely dangerous because it can cause you to stop breathing. The combination can cause death. **Use in pregnancy:** There is a higher rate of babies born with a cleft palate to mothers who took benzodiazepines during pregnancy. **The elderly** are especially sensitive to the effects of benzodiazepines and may experience pronounced side effects at low doses (see chapter 4).

DRUG INTERACTIONS   Don't use if you take: *Itraconazole, ketoconazole,* or *nefazodone,* as they may significantly intensify the effects of triazolam. **Use with extra caution if you take:** *Anticonvulsants, antidepressants, antihistamines, antipsychotics, barbiturates, benzodiazepines,* or any drug that causes sedation or central nervous system depression, because the combination with triazolam can cause pronounced sedation.

DOSING   **Adults:** The usual dose is 0.125–0.25 mg at bedtime, with a maximum dose of 0.5 mg at bedtime. **Children:** Not FDA-approved for under 18. **The elderly:** The usual starting dose is 0.125 mg at bedtime.

MONITORING YOUR USE   **Time to effectiveness:** 30–60 minutes. **A full trial is:** A few doses, which are generally enough to establish whether it will be helpful. **Half-life of drug and active metabolites:** 1.5–5.5 hours with no active metabolites. **How to monitor dosage:** The optimal dose is determined by its effectiveness in helping you to sleep. **If you miss a dose:** Do *not* try to make up for a missed dose; just continue with your regular dosing schedule. **How to monitor safety:** No specific medical tests are needed to monitor safety.

SIDE EFFECTS   **Common (10–50%):** Daytime fatigue, memory impairment, poor muscle coordination (causing a higher rate of falls in the elderly and a higher risk of motor vehicle accidents in all adults). **Less common:** Dizziness, headache, light-headedness. **Infrequent (less than 1%):** Paradoxical agitation and insomnia. **Those requiring attention from your physician:** Any physical or emotional changes not described here. **Side effects associated with use longer than four weeks:** Use of triazolam longer than four weeks may cause physical and psychological dependence, and you may notice the desire for another dose as each one wears off. Ongoing anxiety, reduced effectiveness of each dose, depression, emotional blunting, and impairment of memory and cognition may occur with use longer than one year.

WHAT TO EXPECT WHEN YOU STOP   You may notice insomnia if triazolam is tapered gradually. Other withdrawal symptoms include anxiety, irritability, headaches, tremors, nausea, diarrhea, sweating, and confusion. The rate of tapering is affected by the duration of your use and the size of your dose but may take months if you have been on it for an extended period of time. **If stopped abruptly:** *Seizures* can occur if triazolam is stopped abruptly, although this is extremely unlikely with routine use at recommended dosages. Seizures are potentially life-threatening. You should always consult with your physician as to how to stop it safely.

Trifluoperazine

GENERAL   **Preparations:** Generic and brand name Stelazine in pills and liquid form. **Class:** Standard antipsychotic of the phenothiazine group. **Used in:** Psychotic disorders, bipolar disorder (Alzheimer's disease, severe anxiety, severe ADHD, developmental disorders). **Mechanism of action:** Blocks postsynaptic dopamine receptors.

PRECAUTIONS   **Warnings:** All antipsychotics can cause *neuroleptic malignant syndrome,* a rare but severe and potentially fatal reaction consisting of fever, muscle rigidity, mental status changes, and alterations in pulse and blood pressure. They can also cause *tardive dyskinesia,* a potentially irreversible disorder of rhythmical, involuntary muscle movements (see chapter 19 for details of both conditions). **Use extra caution if you have:** *Breast cancer,* as trifluoperazine can elevate prolactin, a hormone released by the pituitary which may cause breast cancer to grow faster; *epilepsy,* as trifluoperazine may increase the frequency of seizures; *glaucoma, low blood pressure, prostatic hypertrophy,* or *urinary retention,* as the symptoms may worsen. **Tests before starting:** None. **Alcohol:** Should be avoided, as the simultaneous use of trifluoperazine and alcohol can lower blood pressure significantly and cause confusion. Also, alcohol worsens anxiety and depression and impairs insight and judgment. **Use in pregnancy:** Phenothiazines have been linked with the "floppy infant syndrome," in which the baby has poor muscle tone. The fetus may experience pseudoparkinsonism and dystonia, muscular side effects that may cause fetal distress before, during, and shortly after birth. **Sunlight:** Severe sunburns can occur on trifluoperazine. Avoid sunbathing entirely and avoid casual exposure to the sun for more than thirty minutes. Use a sunblock of a sun protection factor (SPF) of 15 or more if exposure to the sun cannot be avoided.

DRUG INTERACTIONS   **Use with extra caution if you take:** *Tricyclic antidepressants,* as the combination may cause irregular heart rhythms that are potentially fatal; *anticonvulsants, antidepressants, antihistamines, antipsychotics, barbiturates, benzodiazepines,* or any drug that causes sedation or central nervous system depression, because the combination can cause pronounced sedation; *antihypertensive medication,* as trifluoperazine may combine to lower blood pressure excessively; *antihistamines* or *antiparkinsonian agents,* as they may combine to produce pronounced dry mouth, blurry vision, constipation, low blood pressure, rapid heart rate, and mental confusion.

DOSING   **Adults:** The starting dose is 2–10 mg/day with increases every few days of 2–10 mg/day up to a maximum of 40 mg/day. **Children:** Not FDA-approved for under 6. Some child psychiatrists recommend a starting dose of 1 mg/one or two times a day with increases every few days up to a maximum of 15 mg/day for those over 6. Older adolescents may require up to 40 mg/day.

MONITORING YOUR USE   **Time to effectiveness:** Calming effects are often noticed within one to three hours of a dose, but several days may be needed to notice any effect on psychotic symptoms. A pronounced effect may take one to two weeks. Many months may be needed to derive full benefit. **A full trial is:** Four weeks at no less than 20 mg/day. **Half-life of drug and active metabolites:** 20–40 hours with active metabolites. **How to monitor dosage:** The optimal dose is determined by its effectiveness in alleviating the target symptoms. **How to monitor safety:** Examination for the presence of tardive dyskinesia (see below) should be performed twice yearly. **If you miss a dose:**

Take a missed dose if it's the same day. Do not try to make up for a missed dose the next day by doubling your dose; just continue with your regular dosing schedule.

SIDE EFFECTS   **Usual (50–100%):** Dry mouth, constipation, blurry vision. **Common (10–50%):** Low blood pressure (light-headedness, dizziness), fatigue, ataraxia (zombielike feeling), weight gain, menstrual irregularities, akathisia (restlessness), pseudoparkinsonism (muscular tremor, rigidity, akinesia), and tardive dyskinesia, a form of involuntary muscle movements (see chapter 19 for further details). **Less common (1–10%):** Dystonia (muscle spasms, usually of the head and neck, face, and jaw), galactorrhea (milk leaking from breasts), sedation, sexual dysfunction. **Infrequent (less than 1%):** Cataracts. **Those requiring attention from your physician:** Jaundice (yellow eyes or skin); neuroleptic malignant syndrome, a rare but severe and potentially fatal reaction consisting of fever, muscle rigidity, mental status changes, and alterations in pulse and blood pressure (see chapter 19 for further details). Any other physical or emotional changes not described here.

WHAT TO EXPECT WHEN YOU STOP   You may notice a return of your symptoms if trifluoperazine is tapered gradually. **If stopped abruptly:** There is no acute withdrawal syndrome.

Trihexyphenidyl

GENERAL   **Preparations:** Generic and brand name Artane in pills and liquid form. **Class:** Antiparkinsonian agent. **Used in:** The treatment of side effects induced by antipsychotics: akathisia, dystonia, and pseudoparkinsonism (tremor, rigidity, akinesia). **Mechanism of action:** Blocks postsynaptic acetylcholine receptors.

PRECAUTIONS   **Use extra caution if you have:** *Congestive heart failure, edema, epilepsy, glaucoma, low blood pressure, prostatic hypertrophy,* or *urinary retention,* as trihexyphenidyl may worsen the symptoms of the disorder. **Tests needed before starting:** None. **Alcohol:** Should be avoided, as the simultaneous use of trihexyphenidyl and alcohol can lower blood pressure significantly and cause confusion. Also, alcohol worsens anxiety and depression and impairs insight and judgment.

DRUG INTERACTIONS   *Antihypertensives,* as they may combine to lower blood pressure excessively; *antihistamines, phenothiazines,* or *tricyclic antidepressants,* as they may combine to produce pronounced dry mouth, blurry vision, constipation, low blood pressure, rapid heart rate, and even mental confusion.

DOSING   **Adults:** The usual starting dose is 1–5 mg twice daily with a weekly increase of 1–5 mg/day up to 15 mg/day. Some people may need higher dosages. **Children:** 1–2 mg once or twice a day.

MONITORING YOUR USE   **Time to effectiveness:** Effects should be noticeable within an hour or two, but the full effect may take two to three days. **A full trial is:** A few days at the maximum recommended dose. **Half-life of drug and active metabolites:** Unknown, but the effects generally last for 6–12 hours. **How to monitor dosage:** The optimal dose is determined by its effectiveness in alleviating the target symptoms. **How to monitor safety:** No special medical tests are needed. **If you miss a dose:** Take a missed dose if it's within an hour or two. Do not try to make up for a missed dose by doubling your next dose, just continue with your regular dosing schedule.

SIDE EFFECTS   **Usual (50–100%):** Blurry vision, constipation, dry mouth. **Less common (1–10%):** Heart rate elevation, low blood pressure, nausea, vomiting. **Infrequent (less than 1%):** Rash, urinary retention, visual changes. **Those requiring attention from your physician:** Any physical or emotional changes not listed.

WHAT TO EXPECT WHEN YOU STOP   You may notice a return of your symptoms if trihexyphenidyl is stopped. **If stopped abruptly:** There are no acute withdrawal effects.

Trimipramine

GENERAL   **Preparations:** Brand name Surmontil only. **Class:** Tricyclic antidepressant. **Used in:** Depression (bulimia, panic disorder, other anxiety disorders). **Mechanism of action:** Blocks the reuptake of norepinephrine and serotonin into presynaptic neurons.

PRECAUTIONS   **Don't use if you have:** *Heart block* (an abnormal heart rhythm) or if you recently had a *heart attack,* as trimipramine may worsen heart block and dangerously affect heart function. **Use extra caution if you have:** *Bipolar disorder,* as trimipramine may cause a manic episode; *epilepsy,* as trimipramine may increase the frequency of seizures; *glaucoma,* as trimipramine can worsen the symptoms of untreated angle closure glaucoma; *low blood pressure,* as trimipramine may lower blood pressure further; a *psychotic disorder,* as trimipramine may make psychotic symptoms worse; *hyperthyroidism,* as trimipramine may cause irregular heart rhythms; *prostatic hypertrophy* or *urinary retention,* as trimipramine may worsen urinary retention. **Tests needed before starting:** An electrocardiogram (EKG) if you are over 35, to ensure you do not have any form of heart block. **Alcohol:** Should be avoided, as the simultaneous use of trimipramine and alcohol can lower blood pressure significantly and cause confusion. Also, alcohol worsens anxiety and depression, and impairs insight and judgment. **Use in pregnancy:** There is a higher rate of miscarriages born to women who take tricyclics, but no specific defect is associated with their use.

DRUG INTERACTIONS   **Don't use if you take:** *MAOI antidepressants,* as their use with trimipramine can cause pronounced hypertension and the potential for strokes. **Use with extra caution if you take:** *Phenothiazines,* as the combination may cause irregular heart rhythms that are potentially fatal; *antihypertensives,* as they may combine to lower blood pressure excessively; *antihistamines, phenothiazines,* and *antiparkinsonian agents,* as they may combine to produce pronounced dry mouth, blurry vision, constipation, low blood pressure, rapid heart rate, and even mental confusion; *guanethadine* to lower blood pressure, as trimipramine may block its effects.

DOSING   **Adults:** The usual starting dose is 25 mg at bedtime with increases every other day up to 150 mg. The maximum recommended dose is 300 mg/day. **Children:** Not FDA-approved for under 18.

MONITORING YOUR USE   **Time to effectiveness:** Side effects are generally noticeable within a few doses, but the therapeutic effect may take two to four weeks. **A full trial is:** Four weeks at the maximum tolerated dosage. **Half-life of drug and active metabolites:** 16–38 hours, with some active metabolites. **How to monitor dosage:** The optimal dose is determined by its effectiveness in alleviating the target symptoms. A blood level may be useful to assist in determining the best dosage if you do not respond or if your side effects are more pronounced than expected. **How to monitor safety:** A blood level should be obtained if doses go over 150 mg/day. An EKG may be useful to ensure that heart function is not impaired. **If you miss a dose:** Take a missed dose if it's within an hour or two. Do not try to make up for a missed dose by doubling your next dose; just continue with your regular dosing schedule.

SIDE EFFECTS   **Usual (50–100%):** Blurry vision, constipation, dizziness, dry mouth, fatigue, increased heart rate, low blood pressure. **Common (10–50%):** Agitation, sweating, weight gain. **Less common (1–10%):** Insomnia, sexual dysfunction, urinary retention. **Those requiring attention from your physician:** Physical or emotional changes not listed, such as suicidal thoughts or behavior.

WHAT TO EXPECT WHEN YOU STOP   You may notice a return of your symptoms if trimipramine is stopped. **If stopped abruptly:** You may experience agitation, headaches, insomnia, and nausea, as well as depression. Trimipramine should be slowly tapered if you decide to stop it. The rate of discontinuation is different for each person and is determined by the clinical situation necessitating the change, your age, severity of symptoms, dosage size, and your duration of use.

Valproate

GENERAL   **Preparations:** Generic, brand names Depakote and Depakote ER (extended release) in pills and sprinkles, and Depakene in liquid form. **Class:** Mood stabilizer. **Used in:** Bipolar disorder. **Mechanism of action:** Valproate has many actions in the brain on receptors, neurotransmitter concentrations, ion channels, and second messenger systems, but it is unknown which effect stabilizes mood.

PRECAUTIONS   **Warnings:** Rarely, *liver failure, pancreatitis* (inflammation of the pancreas), and *thrombocytopenia* (low blood platelets, which are necessary for blood clotting) can be caused by valproate. These conditions are potentially life-threatening (see chapter 19). **Use extra caution if you have:** *Glaucoma* or *polycystic ovary syndrome,* as valproate can worsen the symptoms. **Tests needed before starting:** Complete blood count (CBC), liver function tests. **Alcohol:** Should be avoided as it may impair the effectiveness of valproate. Alcohol should also be avoided because it can worsen depression in bipolar disorder. **Use in pregnancy:** It may cause spina bifida, a defect in the spinal cord. There may be seizures, vomiting, and diarrhea in babies born to mothers who took valproate during pregnancy. These symptoms may be due to a withdrawal syndrome.

DRUG INTERACTIONS   **Use with extra caution if you take:** *Anticonvulsants, antidepressants, antihistamines, antipsychotics, barbiturates, benzodiazepines,* or any drug that causes sedation or central nervous system depression, because the combination can cause pronounced sedation.

DOSING   **Adults:** The usual starting dose is 250 mg two to three times daily, with weekly increases of 250–500 mg/day up to a maximum of 2000 mg/day. Rarely, higher doses are used. **Children:** Not FDA-approved for under 18. Some child psychiatrists recommend a starting dose of 15 mg/kg day, with weekly increases of 5 mg/kg/day up to a maximum of 60 mg/kg/day.

MONITORING YOUR USE   **Time to effectiveness:** You may notice some side effects within one to two days, but any improvement in symptoms generally takes one to two weeks if you are manic. **A full trial is:** Three weeks at the maximum therapeutic level if you are manic. There is no set period of time within which to determine effectiveness if you start valproate when your mood is stable, as manic symptoms are often absent for extended periods of time. Essentially, you stay on the drug and watch for any symptoms of mania. If none appear, or if they are milder than usual, then valproate is at least partially effective. **Half-life of drug and active metabolites:** 9–16 hours with no active metabolites. **How to monitor dosage:** The optimal dose is determined by a blood level of 50–125 micrograms/ml of blood. Improved effectiveness can sometimes be achieved by maintaining the level at the higher end of the therapeutic range. **How to monitor safety:** Periodic CBCs and liver function tests when you first begin are essential to screen for liver failure and thrombocytopenia. **If you miss a dose:** Take a missed dose if it's within a few hours. Do not try to make up for a missed dose by doubling your next dose; just continue with your regular dosing schedule.

SIDE EFFECTS   Common (10–50%): Mild sedation, dizziness, impaired muscular coordination, an unsteady gait, and nausea and vomiting may occur when you first start, but tend to go away within the first week. Apparent hair loss can occur in the first few months, but this is generally transient (see chapter 19). Significant weight gain is common. **Those requiring attention from your physician:** You should consult your physician immediately if you notice abdominal pain, yellow skin or eyes, or any sign of liver impairment. You should consult your physician immediately if you notice unusual bleeding or bruising, which may suggest thrombocytopenia, or any physical or emotional changes not listed.

WHAT TO EXPECT WHEN YOU STOP   You may notice a return of your symptoms if valproate is tapered gradually. **If stopped abruptly:** You may develop withdrawal seizures. Valproate should not be stopped abruptly, but needs to be gradually tapered in consultation with your physician.

Vardenafil

GENERAL   **Preparations:** Brand name Levitra only in pills. **Used in:** Impotence from any etiology, including that caused by psychiatric medications. **Mechanism of action:** Inhibits phosphodiesterase type 5, causing increased levels of guanosine monophosphate, relaxation of smooth muscle, and greater blood flow to the penis, enhancing erection during sexual stimulation.

PRECAUTIONS   **Warnings:** Deaths have been associated with the simultaneous use of this type of medication and nitrates (used in prescription medicines for heart disease such as nitroglycerin, Nitrobid, or Isordil, and recreational drugs such as amyl nitrate). Decreased or a loss of vision can occur with vardenafil due to nonarteritic anterior ischemic optic neuropathy (NAION). **Don't use if you have:** *Heart disease,* as there is a degree of heart risk associated with sexual activity. **Use with extra caution if you have:** *Kidney or liver problems,* as vardenafil is not cleared from the body as efficiently; *retinitis pigmentosa,* as there is the potential for adverse effects with the use of vardenafil. **Tests needed before starting:** None. **Alcohol:** The combination can cause low blood pressure, elevated heart rate, headaches, and dizziness.

DRUG INTERACTIONS   **Don't use if you take:** *Nitrates,* or *alpha-adrenergic blocking agents* (used in high blood pressure) *such as doxazosin or terazosin,* as blood pressure can go too low. **Use with extra caution if you take:** *Erythromycin,* *indinavir, itraconazole, ketoconozole,* or *ritonivir,* as these drugs decrease the breakdown of vardenafil and blood pressure can go too low.

DOSING   Adults: The usual starting dose is 10 mg at least 60 minutes before sexual activity, no more than once a day. Subsequent doses up to a maximum of 20 mg/day can be used. People over 65 should start with 5 mg. Those with liver problems should take no more than 10 mg in a 24-hour period.

MONITORING YOUR USE   Time to effectiveness: 60 minutes. **A full trial is:** 2–3 tries at the maximum dose. **Half-life of drug and active metabolites:** 4–5 hours with one active metabolite. **How to monitor dosage:** The optimal dose is determined by its effectiveness in enhancing potency. **How to monitor safety:** No tests needed.

SIDE EFFECTS   Common (10–50%): Headache, flushing. **Less common (1–10%):** Indigestion, nasal congestion, color-tinged visual changes. **Those requiring attention by your physician:** Erections lasting more than four hours require immediate medical attention, as damage to the penis can result.

Venlafaxine

GENERAL   Preparations: Brand name Effexor and Effexor XR (extended release) in regular and sustained-release. **Class:** Antidepressant. **Used in:** Depression. **Mechanism of action:** Blocks the reuptake of norepinephrine and serotonin into presynaptic neurons.

PRECAUTIONS   Use extra caution if you have: *Bipolar disorder,* as venlafaxine can cause a manic episode; *epilepsy,* as venlafaxine may increase the frequency of seizures; *high blood pressure,* as venlafaxine can increase blood pressure; a *psychotic disorder,* as venlafaxine can worsen psychotic symptoms. **Tests needed before starting:** None. **Alcohol:** The simultaneous use of venlafaxine and alcohol causes no specific adverse consequences, but alcohol should be avoided because it worsens anxiety and depression.

DRUG INTERACTIONS   Do not use if you take: *Other SSRIs, St. John's wort,* or *tryptophan* or other serotonin reuptake inhibitors, as their use with venlafaxine can cause the *serotonin syndrome,* which consists of potentially dangerous alterations in pulse, blood pressure, hyperactivity, and mental status changes (see chapter 19); *MAOI antidepressants,* as their use with venlafaxine can cause a serious, sometimes fatal, reaction of agitation, fever, cardiovascular changes, and mental status changes.

DOSING   Adults: The usual starting dose is 37.5 mg twice daily with weekly increases of 37.5–75 mg/day up to a maximum of 175 mg twice daily. Doses of the sustained-release preparation are the same but can be taken as a single daily dose. Ingestion with meals may minimize indigestion and does not impair absorption. **Children:** Not FDA-approved for under 18.

MONITORING YOUR USE   **Time to effectiveness:** You may notice some side effects within one to two days, but any improvement in symptoms generally takes two to four weeks. **A full trial is:** Four weeks at the maximum dose. **Half-life of drug and active metabolites:** 3–7 hours with one active metabolite with a half-life of 9–13 hours. **How to monitor dosage:** The optimal dose is determined by its effectiveness in alleviating the target symptoms. **How to monitor safety:** Pulse and blood pressure should be monitored regularly until the dose is stabilized. **If you miss a dose:** Take a missed dose if it's within an hour or two. Do not try to make up for a missed dose the next day by doubling your dose; just continue with your regular dosing schedule.

SIDE EFFECTS   **Common (10–50%):** Decreased appetite, anxiety, constipation, dizziness, dry mouth, fatigue, headache, insomnia, nausea, sweating, sexual dysfunction, and weight loss. **Less common (1–10%):** Blurry vision, tremor. **Those requiring attention from your physician:** Hyperactivity, mental status changes, or alterations in your pulse or blood pressure, which suggest the *serotonin syndrome;* any physical or emotional changes not listed, such as suicidal thoughts or behavior.

WHAT TO EXPECT WHEN YOU STOP   You may notice a return of your symptoms if venlafaxine is tapered gradually. **If stopped abruptly:** You may notice a flulike syndrome of nausea, vomiting, diarrhea, dizziness, as well as anxiety and depression. Venlafaxine should not be stopped abruptly but needs to be gradually tapered in consultation with your physician.

Yohimbine

GENERAL   **Preparations:** Brand name Yocon only. **Class:** Aphrodisiac. **Used in:** Medication-induced sexual dysfunction. **Mechanism of action:** Unknown effects in the brain. In the peripheral nervous system, it changes the muscle tone of blood vessels, resulting in enhanced blood flow to the genitals during sexual activity.

PRECAUTIONS   **Warnings:** Yohimbine is found in rubacae and related trees. It has been used as an aphrodisiac for many years in many cultures. It has been helpful in some people to reverse the sexual dysfunction caused by antidepressants and other psychiatric drugs. It has not been extensively studied and specific information is therefore limited. **Tests needed before starting:** None. **Alcohol:** No information available.

DRUG INTERACTIONS   None described by the manufacturer.

DOSING **Adults:** To restore sexual desire: half of a 5.4 mg tablet daily, with an increase up to half a tablet three times a day after a few days and then an increase up to a maximum of 5.4 mg three times daily. To improve sexual arousal and ability to achieve orgasm: one half to one tablet one to two hours prior to sexual activity.

MONITORING YOUR USE **Time to effectiveness:** One to two hours. **A full trial is:** One to two weeks at the maximum dose. **Half-life of drug and active metabolites:** Unknown. **How to monitor dosage:** The optimal dose is determined by its effectiveness in improving sexual functioning. **How to monitor safety:** No specific tests are needed. **If you miss a dose:** Take a missed dose if it's within an hour or two. Do not try to make up for a missed dose the next day by doubling your dose, just continue with your regular dosing schedule.

SIDE EFFECTS **Common (10–50%):** Anxiety, elevation of pulse and blood pressure, hyperactivity, tremor. **Less common (1–10%):** Nausea, sweating. **Those requiring attention from your physician:** Physical or emotional changes not listed.

WHAT TO EXPECT WHEN YOU STOP The manufacturer describes no withdrawal effects.

Zaleplon

GENERAL **Preparations:** Brand name Sonata only. **Class:** Hypnotic (sleeping aid). **Used in:** Insomnia. **Mechanism of action:** Intensifies the effects of gamma-aminobutyric acid (GABA).

PRECAUTIONS **Warnings:** *It may be habit-forming.* Zaleplon is different structurally from benzodiazepines but has similar pharmacological properties, and may share their tendency to be physically and psychologically habit-forming. This issue is not resolved. **Use with extra caution if you have:** Liver damage, as the metabolic breakdown of zaleplon will be reduced, increasing the intensity and duration of its effects. **Tests needed before starting:** None. **Alcohol:** Alcohol must be avoided entirely. The simultaneous use of zaleplon and alcohol is extremely dangerous because it may cause you to stop breathing. The combination may cause death. **The elderly** are especially sensitive to the effects of hypnotics and may experience pronounced side effects at low doses (see chapter 4).

DRUG INTERACTIONS **Use with extra caution if you take:** *Anticonvulsants, antidepressants, antihistamines, antipsychotics, barbiturates, benzodiazepines,* or any drug that causes sedation or central nervous system depression, because the combination with zaleplon can cause pronounced sedation; *cimetidine (Tagamet),* because the breakdown of zalplon will be significantly slowed, increasing the duration and intensity of its effects.

DOSING   **Adults:** The usual starting dose is 5–10 mg at bedtime with increases up to 20 mg if necessary. **Children:** Not FDA-approved for under 18. **The elderly:** The usual starting dose is 5 mg at bedtime. Doses over 10 mg are not recommended.

MONITORING YOUR USE   **Time to effectiveness:** 30–60 minutes. **A full trial is:** A few doses, which are generally enough to establish whether it will be helpful. **Half-life of drug and active metabolites:** One hour with no active metabolites. **How to monitor dosage:** The optimal dose is determined by its effectiveness in helping you sleep. **If you miss a dose:** Do not try to make up for a missed dose, just continue with your regular dosing schedule. **How to monitor safety:** No specific medical tests are needed to monitor safety.

SIDE EFFECTS   **Common (10–50%):** Headache. **Less common (1–10%):** Fatigue, memory impairment, nausea, poor muscle coordination (which may cause a higher rate of falls in the elderly and a higher risk of motor vehicle accidents in all adults). **Those requiring attention by your physician:** Any physical or emotional changes not described here.

WHAT TO EXPECT WHEN YOU STOP   You may notice insomnia if zaleplon is tapered gradually. There may be other physical symptoms during withdrawal.

Ziprasidone

GENERAL   **Preparations:** Brand name Geodon only in pills and short-acting injectable. **Class:** Atypical antipsychotic. **Used in:** Bipolar disorder, psychotic disorders (Alzheimer's disease, severe anxiety, developmental disorders). **Mechanism of action:** Blocks a subset of dopamine and serotonin receptors.

PRECAUTIONS   **Warnings:** Because ziprasidone can cause *QTc prolongation* of the heart, it should not be used if you have had a recent heart attack, heart failure, or irregular heartbeats. All antipsychotics can cause *neuroleptic malignant syndrome,* a rare but severe and potentially fatal reaction consisting of fever, muscle rigidity, mental status changes, and alterations in pulse and blood pressure. They can also cause *tardive dyskinesia,* a potentially irreversible disorder of rhythmical, involuntary muscle movements. Ziprasidone and other atypical antipsychotics are associated with the development of *weight gain, high cholesterol, and diabetes mellitus.* Ziprasidone and other atypical antipsychotics are also associated with a higher incidence of *strokes* and *sudden death* in elderly people with dementia. **Don't use if you have:** Known prolongation of QT interval on your EKG, or if you take other drugs that can prolong the QT interval (such as quinidine, chlorpromazine, thioridazine, pimozide, and others). **Use extra caution if you have:** *Breast cancer*, as ziprasidone may elevate prolactin, a hormone released by the pituitary that may cause breast cancer to grow faster; *epilepsy,* as ziprasidone may increase the frequency of seizures; *heart problems,* as ziprasidone can worsen heart function further; *low blood pressure,* as ziprasidone can lower blood pressure even further. **Tests before starting:** Weight measurement. **Alcohol:** It should be avoided, as the simultaneous use of ziprasidone and alcohol can lower blood pressure significantly and cause confusion. Also, alcohol worsens anxiety and depression and impairs insight and judgment.

DRUG INTERACTIONS   Use with extra caution if you take: *Anticonvulsants, antidepressants, antihistamines, antipsychotics, barbiturates, benzodiazepines,* or any drug that causes sedation or central nervous system depression, because the combination can cause pronounced sedation; *antihypertensives,* as ziprasidone may combine to lower blood pressure excessively; *antihistamines* or *antiparkinsonian agents,* as they may combine to produce pronounced dry mouth, blurry vision, constipation, low blood pressure, rapid heart rate, and mental confusion.

DOSING   Adults: The starting dose is 40 mg twice daily, with increases every few days of 40 mg twice daily up to a maximum of 160 mg twice daily. Doses need to be taken with food to enhance absorption. **Children:** Not FDA-approved for under 18.

MONITORING YOUR USE   Time to effectiveness: The first effects may be noticed within some days, but it may be one to three weeks to notice a pronounced change. It may take several months to derive full benefit. **A full trial is:** Four weeks at no less than 160 mg/day. **Half-life of drug and active metabolites:** Seven hours with no active metabolites. **How to monitor dosage:** The optimal dose is determined by its effectiveness in alleviating the target symptoms. **How to monitor safety:** Pretreatment and periodic weight measurements should be performed to assess weight gain; blood glucose, cholesterol, and lipid profiles should be obtained within three months and yearly thereafter to check for diabetes and elevations in cholesterol or triglycerides; a physical examination for the presence of tardive dyskinesia should be done twice yearly. **If you miss a dose:** Take a missed dose if it's within an hour or two. Do not try to make up for a missed dose the next day by doubling your dose; just continue with your regular dosing schedule.

SIDE EFFECTS   Common (10–50%): Low blood pressure (light-headedness, dizziness), fatigue, headaches. **Less common (1–10%):** Akathisia (restlessness), constipation, menstrual irregularities, nausea, sedation, sexual dysfunction, pseudoparkinsonism (muscular tremor, rigidity, akinesia), rash, tardive dyskinesia, weight gain. **Those requiring attention by your physician:** Symptoms of fever, muscular rigidity, and mental status changes, as you may have neuroleptic malignant syndrome, a potentially severe reaction; a rash; any abnormal involuntary movements that suggest tardive dyskinesia; any irregular heartbeats, as you need an EKG to determine if you're having a dangerous abnormal heart rhythm; any other physical or emotional changes not described here.

WHAT TO EXPECT IF YOU STOP You may notice a return of your symptoms if ziprasidone is tapered gradually. **If stopped abruptly:** There is no acute withdrawal syndrome, but symptoms may return quickly.

Zolpidem

GENERAL **Preparations:** Brand name Ambien only. **Class:** Hypnotic (sleeping aid). **Used in:** Insomnia. **Mechanism of action:** Intensifies the effects of gamma-aminobutyric acid (GABA).

PRECAUTIONS **Warnings:** *It may be habit-forming.* Zolpidem is different structurally from benzodiazepines but has similar pharmacological properties, and may share their tendency to be physically and psychologically habit-forming. This issue is not resolved. **Tests needed before starting:** None. **Alcohol:** Alcohol must be avoided entirely. The simultaneous use of zolpidem and alcohol is extremely dangerous because it can cause you to stop breathing. The combination may cause death. **The elderly** are especially sensitive to the effects of hypnotics and may experience pronounced side effects at low doses (see chapter 4).

DRUG INTERACTIONS **Use with extra caution if you take:** *Anticonvulsants, antidepressants, antihistamines, antipsychotics, barbiturates, benzodiazepines,* or any drug that causes sedation or central nervous system depression, because the combination with zolpidem can cause pronounced sedation.

DOSING **Adults:** The usual starting dose is 5–10 mg at bedtime. Doses of 20 mg are sometimes needed. **Children:** Not FDA-approved for under 18. **The elderly:** The usual starting dose is 5 mg at bedtime.

MONITORING YOUR USE **Time to effectiveness:** 30–60 minutes. **A full trial is:** A few doses, which are generally enough to establish whether it will be helpful. **Half-life of drug and active metabolites:** 1.4–4.5 hours with no active metabolites. **How to monitor dosage:** The optimal dose is determined by its effectiveness in helping you sleep. **If you miss a dose:** Do not try to make up for a missed dose; just continue with your regular dosing schedule. **How to monitor safety:** No specific medical tests are needed to monitor safety.

SIDE EFFECTS **Less common (1–10%):** Daytime fatigue, headache, memory impairment, nausea, poor muscle coordination (which may cause falls in the elderly and motor vehicle accidents in all adults) and sleepwalking. **Those requir-**

ing attention from your physician: Any physical or emotional changes not described here.

WHAT TO EXPECT WHEN YOU STOP   You may notice insomnia if zolpidem is tapered gradually. Other withdrawal symptoms may include anxiety, cramps, crying, fatigue, flushing, insomnia, light-headedness, and vomiting.

CHAPTER 18

Alternative Remedies

There is a great deal of interest in herbal remedies, vitamins, dietary supplements, and "natural" medicines for a wide variety of psychiatric and medical problems. In recent years, the possible benefits of St. John's wort, vitamin E, zinc supplements, and other alternative remedies have captured the attention of the media and the public and become the focus of intense interest.

Alternative remedies are advertised and marketed differently from standard prescription drugs because of regulations put out by the Food and Drug Administration (FDA). The FDA allows a company to advertise and sell a drug only if the company's claims are backed up with research. A rigorous series of trials must prove that a drug has some beneficial effect before the FDA will permit a company to advertise a drug and make claims for its effectiveness.

It is very expensive for a company to perform these trials and bring a drug to market. As a result, a company will perform this work only if it can get a patent on a drug, allowing the company to be the only supplier to the public. This permits it to set a price that no one can undercut and thereby make a large profit. They spend a great deal of time and money developing new compounds on which they can hold the patent.

The vast majority of alternative remedies are naturally occurring compounds for which the FDA does not issue patents. Any company can package and sell these drugs, so no individual company bothers to fund rigorous (and expensive) clinical trials to determine the effectiveness and side effects of a particular remedy. As a result, most of these remedies have not been formally studied.

Evaluating Alternative Remedies

Because there is a general lack of reliable information about many alternative treatments, people shape the little data available to promote their own agendas. Proponents strongly advocate their use but ignore the lack of evidence supporting their position and the potential for side effects. The medical establishment derides them as useless, handily promoting their own treatments, but minimizing the undeniable benefit many people derive. Stores do a booming business selling remedies that even some of their owners admit provide little aid. There are large companies that make and sell alternative remedies without regard to their genuine value. The lack of reliable information and the conflicting claims of competing groups generate even more misinformation about alternative treatments.

There are seven issues to keep in mind if you consider using an alternative remedy.

Realize that a drug is a drug. A drug is *any* chemical compound you take to alter your physical or mental state. Penicillin, codeine, and fluoxetine are drugs. So are caffeine, alcohol, and nicotine. The vitamin C many people take to ward off colds is a drug. Herbs are drugs. Multivitamins, "stress" pills, and minerals like zinc supplements are drugs, too. All of these are drugs, with the possible benefit of changing your physical or mental state, *and* the potential for bad reactions.

Realize that "natural" is neither good nor bad. Many people believe that a drug is somehow "safe" if it comes more or less directly from nature. "Synthetic" drugs made by pharmaceutical companies, especially those with known problems, seem scarier and more harmful than drugs derived from nature.

The source of a drug does not determine whether a drug is "safe" or whether its use makes sense. Just because a drug is derived from nature doesn't make it safe. Many poisons are made by Mother Nature. Curare, a muscle paralyzer used by native South Americans for hundreds of years to kill animals, is derived from plants. Opium, morphine, and heroin are synthesized from the poppy plant. Alcohol is synthesized from grapes or grain. Marijuana leaves are smoked without any preparation at all besides drying. Hormones for menopause or birth control can cause strokes, blood clots, and mood swings. Tryptophan, a naturally occurring amino acid promoted as a sleep aid causes a potentially fatal disorder called eosinophilia-myalgia syndrome in some people who take it.

Whether a drug is safe and sensible to use depends on the same kind of assessment and decision-making process outlined in the main text for psychiatric drugs: Make a *full* diagnosis, consider all possible treatments, choose an agent that may improve some target symptoms, educate yourself about the drug you choose, and monitor your use carefully.

Educate yourself about the evidence. Educate yourself about the evidence supporting the value of *any* drug you try. Some drugs, like St. John's wort, have been studied extensively, while others derive their popularity merely from clever advertising, without any valid foundation for the claims for effectiveness.

In 1978, the Minister of Health of Germany established a series of commissions to evaluate the safety and effectiveness of all drugs. Commission E reviewed the scientific literature of herbal preparations. It created a list of "approved" herbs, those for which there was scientific evidence of effectiveness and an absence of documented risk. In the opinion of most experts, Commission E set a reasonable standard for determining the safety and effectiveness of herbal preparations. The herbs listed below all have the approval of German Commission E.

Don't fall for "It worked for him, it'll work for me." There is something compelling when someone says, "This drug helped me. Maybe it'll help you." You may be looking for relief and inquiring among friends, a health care practitioner, or a store owner about what might help you. However, it is not useful, or safe, to generalize from the experience of another person. For example, penicillin (derived from a "natural" mold) has saved many lives from pneumonia and other life-threatening infections, but a very small proportion of people of those taking it have died from an allergic reaction. If you based your use on a person who was helped, you might be unaware of how harmful it could be. On the other hand, if you heard only a disaster story, you might refuse a treatment that could save your life.

When you hear a story about one person improving, it is not safe to conclude that you will be helped, too. Maybe your problems aren't all that similar. Maybe their improvement was due to something other than the drug they're recommending. Maybe you'll respond to the drug differently. As we discussed previously, make a *full* diagnosis, learn about *all* possible treatments (not just those that you hear about from friends or the media), choose an agent that may improve some target symptoms, and monitor your use carefully.

Know that alternative remedies have side effects. Although drugs from a doctor are expected to have side effects, alternative remedies also carry this same risk. Any substance that can cause an alteration in one body system can cause alterations in others. There is no drug that has only beneficial effects.

One of the differences between most alternative remedies and traditional Western medicines is in the amount of information available about possible side effects. The FDA requires any company who wants to advertise and market a drug to thoroughly document all side effects experienced by people enrolled in the pre-marketing trials. Periodic blood work, EKGs, physical exams, and patient questioning are done regularly to ferret out any and all possible side effects. Each side effect is then evaluated to determine whether further investigation or treatment is necessary. Occasionally, a trial is even halted because a serious and potentially dangerous side effect is discovered by this process. Most, though not all, side effects are discovered in this fashion *before* the FDA permits the marketing of a drug. This permits health care providers and patients to use them with some preparation for the potential side effects of a drug.

Since these trials aren't performed on most alternative remedies, there is no reliable database about the occurrence and frequency of side effects. As a result, you won't know which side effects to expect, which ones to worry about, and what you should do about them if you experience one. For example, I know one person who developed palpitations on St. John's wort, and another developed a rash. Both people discontinued the drug, but what was their risk? Were the palpitations just an intermittent increase in heart rate, or was it a sign of a potentially more serious reaction? Was the rash merely an unpleasant itch or a sign of a serious allergic reaction that needed medical treatment? These questions can't be answered because the frequency and severity of most side effects have not been systematically evaluated.

When you take an alternative remedy, therefore, you should monitor your physical and mental health and note any changes. You should contact your physician about any effect that concerns you.

Pick the right dosage. There are two problems with determining dosages for herbal remedies. First, the dosage that is most likely to help you has not been objectively established. Many drugs, especially those used for psychiatric problems, can be effective at one dose but not at another. Sometimes different people respond to different dosage sizes. As a result, you are more or less on your own. If one cup of chamomile tea will help you to sleep, will two be stronger? Will ten cups be stronger, or could that much possibly pose a danger?

It's important to know that a remedy can be therapeutic at one dose but cause problems if the dose is too high. Just because it's "natural" doesn't mean that you can't take too much. For example, in small doses, vitamin A is essential for proper metabolic function, especially aiding vision, but large doses can cause yellowing of the skin. Large doses of vitamin B_6 can cause clumsy hands and feet and numbness around the mouth. The high doses of vitamin C used by some people in the mistaken belief that it wards off colds can interfere with the absorption of vitamin B_{12}, increase estrogen levels, and increase the possibility of kidney stones. Calcium supplements can help osteoporosis, but too much may cause kidney stones and induce a zinc deficiency. Zinc is touted to help sexual functioning, but an excess can cause ulcers, anemia, and inflammation of the pancreas.

The second problem with many alternative remedies is that preparations by different companies do not always contain the same amount. Dried herbs probably vary the most, but even pills are not uniform. This is less of a problem with vitamins and mineral supplements, which are easily measured, than with the dried leaves, flowers, or roots of herbal remedies.

There is no easy solution to either of these problems. You have to educate yourself about the different preparations on the market and the doses recommended by people who promote the use of whatever remedy you want to try.

Inform your physician. If you decide you want to take an alternative remedy, you should inform your physician (and psychiatrist). It's possible that any remedy you take can impair your functioning or interact with another medication that you are on. Green tea is touted as a health aid, but the caffeine can worsen anxiety and insomnia. St. John's wort may aid mild depression, but can cause the serotonin syndrome (a potentially dangerous reaction with symptoms of fever, hyperactivity, and alterations in mental status, pulse, and blood pressure) if taken in combination with SSRIs.

Alternative Remedies

Although there are myriad remedies touted to aid your mental health and well-being, I will discuss only those that are widely used or for which there is evidence for their effectiveness. You should take the same precautions with these remedies that were outlined in chapter 16. Remember—a drug is a drug.

S-adenosylmethionine (SAMe)   General: SAMe is produced in most cells of the body by combining adenosine triphosphate and methionine, an amino acid. It serves as a methyl donor in transmethylation reactions, a process essential to many cellular processes, including the regulation of genes and neurotransmitters. **Used**

in: Depression. **Mechanism of action:** Although the role of SAMe in chemical re-actions in the body is well understood, it is not known how it may improve mood. **Evidence for effectiveness:** A number of studies, some placebo-controlled, have demonstrated its effectiveness in alleviating depression in some people. No long-term studies have been performed. **Precautions:** It may cause a manic episode in people with bipolar disorder. **Dosing:** The manufacturer suggests a starting dose of 200 mg twice a day, but recommends 200 mg/day for the first week if you are sensitive to medications. It should be taken on an empty stomach, such as before meals. Doses of up to 1600 mg/day may be needed. **Side effects:** Stomach upset.

Chamomile   General: Chamomile (*Matricaria recutita*) is derived from the flower of the herb. The active ingredient is believed to be apigenin. **Used in:** Anxi-ety, nervous stomach. **Mechanism of action:** It may interact with the benzodi-azepine receptor and the histamine system. **Evidence for effectiveness:** It is approved by the German Commission E. **Precautions:** None. **Dosing:** 3 g of dried flower heads three to four times daily as tea. **Side effects:** Allergic reactions.

Ginkgo   General: *Ginkgo biloba* is a tree. Once native to China, it is now com-mon in many areas of the world. It has been used in China for several thousand years. The active ingredients are believed to be flavonone glycosides, or hetero-sides, and terpene molecules found in the leaves. Organic acids, which are also present in ginkgo extract, permit the active ingredients to be water-soluble, im-proving absorption. **Used in:** Vascular insufficiency (poor blood flow) in the brain. It has also been used in depression and sexual dysfunction. **Mechanism of action:** It is believed that ginkgo acts by stabilizing the outer coating of nerve cells, called the cell membrane. Additionally it appears to improve circulation. **Ev-idence for effectiveness:** There are many studies that demonstrate that ginkgo im-proves the symptoms associated with poor circulation, including poor memory. There are some reports of improvement in mood and improved sexual functioning. Commission E approves only the dry extract of the leaf. **Precautions:** Use with extra caution with anticoagulants such as aspirin and warfarin (Coumadin). **Dos-ing:** The dose is 120–240 mg dry extract in two or three doses a day. It generally takes some weeks to work, although the full effect may take 12 weeks. **Side ef-fects:** Indigestion, headaches, dizziness, and allergic reactions.

Hops   General: Hops (*Humulus lupulus*) is a vine that grows in Europe and North and South America. The active ingredient may be an oil found in the plant, 2-methyl-3-butene-2-ol. The oil itself is quite volatile, which means that any preparation may lose its effectiveness if it is stored for any length of time. **Used in:** Anxiety and insomnia. **Mechanism of action:** Unknown. **Evidence for effective-ness:** There are some studies documenting its effectiveness as a mild sedative, and Germany's E commission has approved its use. **Precautions:** Use with extra cau-tion in combining with other sedatives such as alcohol. **Dosing:** 0.5 g as a single dose. **Side effects:** None reported.

Kava   General: Kava (*Piper methysticum*) is a member of the pepper family. The kava extract was originally used by natives of the South Pacific islands. The active ingredients of the kava extract are believed to be *kavalactones,* which are found primarily in the root. **Used in:** Anxiety. **Mechanism of action:** The mechanism of action is unknown. Kavalactones do not bind to GABA receptors as do benzodiazepines. **Evidence for effectiveness:** There are many studies that demonstrate that kava is more effective than placebo in the treatment of different forms of anxiety. It has been approved in the treatment of anxiety in England and Switzerland and by Germany's Commission E. **Precautions:** It can worsen the symptoms in Parkinson's disease. It must be used with extra caution with alcohol or other drugs that cause sedation as they may combine to cause pronounced sedation. Commission E recommends against its use if you are depressed. **Dosing:** The usual starting dose is 60–120 mg of kavalactones one to three times a day. It generally takes some weeks to work. It should not be used for more than three months without medical advice. **Side effects:** Kava has caused severe liver damage in some people. Symptoms of liver damage include yellow skin, yellow eyes, and abdominal pain. Contact your physician immediately if you notice any of these symptoms.

Lemon Balm   General: Lemon balm (*Melissa officinalis*) is a member of the mint family. **Used in:** Anxiety, nervous stomach. **Mechanism of action:** Unknown. **Evidence for effectiveness:** There are no studies demonstrating its effects in humans. **Precautions:** Use with caution in combination with other sedative drugs such as alcohol. **Dosing:** 1.5–4.5 grams daily. **Side effects:** None reported.

Omega 3 Fatty Acids   General: Omega 3 fatty acids (O3FA) are compounds of carbon, hydrogen, and oxygen essential to healthy functioning in all cells of the body. They are found in high proportion in salmon and some other fish. Examples of O3FA include eicosapentanoic acid and docosahexanoic acid. **Used in:** Bipolar disorder. **Mechanism of Action:** Unknown. **Evidence for effectiveness:** One report of thirty patients with bipolar disorder demonstrated some effectiveness. **Precautions:** It may affect blood clotting and should be used *only with your doctor's knowledge and consent,* especially if you have had heart problems, a stroke, or clotting or bleeding disorder. **Dosing:** 6.2 grams of eicosapentanoic acid and 3.4 grams of docosahexanoic acid daily. **Side Effects:** O3FA may impair blood-clotting, which may cause nosebleeds. You should contact your physician immediately if you notice a nosebleed or any unusual bleeding while taking O3FA.

Passion Flower   General: Passion flower (*Passiflora incarnata*) is a vine native to North and South America. The active ingredient is believed to be isovitexin. **Used in:** Anxiety, insomnia. **Mechanism of action:** Unknown. **Evidence for effectiveness:** There are reports that document its sedative qualities. It is approved by Commission E. **Precautions:** Use with extra caution with other sedatives such as alcohol. **Dosing:** 3–6 grams of the leaf; 5–15 grams of the tincture before bedtime. **Side effects:** Allergic reactions.

St. John's Wort (Hypericum)   General: St. John's wort (*Hypericum perfora-tum*) is a plant found in Europe and the United States. The active ingredient is be-lieved to be hypericin, which is derived from the leaves and flowers. **Used in:** Primarily used in depression, it has also been tried for anxiety. **Mechanism of ac-tion:** Hypericum affects many different neurotransmitter systems, including sero-tonin, norepinephrine, dopamine, and GABA, and lowers the level of the hormone cortisol. **Evidence for effectiveness:** There are a wealth of studies that document the effectiveness of St. John's wort in relieving mild to moderate depression. It is approved by Germany's Commission E. There are some reports that it can aid anx-iety. **Precautions:** Don't use if you take other antidepressants, as the combination can lead to the serotonin syndrome (see chapter 19) and other potentially negative reactions. Be careful in the sun, as St. John's wort can cause you to sunburn easily. **Dosing:** The usual dose is 300 mg of 0.3 percent hypericin three times a day, al-though some people take a higher dose. It generally takes some weeks to work. **Side effects:** Known side effects include photosensitivity (excessive sensitivity to the sun), indigestion, dizziness, dry mouth, sedation, restlessness, and constipation.

Valerian   General: Valerian (*Valeriana officinalis*) is a plant found in Europe and the United States. The active ingredients are believed to be valepotriates and valeric acid, found in the root. **Used in:** Insomnia. **Mechanism of action:** Valer-ian binds with GABA, the same receptor upon which benzodiazepines exert their effects. **Evidence for effectiveness:** Many studies document the effective-ness of valerian in the treatment of insomnia. It is approved for anxiety and in-somnia by Commission E. **Precautions:** None. **Dosing:** 2-3 grams one to four times per day. **Side effects:** There is no documented evidence that valerian is habit-forming, in spite of its similarity to benzodiazepines. Daytime sedation, depression, and impairment of memory and motor performance are not com-mon, as they are with benzodiazepines. There have been reports of headaches and paradoxical stimulant-like effects.

Vitamin E (alpha-tocopherol)   General: Vitamin E is a fat-soluble vitamin found in vegetable oils. **Used in:** Alzheimer's disease, tardive dyskinesia. **Mecha-nism of action:** Vitamin E prevents the breakdown of nerve cell membranes. **Evi-dence for effectiveness:** Studies document that vitamin E slows the rate of deterioration in Alzheimer's disease and lessens the severity of tardive dyskinesia in some people. **Precautions:** It can alter the effectiveness of anticoagulants like warfarin (Coumadin). **Dosing:** The usual dose is 400 international units three times daily. **Side effects:** The use of vitamin E at dosages helpful for Alzheimer's disease and tardive dyskinesia (1000 international units or more per day) has caused heart problems in some people. Although it is available without a prescrip-tion, you should only use it in consultation with your primary care physician.

Yohimbine   Discussed in chapter 17, as it is FDA-approved.

CHAPTER 19

Managing Side Effects

A ll psychiatric drugs have side effects. Some are mild and not distressing. Some are annoying and may interfere with some aspect of your functioning. Some can be dangerous and require immediate medical attention. This chapter discusses the side effects that you may experience when you take a psychiatric drug.

Each side effect is associated with one or more drugs. Following each drug name is a number that estimates the seriousness of the side effect and what you should do about it: (1) denotes medications for which side effects are generally mild, though they may be annoying, and will not cause you any harm. Discussion with your doctor at the next appointment is generally sufficient, although you may want to consult sooner if you have any specific concerns that you don't feel should wait. (2) denotes medications for which side effects are more severe, though not dangerous; these side effects may worsen with continued use of the drug. You should contact your physician within a day or two to discuss the best way of managing it. (3) denotes a medication side effect that requires immediate intervention to prevent any further harm. You should contact your doctor immediately to discuss whether you should continue on any of these medications and the need for any emergency medical care.

The Side Effects

If you notice a side effect not described here, contact your physician. If you experience a side effect that is listed, but not associated with the drug you take, it is wise to contact your physician to ensure your safety. Boldface type indicates side effects described elsewhere in this section.

Abdominal Pain *Nefazodone, phenothiazines, tacrine,* and *valproate* (3) can cause liver damage and failure. If you experience abdominal tenderness, especially if it is accompanied by yellow eyes or skin (signs of **jaundice**), consult your doctor immediately. *Stimulants* (1) commonly cause abdominal pain. Though not medically dangerous, it can be unpleasant. Taking a dose after meals may be helpful, although this may reduce effectiveness. A medication change is another option.

Acne *Disulfiram and lithium* (1) cause acne. It generally persists as long as you are on the drug. Topical tetracycline may improve it somewhat. Dosage reduction is generally ineffective. If it is from lithium and it is severe, consider other mood stabilizers.

Agitation *Antihistamines, antidepressants, stimulants, SSRIs,* and *other antidepressants* (2) can cause agitation. Agitation generally persists, and most people do not become used to it. Dosage reduction or a medication change are options. If the agitation is accompanied by rapid speech, hyperactivity, racing thoughts, euphoric or irritable mood, and insomnia, you may be experiencing a manic episode (see chapter 8), an uncommon, but potentially serious reaction that requires immediate attention from your physician. *Antipsychotics* (1) can cause a feeling of restlessness or agitation. This can be **akathisia.** Rarely, *benzodiazepines* (2) can cause agitation. Though not dangerous, it is unpleasant. Stopping the benzodiazepine is usually the best course of action. *Buprenorphine* and *methadone* (1) can cause agitation that is not serious, but can be unpleasant. A dosage reduction or stopping the drug are the only remedies.

Agranulocytosis *Clozapine, carbamazepine,* and *mirtazapine* (3) can cause this extremely serious problem. Agranulocytosis is a medical condition in which your bone marrow doesn't produce enough white blood cells, which are necessary for your body to fight infection. It is possible to develop an infection severe enough to cause death.

Carbamazepine causes agranulocytosis at a fairly low rate: 3–5/100,000. The rate for mirtazapine is 1/1500. Monitoring your blood for a few months after you start carbamazepine or mirtazapine is generally sufficient to ensure your safety. In the first six months of use, the time of greatest danger, you should contact your physician and consider getting a blood test to measure your white blood cells if you notice any sign of an infection, such as fever or sore throat.

Clozapine causes agranulocytosis in 1 percent of those who try it. A monitoring system was developed in order to ensure early detection of agranulocytosis for those on clozapine. This system requires weekly blood counts for six months (the time of greatest risk) and every other week thereafter. While this system has detected many cases of agranulocytosis, permitting immediate discontinuation of clozapine with no long-lasting effects, some people have died. The rate of death is approximately 1 percent of those developing agranulocytosis, or 1/10,000 for all patients on clozapine.

The treatment of agranulocytosis requires immediate discontinuation of whichever drug you are on. Consultation with a hematologist, a specialist in blood disorders, is essential, in order to consider the usefulness of drugs to stimulate the bone marrow to produce more white blood cells as rapidly as possible.

Akathisia *Antipsychotics* (2) induce akathisia, an inner restlessness that is very uncomfortable. Dosage reduction is one remedy. Beta-blockers can generally provide significant relief. Benzodiazepines can help as well, though they are habit-forming. Antiparkinsonian agents can sometimes provide some relief.

Akinesia   *Antipsychotics* (2) induce akinesia, one of the symptoms of **pseudoparkinsonism.** Akinesia is a lack of muscle movements. Antiparkinsonian agents provide significant relief.

Anxiety   *Amantadine, amoxapine, bupropion, clomipramine, guanfacine, maprotiline, naltrexone, SSRIs, stimulants, topiramate,* and *yohimbine* (1) can cause anxiety. Though not dangerous, it is unpleasant and unlikely to go away. Either dosage reduction or a change in medications is the most effective remedy.

Aplastic Anemia   *Carbamazepine* (3) causes aplastic anemia at a rate of a 1–2 per hundred thousand people who take it. Aplastic anemia is a potentially fatal medical condition in which your bone marrow does not make the red blood cells that carry oxygen, the white blood cells that fight infection, and platelets to assist in blood clotting. Symptoms of aplastic anemia include unusual bleeding or bruising, sores in the mouth, fever, or sore throat. You should contact your physician immediately and consider getting a blood test to monitor your blood cells if you notice any of these symptoms. Treatment requires immediate discontinuation of the medication. Consultation with a hematologist, a specialist in blood disorders, is essential in order to consider the usefulness of drugs to stimulate the bone marrow to improve as rapidly as possible.

Appetite—Decreased   *Stimulants* (1) can decrease appetite. Children on stimulants need to be closely monitored to ensure adequate weight gain. Drug holidays, periods of time off the medication, are the only remedy. Adults generally don't lose significant amounts of weight unless they take excessive amounts. *Buprenorphine, donepezil, methadone,* and *tacrine* (1) can cause significant weight loss. Monitor your weight to ensure that you maintain your weight. *Bupropion, clomipramine,* and *SSRIs* (1) also decrease appetite, but not enough to induce significant weight loss. *Topiramate* (1) causes weight loss in some people. This may be useful if a person is overweight or if other mood stabilizers have caused weight gain.

Appetite—Increased   *Antidepressants, antipsychotics,* and *mood stabilizers* (1) often increase appetite and cause weight gain. Weight gain is generally slow and gradual, but the amount of weight can be substantial. You may gain as much as 10 to 20 percent of your premedication body weight, some people even more. Dosage reduction is the only remedy for the excessive craving to eat. Obesity can contribute to an increased risk of heart attacks, high blood pressure, and diabetes. These complications can lead to significant illness, impairment of functioning, and increased mortality. It is important, therefore, to plan your diet and maintain your weight as close to your ideal weight as possible. It is easier to keep weight off than to lose it, so address this as soon as you realize your weight is increasing.

Ataraxia   Induced by *standard antipsychotics* (1), ataraxia is an unpleasant zombielike feeling in which you are aware of your surroundings but have little reaction to them. Atypical neuroleptics generally do not cause this side effect. Consider changing to them if you experience ataraxia. Dosage reduction is the only other remedy.

Bedwetting   *Clozapine* (1) often causes bedwetting due in part to its tendency to cause pronounced sedation. Eliminating caffeine, which increases urination, restricting fluids for three hours before bedtime, and emptying your bladder just before sleeping are usually sufficient to stop bedwetting. If it persists after doing this, consider consultation with a urologist, who may recommend administration of oxybutinin (Ditropam) tablets or desmopressin spray (DDAVP), drugs that treat urinary incontinence.

Bleeding   *Carbamazepine* (3) can cause bleeding from **aplastic anemia,** and *valproate* can cause bleeding from **thrombocytopenia.** Both are potentially life-threatening reactions. If you notice unusual bleeding, contact your physician immediately.

Blood Pressure—High   In combination with certain foods or medicines, *MAOIs* (3) can cause elevations in blood pressure that can be severe enough to cause strokes and brain damage. Possible symptoms of elevated blood pressure include headaches, heart palpitations, neck stiffness, nausea, vomiting, sweating, dilated pupils, and changes in heart rate. If you suspect that your blood pressure is too high, it is essential that you be evaluated immediately. Treatment will include stopping the MAOI and lowering your blood pressure with other drugs. *Stimulants* and *venlafaxine* (1) can also cause an elevation in blood pressure. The rise is usually mild and not clinically significant. Monitor your blood pressure until a maintenance dose is attained and you know your blood pressure is in the normal range.

Blood Pressure—Low   *Tricyclic antidepressants, antihistamines, antiparkinsonian agents, antipsychotics, beta-blockers, nefazodone,* and *trazodone* (1) can all lower your blood pressure. Symptoms include light-headedness, especially when you arise from sitting or lying down, becoming easily fatigued, and rapid heart rate (except for beta-blockers). The symptoms of low blood pressure are generally mild and don't require intervention, although the elderly are more sensitive to these effects and may have a higher rate of falls. Ensure adequate fluid intake and eliminate caffeine, which acts as a diuretic and causes you to excrete water excessively. Dosage reduction is the only remedy, but it is rarely needed.

Blurry Vision   Many *antidepressants, antipsychotics, antihistamines,* and *antiparkinsonian agents* (1) may cause mild blurry vision when you first begin taking them. Your eyes will gradually improve as your dose stabilizes, although some slight impairment may remain. Though unpleasant, blurry vision isn't dangerous. Dosage reduction is the only remedy. Obtaining a new or different prescription for eyeglasses may be helpful. See also **Vision Changes.**

Breathing—Difficulty   *Beta-blockers* (3) can sometimes worsen asthma and may making breathing more difficult. Consider changing to antiparkinsonian agents if you take beta-blockers for antipsychotic-induced akathisia. *Clozapine* (3) can rarely cause sudden shortness of breath due to **pulmonary embolism,** a potentially life-threatening reaction requiring immediate medical attention. It can also impair breathing at night due to the pooling of saliva and the sensation of choking. This is unpleasant, though not dangerous.

Breathing—Slowed   *Benzodiazepines* (3) can sometimes slow the rate of breathing. Generally this effect is unnoticeable. Ingested with alcohol, however, it may be severe and potentially life-threatening. The combination of *clozapine* and *benzodiazepines* (3) can sometimes lower the rate of breathing to dangerous levels and has been associated with some deaths.

Bruising—Frequent   *Frequent bruising can be a sign of* **aplastic anemia** or **thrombocytopenia** rare side effects of *carbamazepine* and *valproate* (3), respectively. If you notice bruising with any other medication, however, you should consult your physician immediately to discuss a formal evaluation of your blood counts and the ability of your blood to clot.

Cataracts   *Phenothiazines* (1) can cause tiny cataracts after years of use. They are generally of no significance and do not significantly impair vision. Premarketing testing of *quetiapine* (2) on dogs revealed cataracts. It is not clear whether or not quetiapine causes cataracts in humans. If you take quetiapine for more than a few months, periodic examination of your eyes (once a year) by an ophthalmologist or optometrist appears prudent until this matter is resolved.

Choking   *Clozapine* (1) can lead some people to feel a choking sensation at night. This is probably due to the pooling of saliva that occurs because people swallow less on clozapine. Though uncomfortable, this is generally not dangerous.

Cholesterol Elevations   *Atypical antipsychotics* (2) can cause elevations in cholesterol and triglycerides (another form of fat in your blood). Elevations in cholesterol and triglycerides put you at greater risk for heart attacks, strokes, and gallbladder problems, even if you are not overweight. Careful dieting, exercise, and cholesterol-lowering medications can be helpful to lower cholesterol and/or triglycerides to normal levels. It is not clear if low doses are less likely to cause elevations in cholesterol or triglycerides. Aripiprazole and ziprasidone may be less likely to cause elevations in cholesterol and triglycerides than other atypical antipsychotics. Standard antipsychotics are less likely to cause elevations in cholesterol and triglycerides.

Cognition Impairment   *Benzodiazepines* (1) impair cognition (thinking processes). Memory impairment is generally the most noticeable effect, but attention span and visual perceptual analysis are also compromised. *Lithium* (1) may cause a decrease in creativity in some people. *Antiparkinsonian agents, antidepressants, antipsychotics,* and *topiramate* (1) may impair your ability to think clearly, although the effect is generally quite mild.

Confusion   Toxic amounts of *any drug* (3) can cause confusion. Therapeutic doses of antiparkinsonian agents may combine with other medications to cause confusion. No matter what the cause, however, confusion is a matter of great concern, and you should call your physician immediately.

Constipation   *Antidepressants, antihistamines, antiparkinsonian agents, antipsychotics,* especially *clozapine, buprenorphine,* and *methadone* (1) commonly cause or worsen constipation. They generally do this by absorbing water from the stool in the large intestine. It is generally uncomfortable and frustrating. It can also require intrusive medical intervention if it becomes severe, so it's important to address as soon as you notice it. Although you should avoid water restriction, drinking large amounts of water generally provides minimal improvement. The most effective remedy is to alter your diet. Minimize your intake of foods that are likely to worsen constipation, such as white rice, bananas, cheese, white bread, and peanut butter. Make sure that you include adequate fiber in your diet by eating fruits, vegetables, and whole-grain breads and muffins. A bowl of bran cereal every day can help, though you may want to spice up the taste with fruit or another cereal.

Try to avoid laxatives if you can, as your system will come to rely on them and you will need them indefinitely to induce a bowel movement. Docusate (Colace) and psyllium (Metamucil) are stool softeners that promote the retention of water in the stool. They provide significant aid without harming the bowel. Senna (Senakot) and casanthronol (sold in combination with docusate as Peri-Colace) are mild laxatives, which some people require on a daily basis. Stronger laxatives should be taken only in consultation with your physician.

Depression   *Amantadine, antipsychotics, benzodiazepines,* and *guanfacine* (1) can cause depression when taken for extended periods of time. The effect may be gradual, and there may be so many other things going on that depression goes unnoticed. Undiagnosed, it can substantially impair your ability to lead a satisfying and meaningful life. You should not settle for being depressed if you take any class of drug. Benzodiazepines can be gradually tapered and stopped, though it may take a great deal of effort. Your mood, and other aspects of your life, will likely improve once you get off them. Reducing the dose of your antipsychotic or switching to an atypical antipsychotic can both help. You might consider antidepressants if you remain depressed on antipsychotics. *Topiramate* (1) may cause depression. There has not been sufficient experience with it to know how severe this effect is, or the best way to manage depression if it occurs.

Diabetes Mellitus   *Atypical antipsychotics* (2) are associated with weight gain and the emergence of diabetes mellitus. Diabetes is an illness in which your body is no longer able to control levels of glucose, the body's main source of sugar and energy. High levels of glucose over some years, the main problem in diabetes, can damage your heart, kidneys, eyes, brain, and extremities. Abnormally high levels can cause coma and even death. It is not clear if atypical antipsychotics cause changes in metabolism directly or whether the changes result from the weight gain commonly seen with these drugs. In either case, the emergence of diabetes is a serious complication and requires ongoing treatment and monitoring by your primary care practitioner. If you develop diabetes, you may wish to consider changing to aripiprazole, ziprasidone, or one of the standard neuroleptics, as these drugs appear to be less likely to cause diabetes.

Diarrhea   *Lithium* (3,1) can cause diarrhea for two reasons. It can be a sign of lithium toxicity, meaning a level that is too high. Obtain a blood lithium level to ensure that your level and dose are not too high. Sometimes people experience diarrhea at therapeutic levels of lithium. This is most common with generic lithium and Lithonate. Consider switching to Lithobid, Eskalith CR, or liquid lithium citrate. *Donepezil, SSRIs, tacrine,* and *valproate* (1) can cause diarrhea as well. Dosage reduction is the only remedy. If the dose is too low to provide therapeutic benefit, consider switching to another medication.

Dizziness   *Carbamazepine, gabapentin, lamotrigine, topiramate,* and *valproate* (1) can cause dizziness when they are first begun. This generally passes without difficulty once the dose is stabilized. Dizziness can also occur if levels are too high. If you notice the onset of dizziness while on a mood stabilizer, consult your physician and consider obtaining a blood level. A rise in blood level can sometimes accompany a cold or viral illness in which there is some dehydration. *Antidepressants, antiparkinsonian agents, antipsychotics, beta-blockers,* and *guanfacine* (1) can cause **low blood pressure,** of which dizziness is one of the manifestations. The elderly are especially sensitive to changes in blood pressure. The dizziness may be annoying but is rarely dangerous. Measuring your blood pressure is useful if you are troubled by the symptoms. Ensure adequate fluid intake and eliminate caffeine, which acts as a diuretic and causes you to excrete water excessively. Dosage reduction is another remedy but is rarely needed. *Buprenorphine, buspirone, donepezil, naltrexone, sildenafil,* and *tacrine* (1) can cause mild dizziness that is not dangerous, though it may be unpleasant. Dosage reduction is the only remedy.

Drooling   *Antispychotic drugs* (1) can cause decreased muscle movements of the face (part of the syndrome of **pseudoparkinsonism**). This can cause your mouth to remain open and saliva to leak out. Antiparkinsonian agents generally solve this problem. *Clozapine* (1) causes drooling during sleep and a wet pillow because people don't swallow their saliva. Although antiparkinsonian agents can sometimes improve this, most people find the problem remains. There is no good solution for this. Using a vinyl-covered pillow and changing your pillow case every day may make the problem less unpleasant.

Dry Mouth *Antidepressants, antihistamines, antipsychotics, antiparkinsonian agents,* and *stimulants* (1) all cause dry mouth. Some people get dry mouth from other medications as well. Your mouth is dry because the medication decreases the production of saliva, not because you are dehydrated or thirsty. The lack of saliva can lead to dental caries (cavities), so it is important to maintain good dental hygiene with regular brushing and flossing after each meal. Drinking water frequently is generally ineffective because the problem is not due to dehydration. Sugarless gum and hard, nonsugar lozenges can minimize the discomfort of a dry mouth, although they will not prevent tooth decay. Preparations of artificial saliva that do not require a prescription are available in drugstores. Unfortunately, the effect lasts only a few minutes and is generally not worth the inconvenience. Gel-like mouth moisteners last longer and may be useful at night, but many people find them unpleasant.

Dystonia *Amoxapine* and *antipsychotics* (3) cause dystonia, which is a muscle spasm, often of the neck, jaw, mouth, and eyes. Sometimes dystonia occurs in the limbs instead. Standard antipsychotics are much more likely to cause this than the atypical antipsychotics recently marketed. Dystonia is intensely uncomfortable. Rarely, it affects the airway in the throat, in which case it can be dangerous. It is best to get treatment immediately both for your safety and because it will not subside spontaneously. An intramuscular injection of diphenhydramine (Benadryl) or benztropine (Cogentin) usually corrects the problem within an hour. You don't need to stop the antipsychotic if you have a dystonia. Regular doses of benztropine or other antiparkinsonian agents prevent it from occurring again.

Ear Ringing *Any drug* (1) can cause ear ringing, or tinnitus. Though it is unpleasant, it is rarely serious. There is no specific treatment for tinnitus except dosage reduction or changing medications.

Euphoria *Antidepressants* (3) can cause euphoria as part of a manic episode. This is a serious reaction as it may progress to psychotic thinking and poor judgment. Contact your physician immediately. *Buprenorphine* and *methadone* (1) cause euphoria as part of their routine effect. It is generally milder than heroin or other narcotics and tends to decrease in intensity with steady use.

Emotional Blunting *Antipsychotics* and *benzodiazepines* (1) blunt emotions. Although this can usefully decrease the intensity of feelings that are more intense than warranted, the effect can be so pronounced that normal emotions are decreased as well. Antipsychotics are more noticeable in this regard, and many people who take them are distressed by this problem. Atypical antipsychotics are less likely to cause blunting than standard antipsychotics. Dosage reduction is the only remedy, but even subtherapeutic doses can still be troublesome.

You may be unaware of this problem if you take benzodiazepines, or even grateful for the relief from the waxing and waning of anxiety. You may be surprised, if you begin to taper the benzodiazepine, how much of your emotional life you are missing. This may be uncomfortable at first, but you will recapture an important part of your life once you get off the benzodiazepines.

Fainting   *Buprenorphine* and *methadone* (3) can cause fainting. This can be due to low blood pressure or an overdose. In either case you should contact your physician immediately.

Falls   The elderly are especially sensitive to the effects of *antidepressants, antipsychotics, benzodiazepines,* and *mood stabilizers* (2) on their balance and blood pressure. They are likely to experience unsteadiness on their feet and light-headedness. As a result, they have a much higher rate of falls if they take any of these medications. If the symptoms do not gradually improve once the dose is stabilized, the only remedies are dosage reduction or a change in medication.

Fatigue   *Antidepressants, antihistamines, antipsychotics, benzodiazepines, naltrexone, zaleplon,* and *zolpidem* (1) can all cause fatigue. Most people find the fatigue from benzodiazepines eases up after the first week or two. Dosage reduction is the only remedy.

Fever   Fever is generally a sign of infection. It can also be the first sign that the medication you are taking is causing a serious blood problem that makes it hard for your body to fight infection. *Carbamazepine* (3) can cause **aplastic anemia,** *clozapine* and *mirtazapine* (3) can cause **agranulocytosis,** and *amoxapine* and *antipsychotics* (3) can cause **neuroleptic malignant syndrome,** disorders for which immediate medical attention is necessary. If you develop a fever on any of these drugs, consult your physician immediately to consider stopping the medication and the necessity of a physical examination and blood tests.

Flushing   *MAOIs* (3) can cause flushing, a sudden redness of your face, if you are having a hypertensive reaction in which your blood pressure suddenly increases. This is a medical emergency, as elevated blood pressure can cause you to have a stroke, and you should contact your physician immediately to consider the need for immediate treatment to lower your blood pressure. *Clomipramine, sildenafil,* and *SSRIs* (1) can cause flushing as an annoying, but not a serious, reaction.

Gait Unsteadiness   *Lithium* (3) can cause an unsteady gait when the level is too high. Obtain a lithium level immediately if you notice any impairment of your gait or coordination. *Other mood stabilizers* (1) commonly cause an unsteady gait when you first start them or the dose is raised. It generally lasts only a few days, but you shouldn't drive a car or operate heavy machinery until you know that your coordination and gait have returned to normal.

Galactorrhea   *Amoxapine* and *antipsychotics* (1) often cause milk leakage from the breasts in women. It is not dangerous but can be unpleasant. You can use a pad in your bra if it's noticeable. Dosage reduction can improve it as well.

Hair Loss   *Valproate* (1) can cause your hair to fall out at a more rapid rate than usual. Initially, you will notice only that your hair seems to be falling out. This may seem alarming, but the hair is growing back in as fast as it's falling out. Many people notice that their hair is thinner while they remain on valproate. Your hair will resume its normal growth pattern if you stop valproate.

Hallucinations   The excessive combination of medications that block the neurotransmitter acetylcholine can sometimes cause visual hallucinations. These include *tricyclic antidepressants, antihistamines, antiparkinsonian agents,* and *antipsychotics* (3). Hallucinations can occur if you stop *benzodiazepines* (3) abruptly.

Headaches   *MAOIs* (3) can cause headaches if you are having a hypertensive crisis in which your blood pressure suddenly increases. This is a medical emergency, as elevated blood pressure can cause you to have a stroke, and you should contact your physician immediately. *Stimulants* (1) often cause headaches. A mild pain reliever such as acetaminophen can be sufficient. Other remedies involve a dosage reduction or a change in medication. *Antidepressants, antihistamines, amantadine, buprenorphine, guanfacine, clozapine, disulfiram, donepezil, methadone, naltrexone, sildenafil, tacrine, zaleplon,* and *zolpidem* (1) can cause headaches. These are generally mild and not medically dangerous. A mild pain reliever such as acetaminophen, aspirin, or ibuprofen is usually sufficient. Dosage reduction or a change in medication are rarely necessary.

Heart Rate—High   *Tricyclic antidepressants, phenothiazines,* and *clozapine* (1) can cause an elevated heart rate. This is generally not medically significant unless you are elderly or have high blood pressure or heart problems.

Heart Rate—Low   *Buprenorphine, beta-blockers, guanfacine,* and *methadone* (2) lower your heart rate. This is usually not medically significant, although you should contact your physician if it goes below 60 beats per minute. Your pulse should be monitored when you first start until the dose is stabilized. If you notice that you are easily fatigued, your pulse may be too low, and you may need a dosage adjustment.

Hives   Hives from *any drug* (3) are raised red patches of skin that occur rather suddenly. They may be a sign that you are allergic to a medication. If you notice them, you should consult your physician to consider stopping the medication and emergency medical treatment to prevent a more severe reaction.

Hyperactivity   *SSRIs* (3), can cause hyperactivity as a sign of the serotonin syndrome (see below), a serious reaction requiring emergency medical care to stabilize your pulse and blood pressure. Rarely, *antihistamines* and *stimulants* (2) can cause hyperactivity. Though not medically dangerous, hyperactivity as a result of stimulants is a sign of ineffectiveness, and they should generally be stopped. *Bupropion* and *yohimbine* (2) can cause hyperactivity. Depending on how effective the medicine is, you may want to stay on it. Dosage reduction may be somewhat helpful.

Hypertensive Crisis   *MAOIs* (3) slow the breakdown of epinephrine and other chemicals that affect blood pressure. If you ingest any food or medicine that has a substance similar to epinephrine, such as tyramine while you are on an MAOI, your blood pressure can rise dramatically and dangerously. Symptoms of a hypertensive crisis include a headache, neck stiffness, palpitations, nausea, vomiting, sweating, and dilated pupils. A fever may or may not be present. Heart rate may be high or low. High blood pressure can lead to a stroke, in which a blood vessel in your brain bursts, leading to brain damage. It is essential that you follow the diet and avoid the medications outlined in the previous chapter. If you experience symptoms that suggest that you are having a hypertensive crisis, contact your physician immediately, or go to an emergency room for immediate treatment.

Hyponatremia   *Oxcarbazepine, SSRIs* (3) can cause hyponatremia, or low sodium in the blood. You may have no symptoms if you have hyponatremia, but people sometimes experience nausea, headaches, fatigue, mental confusion, or if severe, seizures and even a coma. If you develop hyponatremia, it is generally necessary to stop the medication.

Indigestion   *Antipsychotics, donepezil, naltrexone, quetiapine, sildenafil,* and *tacrine* (1) can cause mild indigestion. It is not medically dangerous. It can be minimized by taking the dose with food or dosage reduction.

Insomnia   *Stimulants* (2) can cause insomnia when taken close to bedtime. All that is usually needed is to take the dose a little bit earlier in the day. *Clomipramine* and *SSRIs* (1) can cause insomnia. Sometimes this occurs only when the medication is first begun. If insomnia persists, there are three options. Dosage reduction can be tried but is rarely effective. Use of a sleeping aid can be helpful. Trazodone is commonly used to aid SSRI-induced insomnia. Zolpidem is another possibility. Benzodiazepines are often helpful at first but are habit-forming and generally lose their effectiveness over some weeks. The last option is to switch medications. Many people who experience insomnia on one SSRI do not experience it on another, so it can be reasonable to try a different one. Tricyclics, especially nortriptyline and amitriptyline, are antidepressants that often improve sleep. Rarely, *benzodiazepines* (2) can cause insomnia. It is unpleasant, though not dangerous. Stopping the benzodiazepine is the only remedy. Discontinuing benzodiazepines can lead to insomnia as part of a withdrawal syndrome. *Buprenorphine, donepezil, methadone,* and *naltrexone* (1) can cause insomnia. This may persist. Dosage reduction is the only remedy.

Jaundice Liver damage caused by *disulfiram, lamotrigine, phenothiazines, tacrine,* or *valproate* (3) can manifest itself by yellow eyes and skin, a condition called jaundice. This is a serious reaction. You should consult your physician immediately about stopping your medication.

Kidney Dysfunction *Lithium* can cause kidney impairment when used on an extended basis. In the vast majority of cases, the impairment is mild and lithium can be continued. Kidney damage is possible but extremely rare. You won't notice any signs of the mild kidney impairment caused by lithium. It is diagnosed by a blood test for creatinine. A creatinine test should be performed every 6–12 months, and more frequently if any impairment is noted.

Light-Headedness *Antidepressants, antipsychotics,* and *beta-blockers* (2) can cause low blood pressure, of which light-headedness is one of the manifestations. The elderly are especially sensitive to changes in blood pressure. The dizziness may be annoying but is rarely dangerous. Measuring your blood pressure is useful if you are troubled by the symptoms. Ensure adequate fluid intake and eliminate caffeine, which acts as a diuretic and causes you to excrete water excessively. Dosage reduction is the only remedy, but it is rarely needed.

Memory Impairment *Benzodiazepines* (1) impair memory for events after you take a dose. If you take them for many months, there may be a lot that is hard for you to remember. *Antiparkinsonian agents, antidepressants, antipsychotics, gabapentin, topiramate, zaleplon,* and *zolpidem* (1) may also impair memory. There is no remedy except changing medications. The impairment resolves after you stop the medication.

Menstrual Irregularities *Antipsychotics* (1) can cause irregular periods and lead some women to stop menstruating altogether. This may accelerate the process of osteoporosis, the decalcification or thinning of bones as you age, and increase the likelihood of bone fractures. If you miss more than an occasional period, obtain a consultation with a gynecologist and consider hormone treatments to induce periods and prevent the exacerbation of osteoporosis. *SSRIs* (1) can cause an occasional missed period, which is generally not significant.

Mental Status Changes *Amantadine, amoxapine,* and *antipsychotics* (3) can cause neuroleptic malignant syndrome (NMS—see below) a dangerous reaction that can cause you to be confused, delirious, and unresponsive. *SSRIs* (3) can cause the **serotonin syndrome,** another dangerous reaction that can also lead to confused and delirious thinking. You should consult your physician or go to an emergency room immediately if you suspect you have either syndrome to receive treatment to reverse the process and stabilize your pulse and blood pressure.

Milk Leakage   *Amoxapine* and *antipsychotics* (1) often cause milk leakage (**galactorrhea**) from the breasts in women. It is not dangerous but can be unpleasant. You can use a pad in your bra if it's noticeable. Dosage reduction can improve it as well.

Muscle Aches   *Clomipramine* can cause mild muscle aches. These are not dangerous but can be unpleasant. Either dosage reduction or a change in medication is the only remedy.

Muscle Coordination, Poor   *Benzodiazepines, mood stabilizers, zaleplon,* and *zolpidem* (1) can impair coordination, especially when first begun. There is a higher rate of car accidents and falls in people who take benzodiazepines. Make sure you know how you react to these medications before you drive a car or operate heavy machinery. Toxic levels of *lithium* (3) can cause an unstable gait and poor coordination. Obtain a blood level of lithium if you notice that your gait is unsteady or that you are poorly coordinated, in order to evaluate the usefulness of temporarily stopping your lithium (for a day or two) and restarting it at a lower dose.

Muscle Cramps   *Antipsychotics* (3) can cause an acute muscle cramp or spasm, called **dystonia.** *Donepezil* (1) can cause muscle cramps. These are uncomfortable, but not dangerous. Dosage reduction is the only remedy.

Muscle Rigidity   *Amantadine, amoxapine,* and *antipsychotics* (3) can cause neuroleptic malignant syndrome (NMS), a dangerous reaction that can cause you to be confused, delirious, and unresponsive. You should consult your physician or go to an emergency room immediately if you suspect NMS. *Antipsychotics* (2) can also cause **pseudoparkinsonism,** of which one of the symptoms is muscle rigidity.

Muscle Twitching   *Antidepressants* and *antipsychotics* (1) can cause muscle twitching. Though uncomfortable, it is not dangerous. Dosage reduction is the only remedy. See also **Dystonia.**

Myocarditis   *Clozapine* (3) can cause myocarditis, a serious and potentially fatal inflammation of the heart in less than 1 percent of people who take it. Symptoms of myocarditis include unexplained fatigue, difficulty breathing, fever, chest pain, and palpitations, any one of which should prompt immediate evaluation by your physician.

Nasal Congestion   *Lamotrigine* and *sildenafil* (1) can cause nasal congestion. Annoying but not dangerous, dosage reduction is the only remedy.

Nausea   *Lithium* (3,1) can cause nausea if the level gets too high. If you notice the onset of nausea after you've been on lithium for awhile, obtain a level to see if the level has risen too high, and whether you should temporarily stop the lithium until the level comes down (this usually takes a day or two). Sometimes people experience nausea at therapeutic levels. This is most common with generic lithium and Lithonate. Consider switching to Lithobid, Eskalith CR, or liquid lithium citrate. *SSRIs* (1) commonly cause nausea when first begun or when the dose is raised. It generally passes within three to fourteen days. *Amantadine, antihistamines, antiparkinsonian agents, antipsychotics, guanfacine, mood stabilizers, naltrexone, tacrine, yohimbine, zaleplon,* and *zolpidem* (1) can also cause nausea. Either dosage reduction or a change to other medications in the same class is an option if nausea significantly troubles you.

Neck Stiffness   *MAOIs* (3) can cause a stiff neck as a symptom of a **hypertensive crisis.**

Neuroleptic Malignant Syndrome   *Amantadine, amoxapine,* and *antipsychotics* (3) can cause neuroleptic malignant syndrome (NMS), a toxic reaction that is potentially fatal. Symptoms of NMS include a high fever, muscle rigidity, mental status changes, irregular pulse, and blood pressure and sweating. Muscle damage and renal failure can occur and lead to death. NMS is a life-threatening emergency that requires immediate medical attention to reverse the process with medication and stabilize your pulse and blood pressure.

Nonarteritic Anterior Ischemic Optic Neuropathy (NAION)   *Phosphodiesterase inhibitors* (3) NAION is a sudden partial or full loss of vision. It occurs in 2.5–10/100,000 people who take this class of medicine for impotence. If you notice any visual changes, contact your physician immediately.

Palpitations   *Stimulants* and *antidepressants* (2) can cause palpitations, or rapid heart beats. It often resolves once your dose stabilizes and your body adjusts to the drug. It is generally not dangerous, but it can be uncomfortable. Either dosage reduction or a change in medication is the only remedy.

Pancreatitis   *Valproate* (3) can cause a potentially life-threatening inflammation of the pancreas in about 0.1 percent (1/1000) of people who take it. Symptoms of abdominal pain, nausea, or vomiting generally occur. Contact your physician immediately if you experience any of these symptoms so blood tests can be ordered that will determine if you have pancreatitis and if you need treatment.

Priapism   *Trazodone* (3) can cause priapism, which is a sustained erection of the penis not due to sexual arousal. Priapism can damage the penis and calls for immediate intervention. Treatment generally consists of an injection into the penis. Though uncomfortable, there are no long-lasting effects. Rarely, surgical intervention has been required, with resultant impotence.

Pseudoparkinsonism   *Amoxapine* and *antipsychotics* (2) can cause pseudo-parkinsonism, a constellation of several symptoms that mimic Parkinson's disease: **akinesia,** a lack of muscle movements, **muscle rigidity,** and **tremor.** Standard antipsychotics are more likely to cause this than atypical antipsychotics. Dosage reduction and the use of antiparkinsonian agents generally provide sufficient relief so that only minimal symptoms remain.

Psychosis   *Amantadine, antidepressants, antiparkinsonian agents,* and *stimulants* (3) can cause psychotic thinking, such as visual or auditory hallucinations (seeing or hearing things that aren't there). Consult your physician immediately about stopping your medication and getting any needed treatment.

Pulmonary Embolism   Rarely, *clozapine* (3) can cause pulmonary embolism, which occurs when a blood clot forms in the leg, breaks off, and travels to the lung. This can be dangerous as it can lower the amount of oxygen in your blood to insufficient levels. If you suddenly become short of breath, the primary symptom of pulmonary embolism, you should consult your physician or go to an emergency room immediately for evaluation and treatment.

QTc Prolongation on EKG   *Tricyclic antidepressants* and *antipsychotics,* especially *mesoridazine, thioridazine,* and *ziprasidone* (3), can cause abnormalities in heart function that can be measured on an electrocardiogram (EKG.) The QTc refers to the period that the heart is recovering from the last beat and preparing for the next one. If this period takes too long, the heart can start beating again before the period of recovery is complete. This can lead to an inability of the heart to beat effectively, fainting, and even cardiac death. Seek immediate evaluation by your primary care practitioner or at an emergency room if you experience irregular heartbeats, periods of fainting, or unexplained dizziness.

Rash   *Lamotrigine* and *oxcarbazepine* (3) can cause a severe rash that is potentially life-threatening. You should contact your physician immediately if you notice a rash while on either drug. *Any other medication* can also cause a rash. This is often a sign of an allergic reaction. You should consult your physician about whether it is safe to stay on the drug.

Respiratory Infections   *Topiramate* (1) can cause respiratory infections (colds) that are not generally serious, though they may be annoying.

Sedation   Some *antidepressants, antihistamines,* and *antipsychotics,* as well as *amantadine* and *disulfiram* (1), cause sedation. By and large, this effect does not go away. Dosage reduction or a change to another drug in the same class are the only remedies. Some *benzodiazepines* (1) cause sedation, which can be useful when they are used to induce sleep but can be problematic during daytime use. *Mood stabilizers* (1) often cause sedation initially. The sedation may persist with gabapentin and topiramate. If it does persist, dosage reduction is the only remedy.

Seizures   A seizure is an epileptic convulsion in which your brain cells all fire at once, causing you to lose consciousness and all your muscles to clench at the same time. Sometimes there is no muscle clenching, and the sole effect is that you lose consciousness. A seizure generally lasts for less than a minute. Abrupt withdrawal of *benzodiazepines, carbamazepine, gabapentin, lamotrigine, topiramate,* and *valproate* (3) can cause a seizure. These drugs should be tapered slowly if you decide to go off them. Rarely, *antidepressants, antipsychotics,* and *stimulants* (3) can cause seizures. If you have a seizure, you should contact your physician to discuss whether you should stop the drug and whether you need any further treatment.

Serotonin Syndrome   *SSRIs* (3) can cause the serotonin syndrome when used together or in combination with other drugs that can increase serotonin, including tryptophan and St. John's wort. Symptoms include fever, hyperactivity, mental status changes, and potentially dangerous alterations in pulse and blood pressure. The serotonin syndrome is a medical emergency for which you need immediate medical attention to ensure stabilization of your pulse and blood pressure.

Sexual Dysfunction   *Antidepressants, antipsychotics, buprenorphine,* and *methadone* (1) can impair sexual function by decreasing your sexual drive and your ability to become aroused and achieve orgasm. *SSRIs* (1) in particular cause these problems, while *tricyclic antidepressants* and *bupropion* (1) are less likely to be troublesome. Some antipsychotics, notably *risperidone* and *thioridazine* (1), can cause retrograde ejaculation in men, which is when the semen is expelled into the bladder during orgasm. Sexual dysfunction may ease up on its own, though this does not usually occur. Dosage reduction can sometimes improve any of these problems. Unfortunately, you may experience a return of your psychiatric symptoms if your dosage is lowered. There are three medications that may help. Yohimbine can sometimes increase sexual drive and desire when taken on a daily basis. When taken prior to sexual activity, it can enhance arousal. Cyproheptadine (Periactin) doesn't enhance desire but may increase arousal and restore the ability to achieve orgasm. Sildenafil restores potency in men. It was initially tested only on men but has restored the capacity for arousal and orgasm in some women as well.

Stuttering   *Olanzapine* (1) can sometimes cause stuttering. Rarely, other *antidepressants, antipsychotics, gabapentin,* and *topiramate* (1) can, too. It is not dangerous, though, it may be frustrating or embarrassing. Dosage reduction is the only remedy.

Suicidal Thoughts or Behavior   *Antidepressants* and *atomoxetine* (3) are associated with the emergence of suicidal thoughts or behavior in some adults and teenagers (less than 1%). This is a complex issue, as suicidal thoughts often occur in depression. It's possible that these thoughts emerge as a direct result of the drugs. It's also possible that the drugs make people more agitated and anxious, giving them more energy and inclination to act on thoughts that were already present as part of the syndrome of depression. No matter what the cause, an emergency evaluation by your physician is necessary if you begin to experience suicidal thoughts or behavior to ensure your safety and make any medication adjustments to help you feel better.

Sunburn   *Phenothiazine antipsychotics* (1), as well as other antipsychotics and antidepressants can cause severe sunburns. It is essential to use suntan lotion with a sun protection factor of 15 or more when you are out in the sun.

Sweating   *Antidepressants* and *yohimbine* (1) can cause sweating as a side effect. Though unpleasant, it is not medically dangerous. *Benzodiazepines* (3) can cause sweating if you are going through withdrawal. *Disulfiram* (3) can cause sweating if you drink alcohol as part of the toxic alcohol-disulfiram reaction. *Antipsychotics* (3) can cause sweating as part of the **neuroleptic malignant syndrome,** and *SSRIs* (3) can cause sweating as part of the **serotonin syndrome,** two serious medical disorders that require immediate medical attention.

Tardive Dyskinesia   *Antipsychotics* and *amoxapine* (1) cause tardive dyskinesia (TD), a disorder that consists of involuntary, rhythmical, nonpainful movements. It most commonly affects the tongue and muscles in the mouth, where it can look like you are chewing gum. It can also affect the trunk, hands, and feet. It can be unsightly, but most people don't find it uncomfortable unless their mouth becomes sore. The movements can be quite pronounced, though they are usually mild. The movements generally occur only after at least one year of use. Women, the elderly, and people with brain damage are more likely to get TD. People who take standard antipsychotics develop TD at the rate of 10 to 20 percent a year. Atypical antipsychotics appear to cause it at a much lower rate: 1 to 5 percent. Once symptoms develop, they usually stay about the same level of severity, although other areas of the body may gradually be affected. Some people find that the symptoms gradually improve after a few years, but some people find that they worsen. Antihistamines, antiparkinsonian agents, and tricyclic antidepressants can make the symptoms worse. There is no cure for TD, although buspirone and vitamin E can sometimes improve the symptoms.

Thirst—Increased   *Lithium* (3, 1) can cause increased thirst. Generally this is not significant but can be a sign of a toxic lithium level. If you have other symptoms of lithium toxicity (pronounced tremor, nausea, diarrhea, an unsteady gait, or confusion), consult your physician and consider obtaining a lithium level. *Antidepressants, antihistamines, antipsychotics,* and *antiparkinsonian agents* (1) all cause dry mouth. Some people get dry mouth from other medications as well. Your mouth is dry because the medication decreases the production of saliva, not because you are dehydrated or thirsty. The lack of saliva can lead to dental caries (cavities), so it is important to maintain good dental hygiene with regular brushing and flossing after each meal. Drinking water frequently is generally ineffective because the problem is not due to dehydration. Sugarless gum and hard, nonsugar lozenges can minimize the discomfort of a dry mouth, although they will not prevent tooth decay. Preparations of artificial saliva that do not require a prescription are available in drugstores. Unfortunately, the effect lasts only a few minutes and is generally not worth the inconvenience. Gel-like mouth moisteners last longer and may be useful at night, but many people find them unpleasant.

Throat Constriction   *MAOIs* (3) can cause throat constriction as part of a **hypertensive crisis,** a reaction that requires immediate medical attention (see above). *Amoxapine* and *antipsychotics* (3) cause **dystonia,** which is a muscle spasm, often of the neck, jaw, mouth, and eyes. Standard antipsychotics are much more likely to cause this than the atypical antipsychotics recently marketed. Dystonia is intensely uncomfortable. Rarely, it affects the airway in the throat, in which case it can be dangerous. It is best to get treatment immediately for safety and because it will not subside spontaneously. An intramuscular injection of diphenhydramine (Benadryl) or benztropine (Cogentin) usually corrects the problem within an hour. You don't need to stop the antipsychotic if you have a dystonia. Regular doses of benztropine or other antiparkinsonian agents prevent it from occurring again.

Thrombocytopenia   *Valproate* (3) can cause thrombocytopenia, which is a medical condition in which you do not make platelets, the blood cells necessary for clotting. Without platelets, any internal or external bleeding will be prolonged and put you at risk for excessive blood loss, low blood pressure, cardiovascular shock, and even death. The symptoms are easy bruisability or prolonged bleeding. Consult your physician immediately should you notice either symptom to consider stopping the medication and the need for medical treatment to restore the platelets.

Thyroid Dysfunction   *Lithium* (1) can cause hypothyroidism, or impaired thyroid function, which can cause lethargy, fatigue, depression, decreased appetite but weight gain, sensitivity to cold, decreased mental and physical activity, and dry hair and skin. *Quetiapine* (1) can impair thyroid function in people with hypothyroidism. In both cases, thyroid function is easily measured by a blood test and easily treated with synthetic thyroid hormone, which has no side effects, since it is identical to the hormone produced by your body.

Tics   *Stimulants* (2) can cause motor or vocal tics, which are more or less involuntary muscle contractions. There can be snorting, sniffing, grunting, barking, or involuntary word vocalizations. As the tics can be permanent, most psychiatrists recommend that the stimulant be stopped at the first sign of tics.

Tingling   *Topiramate* (1) can sometimes cause tingling in the extremities. Vitamin B$_6$ and dosage reduction are possible remedies.

Tinnitus   *Any drug* (1) can cause tinnitus. Though it is unpleasant, it is rarely serious. There is no specific treatment for tinnitus except dosage reduction or changing medications.

Tremor   *Bupropion, gabapentin, lithium,* and *stimulants* (1) can cause an intention tremor, which occurs when your hands are active, such as using a spoon. It is not medically dangerous, but it can be annoying. The beta-blockers propranolol or nadolol can be useful in minimizing it. *Amoxapine* and *antipsychotics* (2) can cause a tremor that occurs when your hand is at rest. This is usually part of the syndrome of **pseudoparkinsonism.** Antiparkinsonian agents generally provide substantial relief. It can also be a symptom of **tardive dyskinesia.**

Urinary—Difficulty   *Tricyclic antidepressants, antihistamines, antiparkinsonian agents, antipsychotics, buprenorphine, maprotiline, methadone, nefazodone,* and *trazodone* (2) can impair urination by preventing the bladder from fully emptying. This can lead you to urinate small amounts frequently and predispose you to infections. It is unpleasant and can be uncomfortable. Either dosage reduction or a change in medications is a remedy.

Urinary—Increased Frequency   *Lithium* (3, 1) can cause increased urination. It may be a sign that your level is too high if this occurs rather quickly with other signs of toxicity, such as nausea, diarrhea, an unsteady gait, slurred speech, and confusion. If this is the case, obtain a blood level of lithium immediately to consider the usefulness of stopping your lithium temporarily (a day or two is generally enough). Sometimes people experience frequent urination on therapeutic levels. If this is the case, ensure adequate fluid intake. Dosage reduction will help some, but this may cause your level to be too low.

Urinary Incontinence   *Tricyclic antidepressants, nefazodone, trazodone, antihistamines, antipsychotics,* and *antiparkinsonian agents* (2) can impair urination by preventing the bladder from fully emptying. This can lead you to urinate small amounts frequently, even when you don't mean to. It may help some to restrict your fluids and eliminate caffeine, which increases urination. Consider dosage reduction or a change in medications. Consider consultation with a urologist, who may recommend administration of oxybutinin (Ditropam) tablets or desmopressin spray (DDAVP), drugs that treat urinary incontinence.

Urinary Retention   *Tricyclic antidepressants, antihistamines, antiparkinsonian agents, antipsychotics, buprenorphine, maprotiline, methadone, nefazodone,* and *trazodone* (3) can impair urination by preventing the bladder from fully emptying. When pronounced, this can prevent urination almost entirely. Men with enlarged prostates are more vulnerable to developing retention. Besides being extremely uncomfortable, this can cause kidney damage. You should consult your physician immediately or go to a hospital emergency room for evaluation and probable catheterization. Consider a dosage reduction or changing medications.

Vision Changes   *Tricyclic antidepressants, nefazodone, trazodone, antihistamines, antipsychotics,* and *antiparkinsonian agents* (1) often cause blurry vision. It is not medically dangerous, and generally improves once the dosage stabilizes. *Sildenafil* (1) can cause color-tinged vision, which is not dangerous. *Topiramate* (1) may cause double vision and other visual abnormalities. Such changes can be annoying but are not dangerous. Dosage reduction is the only option if the effects persist. (See also **Blurry Vision, Cataracts.**)

Weight Gain   *Antidepressants, antipsychotics, lithium, topiramate,* and *valproate* (1) can increase your appetite. This can lead to a gradual but substantial weight gain over a period of time. Obesity can contribute to a high risk of diabetes, high blood pressure, heart disease, and heart attacks. These complications can lead to significant illness, impairment of functioning, and increased mortality. It is important, therefore to maintain your weight as close to your ideal weight as possible. You should weigh yourself a couple of times a month when you are on the medication. If you notice any weight gain, discuss this with your physician. Dosage reduction is generally ineffective. Changing antidepressants to bupropion or an SSRI may be helpful, although these drugs have side effects of their own. Developing and maintaining a strict diet can be a good option, although some people find it hard to stay on a restricted diet.

Weight Loss   *Stimulants* (1) can cause weight loss by decreasing appetite. Children on stimulants need to be closely monitored to ensure adequate weight gain. Drug holidays, periods of time off the medication, are the only remedy. Adults generally don't lose significant amounts of weight unless they take excessive amounts. *Bupropion, SSRIs, topiramate, venlafaxine,* and *other antidepressants* (1) can sometimes decrease appetite and lead to mild weight loss.

Yellow Skin or Eyes   Liver damage caused by *disulfiram, lamotrigine, phenothiazines, tacrine,* or *valproate* (3) can manifest itself by yellow eyes and skin, a condition called **jaundice.** This is a serious reaction. You should consult your physician immediately about stopping your medication.

The Biology of the Brain and How Medications Work

Knowledge of the biology and chemistry of the brain isn't essential to your use of medication, in the same way that knowledge of the inner workings of an engine isn't necessary in order to drive a car. It may be of interest, however, and provide you a more complete understanding of how medications may help you.

The biology of our thoughts, feelings, and behavior is complex. It is directed by the brain, whose anatomy, chemistry, and physiology enable it to perform myriad functions at lightning speeds.

The Brain

The brain is one part of the central nervous system (CNS), the other being the spinal cord. The CNS is composed of billions of individual cells, called *neurons.* *Sensory* neurons take in information from the outside world through the five senses and communicate it to the brain. *Motor* neurons direct the body to respond by making the muscles move. All other neurons communicate only with each other, inside the brain. For example, if you hear an alarm clock in the morning, sensory neurons transmit this information from your ears to your brain. The neurons in the brain access your memory and tell you that it's time to get your body up. Motor neurons direct your arm and hand muscles to turn off the alarm, your body to get out of bed, and your mouth muscles to complain.

Neurons   The main part of each neuron is the *cell body* (see figure 1), which is where the machinery of the cell is located. One part of the wall of the cell body ends in *dendrites,* tiny treelike projections. The other part of the cell body tapers down into a long *axon,* or tail. The tail ends in a number of *terminal buttons.* The terminal buttons of a neuron lie on the dendrites of another neuron, so that each neuron is like a link in a chain. The space between them is called the *synapse.* Each neuron connects with many different other neurons: terminal buttons from many other neurons end on its dendrites, and its terminal buttons end on the dendrites of

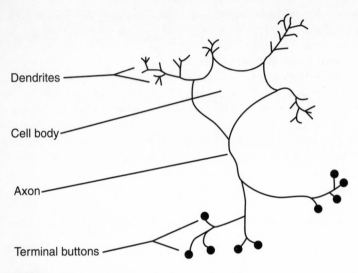

FIGURE 1   The neuron

many different neurons. The entire brain is a series of interconnected groups of cells that affect one another—there is no master cell. Usually a neuron is "at rest," which means it is inactive and is not communicating with other neurons.

Communication between Neurons   It is the communication between neurons that most concerns us, because this is where the generation of emotions, thoughts, and memory occurs. Communication occurs when a neuron "fires." When a neuron fires, it releases chemicals called *neurotransmitters* out of the terminal buttons. Neurotransmitters are small chemical compounds made in the cell body of the neuron. Examples of neurotransmitters include serotonin, dopamine, norepinephrine, acetylcholine, and gamma-amino-butyric acid (GABA). The neurotransmitter crosses the synapse and lands on the dendrites of the postsynaptic neuron. The neurotransmitter is a chemical "messenger" that influences the behavior of the next neuron by interacting with a *receptor* on the postsynaptic neuron. Receptors are proteins made by the cell that sit in the middle of the cell membrane, the cover around the cell, and protrude on both the outside and the inside.

How a Neuron Fires   The excitable nature of a neuron, the ability to be "at rest" and then suddenly "fire," is the product of different concentrations of sodium and potassium inside and outside the cell. At rest, there is a greater concentration of sodium outside the cell compared to the inside, and a lesser concentration of potassium outside the cell compared to the inside. When a neuron is at rest, there is a small electrical charge across the membrane, called the membrane potential, because of the different proportion of ions present. If the total sum of all the neurotransmitters released by other neurons is sufficient to change the membrane potential, there is a sudden inflow of sodium and outflow of potassium. This sudden inflow and outflow travels down the neuron from the cell body to the end of the axon in an *action potential,* or firing. The action potential causes the release of the neurotransmitter from the axon at the end of the neuron.

The release of a single molecule of a neurotransmitter is not enough to determine whether the postsynaptic neuron will fire or not. There must be enough molecules of neurotransmitters present to change the membrane potential. In essence, the postsynaptic neuron adds all the "messages" of neurotransmitters released from all the axons that are resting on its dendrites. If enough excitatory messages are received from presynaptic neurons, the postsynaptic neuron undergoes an action potential and releases its neurotransmitters onto the next neuron and the process starts all over.

Inside a Neuron   The intracellular events that shift the membrane potential and lead to the action potential are due to the change in the physical structure of the receptor caused by the binding of the neurotransmitter. This change has two possible consequences. First, the new shape may open a channel in the receptor through which potassium and sodium can pass. When these ions pass through, an action potential starts, leading to the release of the neurotransmitter.

Besides this fast ion channel, receptors also exert their changes through interaction with G-proteins. G-proteins are located inside the neuron. They do not directly cause the flow of ions through the channel of the receptor in the cell membrane, but they have other effects within cells. First, they alter the behavior of ion channels, thereby affecting the intrinsic excitability of neurons. Also, they regulate enzymes that produce *second messengers.* Neurotransmitters are first messengers, carrying information between neurons. Second messengers are small water-soluble molecules that diffuse throughout the interior of the cell to activate their targets. Second messengers include things such as cyclic adenosine monophosphate (cAMP), inositol triphosphate, calcium, nitric oxide, and prostaglandins.

By and large, second messengers affect enzymes called protein kinases and protein phosphatases. Protein kinases act by transferring a phosphate group (a molecule composed of phosphorus and oxygen) onto a protein; a phosphatase takes it off. Since the function of a protein is highly dependent upon its three-dimensional configuration, the addition or subtraction of a phosphate group produces significant changes in how the protein works. For example, the proteins that produce neurotransmitters can have phosphates put on or taken off, thereby affecting the rate of synthesis of a neurotransmitter.

Besides the direct effect of the second messenger on activity within the cell, second messengers also affect the expression of the DNA genetic material. Regulating the expression of genetic material can also affect the potential excitability of the neuron. Changes in gene expression occur more slowly because of the complex series of events that must occur in the expression of genes, including the transcription of DNA to RNA, the transport of the RNA across the cell to the site of protein production, and the formation of proteins from RNA.

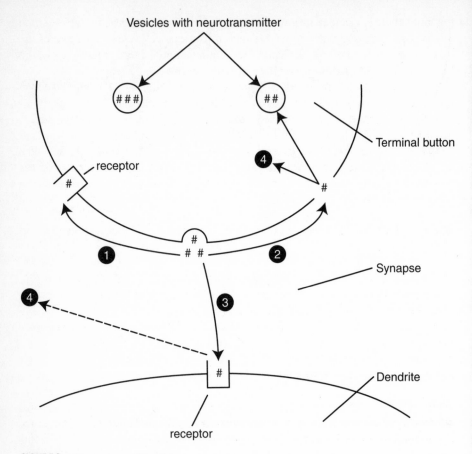

FIGURE 2   Neurotransmitter fate

The Fate of Neurotransmitters   Four things can happen to the neurotransmitter after release into the synapse (see figure 2). It can interact with a receptor on the outside membrane of the cell that it came from ❶. Such stimulation usually starts a negative feedback loop to reduce further synthesis of the neurotransmitter. Second, it can be brought back into the same cell from which it was released in a "reuptake" process ❷. Third, it interacts with a receptor on the postsynaptic neuron ❸. There are many different receptors for each neurotransmitter. For example, there are thirty different receptors for serotonin. Finally, it can be *metabolized,* or broken up into smaller parts to permit excretion. Some neurotransmitters are metabolized in the cell, while others are metabolized in the synapse ❹. In either case, the metabolized parts are eventually carried away in the blood and excreted in the urine.

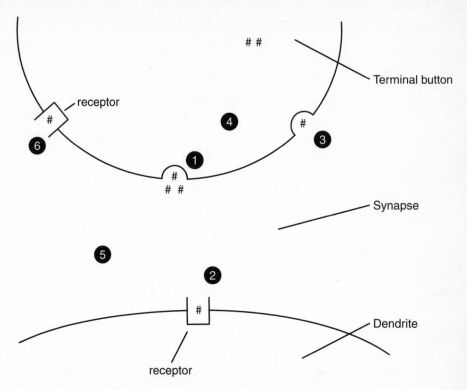

1 Amantadine, dextroamphetamine
2 Acamprosate, antihistamines, antiparkinsonian agents, antipsychotics, benzodiazepines, beta-blockers, buprenorphine, naltrexone
3 Atomoxetine, bupropion, duloxetine, methylphenidate, SSRIs, tricyclic antidepressants, venlafaxine
4 MAOIs
5 Donepezil, galantamine, rivastigmine, tacrine
6 Buspirone, mirtazepine

FIGURE 3   Neurotransmitter sites of action

How Medications Work

Almost all psychiatric medications exert their effects on neurotransmitters. Different ones influence the metabolic breakdown, the reuptake process, or the binding onto the receptor. Figure 3 shows the sites of action for many psychiatric drugs. Amantadine and dextroamphetamine ❶ enhance release of neurotransmitters into the synapse. Antihistamines, antipsychotics, beta-blockers, and antiparkinsonian agents ❷ block the effects of a neurotransmitter on the postsynaptic receptor. Acamprosate, benzodiazepines, and naltrexone ❷, on the other hand, act like a neurotransmitter and stimulate the postsynaptic receptor. Atomoxetine, bupropion, duloxetine, venlafaxine, methylphenidate, SSRIs such as fluoxetine, and tricyclic antidepressants such as imipramine ❸ block the reuptake of the neurotransmitter into the presynaptic neuron. MAOIs ❹ inhibit the breakdown of some neurotransmitters inside the presynaptic neuron. Donepezil, galantamine, and rivastigmine ❺ inhibit the breakdown of acetylcholine, a neurotransmitter, in the synapse. Buspirone and mirtazepine ❻ affect receptors on the presynaptic membrane.

Although the effects of neurotransmitters within the cell are complex, the main effect is to make the postsynaptic neuron either *more* or *less* likely to fire. Neurotransmitters are *excitatory* if they make the postsynaptic neuron more likely to fire and *inhibitory* if they make it less likely to fire.

The Brain as a Whole   Additional complexities in the biology of the brain derive from the presence of many different neurotransmitters in different areas of the brain, multiple receptors for each neurotransmitter, many different second messengers, many different genes that affect the production of the protein enzymes and receptors, and many forces that control the production of those genes. All play a role in whether or not a neuron will fire an action potential. Some of these complexities are beginning to be understood, but there are still areas where we are ignorant.

Brain architecture and functioning are shaped by experiences in life. The brain is not a static organ that is formed in the womb and remains unchanged for the rest of life. The brain continues to develop, grow, and make new connections well into the fourth decade.

Even apart from the incomplete understanding of the events that occur at a cellular level, however, is our almost total lack of understanding of how the brain as a whole is organized. Although we know some of the sites in the brain that are involved in the production of thoughts, feelings, emotions, and memories, we have no understanding at all of how neurons interact with each other to produce these things. Only further research will help us to tease apart the incredible complexity of the brain and its interactions with the outside world.

Sources of Information about Psychiatric Disorders and Treatments

This book has focused primarily on the use of medications in different psychiatric disorders. In order to help yourself the most, it can be useful to educate yourself about whatever disorder you experience. Talking with other people who have the same problem can be enormously helpful and reassuring. Discussion with your doctor can be helpful as well.

There is a wealth of information on the Internet, although the quality varies depending on who is providing it. The American Psychiatric Association has a Web site that you can use as a springboard to other Web sites and find information about all psychiatric disorders. The address is *www.psych.org*. Click first on "Resources for the General Public," then on "Other Mental Health Resources," then on "Internet Mental Health Resources," and then on whatever disorder or topic you are interested in. At *www.amazon.com* you will find many books for each disorder, listed and described. The National Alliance for the Mentally Ill, an organization formed to help people with psychiatric problems and their families cope successfully, can be called at 800-950-6264 or accessed on the Internet at *www.nami.org*.

What follows are the names, addresses, and phone numbers of different organizations that can provide information and support. Books that may be useful are also listed and briefly described.

Alzheimer's Disease and Dementia

Alzheimer's: A Complete Guide for Families and Loved Ones, by Howard Greutzner. This book aids caregivers in the management and understanding of Alzheimer's disease.

The Alzheimer's Sourcebook for Care Givers: A Practical Guide for Getting through the Day, by Frena Gray Davidson. A guide book for caregivers.

Anxiety

Coping with Panic, by George Clum, M.D. An excellent guide to help manage anxiety and panic without drugs by learning and practicing a variety of relaxation techniques and other commonsense ideas.

The Relaxation Response, by Herbert Benson, M.D. The landmark book describing the usefulness of relaxation techniques for anxiety.

Mastery of Your Anxiety and Panic, by David Barlow, M.D. This is a workbook that guides you through a step-by-step series of exercises designed to increase control over the symptoms of anxiety.

Attention Deficit/Hyperactivity Disorder

Books

Attention Deficit Disorder: A Different Perception, by Thomas Hartmann.

Driven to Distraction, by Edward Hallowell, M.D., and John Ratey, M.D. This excellent book describes the symptoms of ADHD and what you can do about them in a readable, intelligent, and fun way.

You Mean I'm not Lazy, Stupid, or Crazy?, by Kate Kelly and Peggy Ramundo. Written by people with ADD for adults, it offers practical advice on how to become more organized and effective.

Organizations

Attention Deficit Disorder Association
PO Box 972
Mentor, Ohio 44061
(800) 487-2282

Children and Adults with Attention Deficit Disorder (CHADD)
499 NW 70th Ave. Suite 308
Plantation, Florida 33317
(305) 587-3700

Bipolar Disorder

Bipolar Disorder: A Guide for Patients and Families, by Francis Mondimore. This is a useful book that describes the symptoms of the disorder, treatments, and how it affects those living with someone who has it. It offers detailed help for living with the disease.

Depression

The Depression Workbook, by Mary Ellen Copeland, M.S. A well-written
practical guide to help anyone with depression to develop skills, habits, and
a lifestyle to improve depression.

Developmental Disorders

Asperger's Syndrome, a Guide for Parents and Professionals, by Tony
Atwood. This guide describes the syndrome and practical approaches to
the day-to-day management in a straightforward easy-to-read style.

The Autism Treatment Guide, by Elizabeth Gerlach. A parent of a child with
autism, Ms. Gerlach has written a resource guide that outlines the basic
facts, research information, and effective treatment options.

Living with Autism, by Kathleen Dillon and Lahri Bond. This book presents the
experiences of six parents who are raising children with autism, and the
strategies they've adopted.

Drug Dependence

Adult Children of Alcoholics, by Janet Woititz, Ed.d. An excellent book
describing the problems you may have if your parents abused alcohol.

The Addiction Workbook, A Step-by-Step Guide to Quitting Alcohol and Drugs,
by Patrick Fanning and John O'Neil. This book helps readers learn about
themselves so that they are able to achieve sobriety.

Eating Disorders

Books

Anorexia Nervosa, A Guide to Recovery, by Lindsey Hall and Monika Ostroff.
A description of Ms. Ostroff's ten-year battle with anorexia, it also offers
factual information and practical advice for others.

Bulimia: A Guide for Families and Friends, by Roberta Sherman and Ron
Thompson. This book describes the symptoms and treatment for people
with bulimia.

Organizations

The National Association of Anorexia Nervosa and Associated Disorders
PO Box 7
Highland Park, Illinois 60035
1-847-831-3438

Psychosis

Surviving Schizophrenia, by E. Fuller Torrey, M.D. A guide for people with schizophrenia and their families, examining all aspects of the disease and treatment, by a pioneer in the field.

When Someone You Love Has a Mental Illness: A Handbook for Families, Friends, and Caregivers, by Rebecca Woolis and Agnes Hatfied. A practical guide about how to interact with a person who is suffering from schizophrenia or bipolar disorder.

NOTES

CHAPTER 1: PSYCHIATRIC DRUGS—POISON OR PANACEA?

1. R. Kessler, K. McGonagle, et al., "Lifetime and 12-Month Prevalence of DSM-III-R Psychiatric Disorders in the United States," *Archives of General Psychiatry 51* (1994): 8–19.

CHAPTER 2: THE TRUTH ABOUT THE "ACCURATE DIAGNOSIS"

1. D. Sheehan, *The Anxiety Disease* (New York: Bantam Books, 1986).
2. M. Laufer, E. Denhoff, and G. Solomons, "Hyperkinetic Impulse Disorder in Children's Behavior Problems," *Psychosomatic Medicine 19* (1957): 38–49.
3. American Psychiatric Association, *Diagnostic and Statistical Manual of Mental Disorders (DSM-IV)* (Washington, D.C.: American Psychiatric Association, 1994).
4. S. Swedo, H. Leonard, et al., "Pediatric Autoimmune Neuropsychiatric Disorders Associated with Streptococcal Infections: Clinical Description of the First 50 Cases," *American Journal of Psychiatry 155* (1998): 264–71.
5. P. Breggin, *Toxic Psychiatry* (New York: St. Martin's Press, 1991).
6. R. Kendell, J. Kemp, "Maternal Influence in the Etiology of Schizophrenia," *Archives of General Psychiatry 46* (1989): 878–82.
7. M. Asberg, L. Traskman, and P. Thoren, "5-HIAA in the Cerebrospinal Fluid: A Biochemical Suicide Predictor?" *Archives of General Psychiatry 33* (1976): 1193–97.
8. K. Kendler, E. Walters, et al., "Childhood Parental Loss and Adult Psychopathology in Women: A Twin Study Perspective," *Archives of General Psychiatry 49* (1992): 109–16.

CHAPTER 4: PEOPLE FOR WHOM PSYCHIATRIC DRUGS POSE EXTRA RISK

1. W. Green, *Child and Adolescent Clinical Psychopharmacology* (Baltimore: Williams and Wilkins, 1995).
2. E. Ettore, *Women and Substance Use* (New Brunswick, N.J.: Rutgers University Press, 1987).
3. M. Jensvold, U. Halbreich, and J. Hamilton, *Psychopharmacology and Women* (Washington, D.C.: American Psychiatric Press, 1996).

4. K. Wisner and J. Perel, "Psychopharmacological Treatment during Pregnancy and Lactation," in Jensvold, Halbreich, and Hamilton, *Psychopharmacology and Women* (Washington, D.C.: American Psychiatric Press, 1996).

5. K. Wisner, J. Perel, et al., "Tricyclic Dose Requirements across Pregnancy," *American Journal of Psychiatry 150* (1993): 1541–42.

6. K. Wisner and J. Perel, "Psychopharmacological Treatment during Pregnancy and Lactation."

7. C. Salzman, A. Satlin, et al., "Geriatric Psychopharmacology," in A. Schatzberg, and C. Nemeroff, *The American Psychiatric Press Textbook of Psychopharmacology* (Washington, D.C.: American Psychiatric Press, 1995).

8. J. Macdonald, "The Role of Drugs in Falls in the Elderly," *Clinics in Geriatric Medicine 1* (1985): 621–36.

9. E. Pi and G. Gray, "A Cross-Cultural Perspective on Psychopharmacology," in *Directions in Psychiatry* (New York: The Hatherleigh Company, 1998), 425–42.

10. Ibid.

CHAPTER 5: ALTERNATIVE TREATMENTS FOR PSYCHIATRIC PROBLEMS

1. M. Copeland, *Wellness Recovery Action Plan* (Brattleboro, Vt.: Peach Press, 1997).

CHAPTER 8: BIPOLAR DISORDER AND MOOD SWINGS

1. A. Stoll, E. Severus, et al., "Omega 3 Fatty Acids in Bipolar Disorder," *Archives of General Psychiatry 56* (1999): 407–12.

INDEX

Page numbers in **boldface** indicate extended discussion of drug.

329